RHEUMATIC DISEASES

Immunological mechanisms and prospects for new therapies

This authoritative review volume provides a wide-ranging account of the immunological mechanisms that underlie many rheumatic diseases. Advances in our understanding of the immunopathology of diseases such as rheumatoid arthritis, ankylosing spondylitis and SLE are paving the way for the development of effective and rational new therapies. This exciting prospect is an important stimulus for groundbreaking research into these diseases and the investigation of new therapeutic options. As the first book to focus exclusively on this burgeoning area of clinical research, this is an invaluable and contemporary account for all rheumatologists, clinical immunologists and those seeking to develop effective new therapies to combat rheumatic diseases.

RHEUMATIC DISEASES

Immunological mechanisms and prospects for new therapies

Edited by

J. S. H. GASTON

Professor of Rheumatology
University of Cambridge School of Medicine

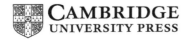

CAMBRIDGE
UNIVERSITY PRESS

PUBLISHED BY THE PRESS SYNDICATE OF THE UNIVERSITY OF CAMBRIDGE
The Pitt Building, Trumpington Street, Cambridge, United Kingdom

CAMBRIDGE UNIVERSITY PRESS
The Edinburgh Building, Cambridge CB2 2RU, UK http:/www.cup.cam.ac.uk
40 West 20th Street, New York, NY 10011–4211, USA http:/www.cup.org
10 Stamford Road, Oakleigh, Melbourne 3166, Australia

First published 1999

Printed in the United Kingdom at the University Press, Cambridge

Typeset in Times 11/14pt, in QuarkXpress™ [SE]

A catalogue record for this book is available from the British Library

Library of Congress Cataloguing in Publication data

Rheumatic diseases / edited by J.S. Hill Gaston
    p. cm.
  Includes Index.
  ISBN 0-521-59327-1 (hardback)
  1. Rheumatism – Immunological mechanisms and prospects for new therapies I. Gaston, J.S.
Hill, (John Stanley Hill), 1952–   .
  [DNLM: 1. Rheumatic Diseases. WE 544R4705 1999]
  RC927.R4522   1999
  616.7'23–dc21   98-11713 CIP
  DNLM/DLC
  for Library of Congress

ISBN 0 521 59327 1 hardback   *£37.50*

Contents

Contributors

J. M. Ahearn
Division of Rheumatology and Clinical Immunology, Department of Medicine, University of Pittsburgh School of Medicine, Pittsburgh, PA, USA

D. R. Alexander
T Cell Laboratory, Department of Immunology, The Babraham Institute, Cambridge, CB2 4AT, UK

J. Hoyt Buckner
Virginia Mason Research Center, 1000 Seneca St, Seattle, WA 98101, USA

K. B. Elkon
Division of Rheumatology, Hospital for Special Surgery, Cornell University Medical Center, New York, NY 10021, USA

J. S. H. Gaston
University of Cambridge School of Clinical Medicine, Addenbrooke's Hospital, Cambridge CB2 2QQ, UK

D. A. Isenberg
Bloomsbury Rheumatology Unit/Department of Rheumatology, Arthur Stanley House, 40–50 Tottenham St, London W1P 9PG, UK

P. Lane
Department of Immunology, Birmingham Medical School, Vincent Drive, Birmingham B15 2TT, UK

D. Mason
MRC Cellular Immunology Unit, Sir William Dunn School of Pathology, Oxford University, Oxford, OX1 3RE, UK

J. McNally
Division of Rheumatology, Hospital for Special Surgery, Cornell University Medical Center, New York, NY 10021, USA

R. J. Moots
Department of Rheumatology, Fazakerley Hospital, Liverpool L9 7AL

G. T. Nepom
Virginia Mason Research Center, 1000 Seneca St, Seattle, WA 98101, USA

C. Pitzalis
Rheumatology Unit UMDS, Guy's, St Thomas and King's College Hospitals, London SE1 9RT, UK

A. Rahman
Bloomsbury Rheumatology Unit/Department of Rheumatology, Arthur Stanley House, 40–50 Tottenham St, London W1P 9PG, UK

F. Ramirez
MRC Cellular Immunology Unit, Sir William Dunn School of Pathology, Oxford University, Oxford, OX1 3RE, UK

A. M. Rosengard
Department of Pathology, Johns Hopkins University School of Medicine, Baltimore, MD, USA

D. M. Sansom
Department of Pharmacology, University of Bath, Bath BA2 7AY, UK

B. Seddon
MRC Cellular Immunology Unit, Sir William Dunn School of Pathology, Oxford University, Oxford, OX1 3RE, UK

F. K. Stevenson
Molecular Immunology Group, Southampton University Hospitals, Tenovus Laboratory, Tremona Road, Southampton SO16 6YD, UK

A. K. Vaishnaw
Division of Rheumatology, Hospital for Special Surgery, Cornell University Medical Center, New York, NY 10021, USA

F. A. J. van de Loo
Department of Rheumatology, University Hospital Nijmegen, Nijmegen, The Netherlands

W. B. van den Berg
Department of Rheumatology, University Hospital Nijmegen, Nijmegen, The Netherlands

L. S. K. Walker
Department of Immunology, University of Birmingham, Birmingham B15 2TT, UK

K. W. Wucherpfennig
Harvard Medical School, Department of Cancer Immunology & AIDS, Dana-Farber Cancer Institute, 44 Binney St, Boston, MA 02115, USA

1

Implications of advances in immunology for understanding the pathogenesis and treatment of rheumatic disease

J. S. H. GASTON

Advances in immunology

This book has been designed to meet the needs of those whose clinical or research interests are in rheumatic diseases. Within rheumatology, there has been a lively debate on the relevance or otherwise of advances in immunology to a better understanding of rheumatic diseases and their treatment. Until relatively recently, it would have to be conceded that treatment of a disease like rheumatoid arthritis (RA) has been based on empirical observation of the usefulness of certain drugs (usually tested originally on the basis of some wholly erroneous idea about pathogenesis); in short, rational therapies based on a new understanding of immunopathology were in short supply. This situation is now changing, with the successful application of 'biologic' treatments, such as antibodies to tumour necrosis factor alpha (TNFα), or recombinant interleukin 1 (IL-1) receptor antagonist in RA (Arend & Dayer, 1995; Maini et al., 1995), and the initial exploration of supplying such therapy by means of gene transfer (Evans & Robbins, 1996). It is very likely that much of the therapeutic effort of rheumatologists in the first part of the 21st century will be directed to defining the place of novel biological therapies in the management of rheumatological disease, while determining in more detail the mode of action of current empirical therapies so that they may be used to best advantage.

In order to participate in this process, it is necessary to have at least some working knowledge of the components of the immune system, and how they might be implicated in rheumatic disease. Although there may have been some dissatisfaction with the relatively small contribution of immunologists to the therapy of rheumatic disease since the late 1960s, it was clearly unrealistic to expect a major therapeutic impact on disease at a time when so little normal immune physiology had been defined. There has been an enormous explosion in knowledge since the late 1970s, and this process continues, fuelled by the power of current molecular techniques. In 1982, three interleukins had been characterized, whereas the number is now approaching 20. To these can be added those cytokines that for some reason do not qualify for interleukin status, such as TNF (three varieties), oncostatin-M, leukaemia inhibitory factor (LIF), and many others, most having names that completely fail to indicate the wide range of their involvement in inflammation and immunity – none of the three examples quoted has effects confined to neoplasia.

To these must be added a plethora of chemokines; around 40 are defined, but there are perhaps as many as 60 additional expressed-sequence tags (ESTs) that have features which make them putative chemokines (Schall & Bacon, 1994). The set of chemokines join IL-8, otherwise a somewhat anomalous member of the interleukin family. There are four major families of chemokines (CKs), classified according to the number and position of cysteine residues at their amino terminus. These are termed the C-X-C, C-C and C families (Baggiolini, Dewald & Moser, 1997), along with the recently described C-X$_3$-C chemokine (Bazan *et al.*, 1997). The predominant actions of chemokines are on neutrophils (C-X-C family) or monocytes and lymphocytes (C-C, C and C-X$_3$-C families). An expanding family of receptors (CCRs and CXCRs) for these factors is also being defined. Faced with so many factors and receptors' it is tempting to assume substantial redundancy, and this is certainly the case for some functions (e.g. neutrophil chemotaxis), but recent investigations in HIV infection clearly show that polymorphisms in single chemokine receptors can have measurable effects on clinical outcome (Garred, 1998). For HIV, these effects probably reflect the fact that the virus hijacks the chemokine receptor to gain access to cells. Nevertheless, it is possible that associations between polymorphisms, in particular chemokine or chemokine receptor genes, will also be discovered with respect to rheumatic diseases when the genetic influences on disease incidence and characteristics are unravelled by current whole genome search strategies.

The most recent chemokines and chemokine receptors to be described are examples of 'reverse genetics', with the first inkling of their existence coming from DNA sequences rather than a biological activity (Forster *et al.*, 1996; Bazan *et al.*, 1997; Gunn *et al.*, 1998a,b). This effectively short-circuits the previous labour-intensive procedure of purifying, sequencing, cloning and expressing new biologically active factors. A similar route has also been used to define new cytokines such as IL-17 (Yao *et al.*, 1995a,b). Amongst newer chemokines are factors that have important roles in establishing the architecture of the immune system, by, for instance, attracting cells into germinal centres (Gunn *et al.*, 1998a). Since the rheumatoid arthritis synovium can take on the architectural appearance of a lymph node, including germinal centre formation, this is likely to reflect chemokine production within the tissue, and the particular stimuli that give rise to this response in chronic inflammation will be of great interest.

Cell surface molecules on lymphoid and myeloid cells are now defined to the extent of more than 160 CD (cluster of differentiation) numbers, where 15 were required in 1982 (Shaw, Turni & Katz, 1998) (http://www.ncbi.nlm.nih.gov/prow/). Some of these can be cleaved from cell surfaces and then act as cytokines or can modulate cytokine action by binding them in solution. The precise function of many of these surface molecules has yet to be defined, but even at our current partial stage of understanding, the cells that make up the immune system are amongst the most thoroughly characterized in the whole body. It is evident that things have changed substantially from the classic description of the lymphocyte as a 'small round cell . . . of which literally nothing of importance is known' (Gowans, 1996).

At one time, the interests of cellular immunologists were almost entirely focused on events at the cell surface, the cell itself being treated as something of a 'black box', but now many signalling pathways have been defined in great detail and shown to be very complex. Examples include signalling from T and B cell receptors, from co-stimulatory molecules and cytokine receptors, and the signalling mechanisms that mediate programmed cell death (apoptosis). Many of the components of the signalling pathways are not used uniquely by the immune system, and signalling pathways used by hormones and growth factors commonly intersect with those of lymphocytes. In addition, many of the transcription factors that are important in lymphocyte activation have a wide spectrum of activity in the activation of other genes (an example would be NFκB). However, signalling components and transcription factors that have a very particular role in the immune system have also been discovered; signalling through the IL-12 receptor is wholly dependent on the signal transducer and activator of transcription STAT-4 (Thierfelder *et al.*, 1996), whereas STAT-6 is required for the actions of IL-4 (Shimoda *et al.*, 1996; Takeda *et al.*, 1996). Deficiency in a single tyrosine kinase, Btk, accounts for Bruton's X-linked agammaglobulinaemia (Vetrie *et al.*, 1993). Increasing knowledge of signalling pathways is likely to be particularly important since it is often more realistic to manipulate the immune system by interfering with signalling pathways using conventional pharmacologic approaches, rather than using biological agents that act primarily on cellular interactions. Even where components of a signalling pathway are used for several biological functions, it is sometimes possible to obtain a useful therapeutic effect on one of the functions without necessarily producing the same phenotype as a genetic knock-out. A recent paper suggested that sulphasalazine, widely used in rheumatology with good efficacy and safety, has its effects by inhibiting the transcription factor NFκB (Wahl *et al.*, 1998), even though NFκB has multiple actions and genetic knock-out of certain NFκB components can be highly deleterious (Baldwin, 1996).

These are just some examples of the exponential growth in knowledge of the immune system; equal attention could be paid to work on the multiple components of the major histocompatibility complex (MHC), the formation and structure of antigen-specific receptors, the components involved in the induction of apoptosis and its role in control of immune responses, and the mechanisms underlying lymphocyte homing and recirculation – to mention only a few areas that have undergone intense scrutiny and are highly likely to be relevant to the pathogenesis of rheumatic diseases.

Faced with the baroque complexity of the immune system, which now genuinely rivals the central nervous system as a finely tuned physiological mechanism, the rheumatologist who has not previously had to grapple with immunology might be tempted to despair. This book is designed to dispel such feelings. Although it would be foolhardy to imply that our current knowledge of immunology is other than partial, a large proportion of the immunological events that are likely to be responsible for rheumatic diseases have already been defined. This is not to say that we know the immunological basis of most rheumatic diseases – from it; rather we have a reasonably comprehensive list of the kinds of thing that might go wrong and can now determine those which actually do cause disease. To take a non-rheumatological example; prior to the discovery of the CD40–CD40-ligand interaction (Disanto et al., 1993), the mechanism of the sex-linked hyperIgM immunodeficiency (HIgM) syndrome was completely unknown. Although it is clearly possible, and indeed likely, that additional co-stimulatory molecules remain to be discovered, deficiencies in these will have some phenotypic similarities with the lack of CD40-ligand (CD40L), which is responsible for HIgM syndrome. Likewise, prior to the description of the cytokine IL-12, certain patients who had difficulty in combating infection by intracellular organisms such as salmonellae and atypical mycobacteria had an immunodeficiency that was unexplained. Recently, patients with just this clinical phenotype have been discovered to have abnormalities in IL-12 (Altare et al., 1998a) or its receptor (Altare et al., 1998b). In keeping with the physiological role of IL-12 in influencing interferon-γ (IFN-γ) production, a somewhat similar phenotype has been seen in patients with defective IFN-γ receptors (Jouanguy et al., 1996). Thus, gradually, clinical phenotypes are being matched with abnormalities in defined components of the immune system. Although this is most easily done where there is the equivalent of a genetic knock-out in humans, more subtle defects that might contribute to the pathogenesis of rheumatic diseases are currently being sought.

Overview of this volume

The objective in each of the remaining chapters of this review is to describe current knowledge of the principal immunological mechanisms in order to provide a physiological 'map', which can then be used to indicate components that might 'go wrong' in rheumatic disease, or components that might in the future be useful targets of therapy. Examples of known defects, and therapies that have been found effective, are provided, but the up-to-date description of the immune system should provide a framework that will facilitate future thinking about the pathogenesis of rheumatological disorders, and an understanding of the rationale behind the novel therapies currently being dreamt up by biotechnology companies.

Specific immune responses begin with antigen recognition and the receptors that mediate this: surface immunoglobulin in the case of B cells, and the different forms of the T cell receptor for antigen. Autoantibodies, which are associated with rheumatic diseases and, in some cases, are directly pathogenic, have now been studied in great detail using molecular techniques, particularly from a structural point of view. The mechanisms whereby specific antibodies are generated, and the properties of particular autoantibodies, are described in Chapter 4.

T cell receptors differ radically from immunoglobulins in their inability to distinguish intact antigen; instead they recognize short peptides that result from processing and which are then presented by means of molecules encoded in the MHC (known as the human leukocyte antigen (HLA) system in humans). This difference has profound implications for our understanding of autoimmune T cell responses, and how these might arise. The concept of 'molecular mimicry' has been put forward for some time in relation to autoimmunity (Oldstone, 1990). Mimicry occurs when antigenic determinants on pathogens (e.g. viruses or bacteria) resemble a determinant on a self-protein, so that an immune response to one cross-reacts with the other. Recently, a first example of this postulated mechanism has been documented in the keratitis induced by infection with herpes simplex virus type 1 (Zhao *et al.*, 1998). Initially, molecular mimicry was considered in relation to cross-reacting antibodies, where, for linear determinants that reflect a particular amino acid sequence, it is possible simply to compare the sequence of an autoantigen with that of a candidate mimic (e.g. a viral protein) to look for regions of sequence conservation. However, for a peptide to be recognized by a T cell there are only two requirements: it must bind to MHC and have appropriate amino acids to contact the T cell receptor. This means that there may be little or no linear sequence conservation between potential mimics, and they have to be sought in other ways. The necessary approaches are described in Chapter 2, having been pioneered by Wucherpfennig and Strominger (1995).

The prominent associations between MHC alleles and various rheumatic disorders represent the most compelling evidence for the involvement of T lymphocytes in pathogenesis: the B27 – ankylosing spondylitis association is still, after 25 years, the strongest for any disease (Brewerton *et al.*, 1973). Despite the strength of these associations for both spondyloarthropathies and RA, and the intense scrutiny of HLA since the associations were first described, the mechanisms underlying them are frustratingly obscure and may well be different for different diseases. Hoyt Buckner and Nepom describe current understanding of the components of the MHC, how they function in immune responses and likely ways in which diseases might be associated with particular alleles (Chapter 3).

The idea that recognition of antigen alone would not be a sufficient signal for activation of B or T cells was predicted early on (Bretscher & Cohn, 1970) and has proved to be the case. Two chapters in this volume (Chapters 5 and 6) deal with important co-stimulatory receptor ligand pairs that have been identified in recent years and that are involved in T cell stimulation. The first of these involves, on the T cell, CD28 and the related molecule CTLA-4, both of which can bind to two other related ligands on antigen-presenting cells, B7.1 and B7.2. The second is CD40L on T cells, which binds to CD40 on antigen-presenting cells, particularly B cells. The importance of these interactions is underlined by the ability to induce allograft acceptance by blocking both pathways – a measure of the severe degree of immunosuppression that is produced (Larsen *et al.*, 1996). However, although CD28 and CD40 were first described as important molecules for T cell and B cell co-stimulation, respectively (prior to the discovery of their ligands), the situation is inevitably more complex. Not only can T cells express B7.1/7.2 and CD40, and B cells CD40L, but in all cases the interaction of these receptor – ligand pairs results in a two-way conversation. Thus, there are important effects on both T and B cells in the CD40L–CD40 interaction, and the same ligand pair is involved in interactions between T cells and antigen-presenting cells, particularly dendritic cells. The same is true for CD28–B7.1, with additional complexity resulting from the inducible expression of CTLA-4 as an alternative ligand for B7.1/7.2 (Thompson & Allison, 1997). The interactions have implications for antibody production, the cytokine programme carried out by activated T cells, and immunity to intracellular pathogens; both co-stimulatory pathways are already being targeted in immunomodulation strategies (Durie *et al.*, 1993; Webb, Walmsley & Feldmann, 1996).

Appropriate engagement of B and T cell receptors by antigen has profound consequences for the cell, such as entering the cell cycle, expressing activation markers on its surface and producing cytokines; in effect, an entirely new genetic programme is initiated and there are multiple differences in gene transcription (involving hundreds of genes) between activated and quiescent T or B cells. To achieve this, intracellular signalling mechanisms are required; in the first instance, both B and T cells are dependent on components of the receptor complex other than those necessary for antigen recognition to initiate cell signalling. Other surface molecules, including the co-stimulatory molecules alluded to in the previous paragraph, can 'fine-tune' the response, again acting through their influence on components of the signalling pathway. Current understanding of these processes, and prospects for modulating intracellular signalling with drugs, are detailed in Chapter 7. It is clear that the notion that encounter with antigen would translate a T or B cell from an 'off' to an 'on' state in some all-or-nothing manner is quite inadequate. The effects of antigen on an antigen-specific cell will reflect the balance of positive and negative signals, in much the same way that a smooth motor action by a limb represents the graded activation of agonist and antagonist muscles rather than unopposed agonists. Indeed, there is an increasing need for such a balance in the interplay of antagonists and agonists in fine accurate movements. In addition to the signalling components involved in this process, the influence of the proportion of receptors on a cell that are activated, and the time for which they are activated, have recently been shown to be critical for the final outcome (Valitutti *et al.*, 1995; Viola & Lanzavecchia, 1996; Iezzi, Karjalainen & Lanzavecchia, 1998).

None of the mechanisms for antigen recognition and the signalling of appropriate responses addresses the question of the geography of the immune system; immune responses take place at certain sites, both within the lymphoid system and in the tissues generally, and ways of ensuring that effector cells are delivered to appropriate locations are an essential component of the immune system. This has been a very active field of research, and an overview is provided by Pitzalis (Chapter 8). Lymphocyte trafficking to appropriate tissue requires expression of ligand on endothelial cells that can be recognized by leukocytes; in fact multiple ligands are involved in the arrest and eventual transmigration of cells across the endothelium into the tissues. More recently recognized components in the process are the chemokines produced by endothelial cells and recognized by specific receptors on the leukocytes (Gunn *et al.*, 1998b); the chemokine–receptor interaction, in turn, modulates the affinity of the integrins required for firm adhesion of cells to the vessel wall. Again there are hopes that it may be possible to modulate leukocyte traffic therapeutically, and attempts to do this have already been made (Kavanaugh *et al.*, 1994).

Having dealt with the principal mechanisms for recognizing and making appropriate responses to antigens, it is important to examine the downstream effects of the antigen-specific responses, since these are the processes that turn immunological recognition into disease. In relation to inflammatory arthritis, it is clear that the synovium is dominated by the presence of macrophage/monocyte-derived rather than T cell-derived cytokines, although the recent description of a novel cytokine, IL-17, exclusively produced by T cells but with monokine-like effects may alter this perception (Spriggs, 1997). However, there is good evidence that the monokines are directly responsible for joint destruction. Much attention has focused on the two principal monokines: TNFα and IL-1. The relative important of each and therapeutic possibilities of inhibiting either or both are discussed by van den Berg and van de Loo (Chapter 10). This review also emphasizes the possible roles of the more recently described proinflammatory monokines such as IL-12 and IL-15, and the production of regulatory monokines such as IL-10 and transforming growth factor beta (TGFβ). It is clear that the effects of blocking one cytokine or adding another are not readily predictable in relation to arthritis, with differing effects depending on the clinical endpoint examined (e.g. joint swelling versus cartilage destruction), and depending on the phase in the evolution of arthritis at which they are applied.

Immune responses have to be controlled at the level of initiation by fine tuning their magnitude and ensuring that their consequences (production of a cytokine or immunoglobulin subclass) are appropriate to the context, e.g. IFN-γ to deal with mycobacterial infection, IgE production for an intestinal helminth. However, it is equally important to have mechanisms for ensuring that appropriate immune responses do not continue indefinitely, and the principal mechanism used by the immune system at all levels involves apoptosis. Apoptosis as a mechanism for the removal of immune or inflammatory effectors after they have performed their required actions is now realised to be of critical importance for normal immunological health. Strains of mice, which were already under scrutiny as examples of spontaneous systemic lupus erythematosus (SLE)-like illness, proved to lack molecules important in one of the major pathways for inducing apoptosis, Fas (in MRL *lpr/lpr* mice) or its ligand (FasL) (in C3H *gld/gld* mice). The mechanisms of apoptosis, the molecules involved (which have rapidly proliferated in recent years) and the regulation of the process are discussed in Chapter 9.

A further level of control in the immune system concerns the recognition of self-antigens. At one time, it was simply assumed that this was forbidden, and indeed mechanisms that allow the deletion of effector T and B cells with high-affinity receptors with self have been worked out in great detail (Kappler, Roehm & Marrack, 1987). However, it has also become apparent that potentially autoimmune effector cells are part of the normal B and T cell repertoire and that, in fact, the functional immune repertoire is selected on the basis of an ability to recognize self MHC–peptide complexes (Blackman et al., 1986). In any case, a repertoire that deleted every cell that could recognize an epitope present on some self molecule would be fatally compromised, since there is considerable (possibly complete) overlap between the set of epitopes comprising self and those expressed by pathogens. Accordingly, mechanisms for the control of potentially autoreactive cells in the periphery after thymic selection are required. These are only just beginning to be delineated; the potential for cells present in the normal T cell repertoire to mediate autoimmune disease is highlighted in Chapter 11, as is the existence in the same repertoire of T cell subsets that are able to control the autoimmune effectors. This has been worked out mainly in relation to organ-specific immune disease (diabetes, thyroiditis) and, more recently, in inflammatory bowel disease, where it may be necessary to tolerate normal intestinal organisms as well as self (Duchmann *et al.*, 1995; 1996). However it is probable that similar mechanisms protect against rheumatic disease or are at fault when it occurs.

The exquisite sensitivity of immune recognition by immunoglobulins and T cell receptors has long fascinated immunologists, and how this is accomplished is now understood in great detail. However, since the process rests fundamentally on chance recombination events to generate receptors of the required specificity, the experience of successfully generating an antibody or T cell to deal with an important pathogen cannot be passed on from generation to generation: the functional receptor is not encoded in the germ-line, only the component genes required for the recombination process. The acquired 'wisdom' of the immune response that is germ-line encoded comprises the innate immune system, which does not require the generation of novel, highly specific receptors (Fearon, 1997). For example, receptors like those that bind mannose are useful for interactions with many bacteria, as are components of the complement system. Having been previously dazzled by the sophistication of the adaptive immune response, immunologists are now paying much more attention to the innate immune system, and in particular to its interactions with the adaptive immune response, which produces the best of both worlds. A good example is the ability of C3d, when complexed to antigen, to boost the antibody response by several orders of magnitude, so that tiny quantities of antigen are rendered immunogenic (Dempsey *et al.*, 1996). This effect depends on a complement receptor, CD21 or CR2; the family of complement receptors is reviewed in detail by Ahearn and Rosengard (Chapter 12), along with an account of how abnormalities in complement components and their receptors are likely to play a part in diseases such as SLE.

Concluding remarks

It can be argued that most rheumatic disorders occur in the context of an immune system that is generally competent – patients are able to protect themselves adequately from pathogens – but has some minor character defect that, as in all the best Greek tragedies, leads ultimately to disaster. These defects have not generally been defined but might include overexuberant responses to environmental antigens in terms of the cytokines produced or the duration of response, or a crucial confusion between similar epitopes on foreign and self antigens. Our therapeutic response to these forgivable errors by the immune system has generally been to shut the whole system down to a substantial extent, with the inevitable consequence of vulnerability to the infectious agents. It is to be hoped that in future more subtle sanctions on the immune system, or a period of re-education, might have the desired effects on autoimmune/chronic inflammatory diseases, while maintaining intact defences against pathogens.

References

Altare, F., Lammas, D., Revy, P., Jouanguy, E., Dvffinger, R., Lamhamedi, S., Drysdale, P., Scheel-Toellner, D., Girdlestone, J., Darbyshire, P., Wadhwa, M., Dockrell, H., Salmon, M., Fischer, A., Durandy, A., Casanova, J.-L. & Kumararatne, D. (1998a). Inherited interleukin 12 deficiency in a child with Bacille Calmette–Guerin and *Salmonella enteritidis* disseminated infection. *J. Clin. Invest.* 102: 2035–2040

Altare, F., Durandy, A., Lammas, D., Emile, J.S., Lahamedi, S., Ledeist, F., Drysdale, P., Jouanguy, E., Doffinger, R., Bernaudin, F., Jeppsson, O., Gollob, J.A., Meinl, E., Segal, A.W., Fischer, A., Kumararatne, D. & Casanova, J.L. (1998). Impairment of mycobacterial immunity in human interleukin-12 receptor deficiency. *Science* 280: 1432–1435.

Drysdale, P., Segal, A., Dvffinger, R., Fischer, A., Kumararatne, D. & Casanova, J.-L. (1998b). IL-12 receptor deficiency selectively impairs mycobacterial immunity. *Science* in press.

Arend, W. & Dayer, J. (1995). Inhibition of the production and effects of interleukin-1 and tumor necrosis factor alpha in rheumatoid arthritis. *Arthritis Rheum.* 38: 151–160.

Baggiolini, M., Dewald, B. & Moser, B. (1997). Human chemokines: an update. *Annu. Rev. Immunol.* 15: 675–705.

Baldwin, A.J. (1996). The NF-kappa B and I kappa B proteins: new discoveries and insights. *Annu. Rev. Immunol.* 14: 649–683.

Bazan, J., Bacon, K., Hardiman, G., Wang, W., Soo, K., Rossi, D., Greaves, D., Zlotnik, A. & Schall, T. (1997). A new class of membrane-bound chemokine with a CX_3C motif. *Nature* 385: 640–644.

Blackman, M., Yague, J., Kubo, R., Gay, D., Coleclough, C., Palmer, E., Kappler, J. & Marrack, P. (1986). The T cell repertoire may be biased in favor of MHC recognition. *Cell* 47: 349–357.

Bretscher, P. & Cohn, M. (1970). A theory of self-nonself discrimination. *Science* 169: 1042–1049.

Brewerton, D., Caffrey, M., Hart, F., James, D., Nicholls, A. & Sturrock, R. (1973). Ankylosing spondylitis and HL-A27. *Lancet* i: 996–999.

Dempsey, P.W., Allison, M.E.D., Akkaraju, S., Goodnow, C.C. & Fearon, D.T. (1996). C3d of complement as a molecular adjuvant: bridging innate and acquired immunity. *Science* 271: 348–350.

Disanto, J.P., Bonnefoy, J.Y., Gauchat, J.F., Fischer, A. & Desaintbasile, G. (1993). CD40 ligand mutations in X-linked immunodeficiency with hyper-IgM. *Nature* 361: 541–543.

Duchmann, R., Kaiser, I., Hermann, E., Mayet, W., Ewe, K. & Meyer zum Buschenfelde, K. (1995). Tolerance exists towards resident intestinal flora but is broken in active inflammatory bowel disease. *Clin. Exp. Immunol.* 102: 448–455.

Duchmann, R., Schmitt, E., Knolle, P., Zumbuschenfelde, K.H.M. & Neurath, M. (1996). Tolerance towards resident intestinal flora in mice is abrogated in experimental colitis and restored by treatment with interleukin-10 or antibodies to interleukin-12. *Eur. J. Immunol.* 26: 934–938.

Durie, F.H., Fava, R.A., Foy, T.M., Aruffo, A., Ledbetter, J.A. & Noelle, R.J. (1993). Prevention of collagen-induced arthritis with an antibody to gp39, the ligand for CD40. *Science* 261: 1328–1330.

Evans, C. & Robbins, P. (1996). Pathways to gene therapy in rheumatoid arthritis. *Curr. Opin. Rheumatol.* 8: 230–234.

Fearon, D. (1997). Seeking wisdom in innate immunity. *Nature* 388: 323.

Forster, R., Mattis, A.E., Kremmer, E., Wolf, E., Brem, G. & Lipp, M. (1996). A putative chemokine receptor, BLR1, directs B cell migration to defined lymphoid organs and specific anatomic compartments of the spleen. *Cell* 87: 1037–1047.

Garred, P. (1998). Chemokine-receptor polymorphisms: clarity and confusion for HIV-1 prognosis? *Lancet* 351: 2–3.

Gowans, J. (1996). The lymphocyte – a disgraceful gap in medical knowledge. *Immunol. Today* 17: 288–291.

Gunn, M.D., Ngo, V.N., Ansel, K.M., Ekland, E.H., Cyster, J.G. & Williams, L.T. (1998a). A B-cell-homing chemokine made in lymphoid follicles activates Burkitt's lymphoma receptor-1. *Nature* 391: 799–803.

Gunn, M.D., Tangemann, K., Tam, C., Cyster, J.G., Rosen, S.D. & Williams, L.T. (1998b). A chemokine expressed in lymphoid high endothelial venules promotes the adhesion and chemotaxis of naive T lymphocytes. *Proc. Natl. Acad. Sci. USA* 95: 258–263.

Iezzi, G., Karjalainen, K. & Lanzavecchia, A. (1998). The duration of antigenic stimulation determines the fate of naive and effector T cells. *Immunity* 8: 89–95.

Jouanguy, E., Altare, F., Lamhamedi, S., Revy, P., Emile, J., Newport, M., Levin, M., Blanche, S., Seboun, E., Fischer, A. & Casanova, J. (1996). Interferon-gamma-receptor deficiency in an infant with fatal bacille Calmette–Guerin infection. *N. Engl. J. Med.* 335: 1956–1961.

Kappler, J., Roehm, N. & Marrack, P. (1987). T cell tolerance by clonal elimination in the thymus. *Cell* 49: 273–280.

Kavanaugh, A.F., Davis, L.S., Nichols, L.A., Norris, S.H., Rothlein, R., Scharschmidt, L.A. & Lipsky, P.E. (1994). Treatment of refractory rheumatoid arthritis with a monoclonal antibody to intercellular adhesion molecule 1. *Arthritis Rheum.* 37: 992–999.

Larsen, C.P., Elwood, E.T., Alexander, D.Z., Ritchie, S.C., Hendrix, R., Tuckerburden, C., Cho, H.R., Aruffo, A., Hollenbaugh, D., Linsley, P.S., Winn, K.J. & Pearson, T.C. (1996). Long-term acceptance of skin and cardiac allografts after blocking CD40 and CD28 pathways. *Nature* 381: 434–438.

Maini, R.N., Elliott, M.J., Brennan, F.M., Williams, R.O., Chu, C.Q., Paleolog, E., Charles, P.J., Taylor, P.C. & Feldmann, M. (1995). Monoclonal anti-TNF alpha antibody as a probe of pathogenesis and therapy of rheumatoid disease. *Immunol. Rev.* 144: 195–223.

Oldstone, M. (1990). Molecular mimicry and autoimmune disease. *Cell* 50: 819–820.

Schall, T. & Bacon, K. (1994). Chemokines, leukocyte trafficking, and inflammation. *Curr. Opin. Immunol.* 6: 865–873.

Shaw, S., Turni, L. & Katz, K. (1998). Protein reviews on the web: controlling the flood of biological information. *Immunol. Today* 18: 557–558.

Shimoda, K., Vandeursen, J., Sangster, M.Y., Sarawar, S.R., Carson, R.T., Tripp, R.A., Chu, C., Quelle, F.W., Nosaka, T., Vignali, D.A.A., Doherty, P.C., Grosveld, G., Paul, W.E. & Ihle, J.N. (1996). Lack of IL-4-induced Th2 response and IgE class switching in mice with disrupted Stat6 gene. *Nature* 380: 630–633.

Spriggs, M. (1997). Interleukin-17 and its receptor. *J. Clin. Immunol.* 17: 366–369.

Takeda, K., Tanaka, T., Shi, W., Matsumoto, M., Minami, M., Kashiwamura, S., Nakanishi, K., Yoshida, N., Kishimoto, T. & Akira, S. (1996). Essential role of Stat6 in IL-4 signalling. *Nature* 380: 627–630.

Thierfelder, W.E., Vandeursen, J.M., Yamamoto, K., Tripp, R.A., Sarawar, S.R., Carson, R.T., Sangster, M.Y., Vignali, D.A.A., Doherty, P.C., Grosveld, G.C. & Ihle, J.N. (1996). Requirement for Stat4 in interleukin-12-mediated responses of natural killer and T cells. *Nature* 382: 171–174.

Thompson, C.B. & Allison, J.P. (1997). The emerging role of CTLA-4 as an immune attenuator. *Immunity* 7: 445–450.

Valitutti, S., Muller, S., Cella, M., Padovan, E. & Lanzavecchia, A. (1995). Serial triggering of many T-cell receptors by a few peptide-MHC complexes. *Nature* 375: 148–151.

Vetrie, D., Vorechovsky, I., Sideras, P., Holland, J., Davies, A., Flinter, F., Hammarstrom, L., Kinnon, C., Levinsky, R., Bobrow, M., Smith, C.I.E. & Bentley, D.R. (1993). The gene involved in X-linked agammaglobulinaemia is a member of the *src* family of protein-tyrosine kinases. *Nature* 361: 226–233.

Viola, A. & Lanzavecchia, A. (1996). T cell activation determined by T cell receptor number and tunable thresholds. *Science* 273: 104–106.

Wahl, C., Liptay, S., Adler, G. & Schmid, R. (1998). Sulfasalazine: a potent and specific inhibitor of nuclear factor kappa B. *J. Clin. Invest.* 101: 1163–1174.

Webb, L.M.C., Walmsley, M.J. & Feldmann, M. (1996). Prevention and amelioration of collagen-induced arthritis by blockade of the CD28 co-stimulatory pathway: requirement for both B7-1 and B7-2. *Eur. J. Immunol.* 26: 2320–2328.

Wucherpfennig, K.W. & Strominger, J.L. (1995). Molecular mimicry in T cell-mediated autoimmunity: viral peptides activate human T cell clones specific for myelin basic protein. *Cell* 80: 695–705.

Yao, Z., Fanslow, W., Seldin, M., Rousseau, A.-M., Painter, S., Comeau, M., Cohen, J. & Spriggs, M. (1995a). Herpes saimiri encodes a new cytokine, IL-17, which binds to a novel cytokine receptor. *Immunity* 3: 811–821.

Yao, Z.B., Painter, S.L., Fanslow, W.C., Ulrich, D., Macduff, B.M., Spriggs, M.K. & Armitage, R.J. (1995b). Human IL-17: a novel cytokine derived from T cells. *J. Immunol.* 155: 5483–5486.

Zhao, Z.S., Granucci, F., Yeh, L., Schaffer, P.A. & Cantor, H. (1998). Molecular mimicry by herpes simplex virus type 1: autoimmune disease after viral infection. *Science* 279: 1344–1347.

2

The role of T cells in autoimmune disease

R. J. MOOTS and K. W. WUCHERPFENNIG

Introduction

Knowledge about T lymphocyte function has expanded dramatically in the 1990s, resulting in many advances in the understanding of the mechanisms underlying autoimmune diseases. T lymphocytes, initially believed to play a small role, if any, in autoimmune disease, are now implicated even in 'antibody-mediated' conditions such as pemphigus vulgaris. The undoubted advances in understanding autoimmune diseases have not, however, developed at the same pace for all conditions. More is known about T cell behaviour in multiple sclerosis and myasthenia gravis than in rheumatological conditions such as Sjögren's syndrome, SLE and RA. Indeed there are still claims, with some evidence, that T cells do not play a significant role at all in RA (Fox, 1997). In this chapter, we shall present some of the evidence implicating a pathological role for T cells in autoimmune rheumatic diseases particularly RA and discuss this in the context of recent advances in knowledge of T cell function. We will focus on the potential mechanisms triggering the activation of T cells, and on effector mechanisms. Finally, we will discuss potential strategies for the modulation of the autoimmune response in therapy.

Are T cells involved in autoimmune disease?

Genetic predisposition

Many population, family and twin studies have clearly demonstrated that genetic factors exert a major influence on predisposition to autoimmune disease. Reviewed in detail elsewhere (Theofilopoulos, 1995), the best-defined association is with genes from the class II region of the MHC. These highly polymorphic genes encode cell surface glycoproteins, which present peptides to CD4+

T lymphocytes (Trowsdale, 1993). Potential mechanisms whereby MHC molecules may be involved in immune system dysfunction range from thymic selection, and generation of an immune repertoire, to presentation of disease-specific peptides to autoreactive T cells in the periphery.

Some of the clearest examples of HLA class II disease associations are seen with insulin-dependent diabetes mellitus (IDDM), pemphigus vulgaris and RA. Firstly, resistance to IDDM was found to correlate with the presence of the negatively charged amino acid aspartic acid at position 57 of the HLA-DQ β chain (Todd, Bell & McDevitt, 1987; Morel *et al.*, 1988). HLA-DQ β chains with serine, valine or alanine at position 57 were then found to be associated with an increased susceptibility to IDDM (Nepom & Erlich, 1991). The profound effect of key residues within MHC alleles on susceptibility to autoimmune disease was confirmed by the discovery that patients with pemphigus vulgaris had a unique *HLA-DQβ* allele, differing from closely related alleles at position 57 (Scharf *et al.*, 1989). Subsequent structural analyses of MHC class II molecules by X-ray crystallography clearly illustrated the importance of position 57 in the class II β chain. This lies at one end of the peptide-binding groove, interacts intimately with the α chain and contributes to a peptide side-chain specificity pocket (Brown *et al.*, 1993; Stern *et al.*, 1994). Such a structure would limit potential auto-antigens to those with appropriate size, shape, hydrophobicity and charge – implying that presentation of peptide to CD4+ T cells is important in the development of autoimmunity (Wucherpfennig & Strominger, 1995b).

The association between RA and class II MHC is also strong. Approximately 70% of patients with RA express HLA-DR4, increasing to over 90% in severe disease (Salmon *et al.*, 1993), and nearly 100% in the subgroup Felty's syndrome. Furthermore, expression of *HLA-DR4* (and other RA-related alleles) is a predictor of disease progression (Gough *et al.*, 1994). A number of other *HLA-DR* alleles are also linked to RA. All of these share a common short sequence of amino acids (QKRAA), residues 67 to 71 in the polymorphic α helix of the HLA-DR β chain forming the third allelic hypervariable region or shared epitope (Gregersen, Silver & Winchester, 1987). Structural analysis of these disease-linked MHC molecules reveals that this region is intimately concerned with binding peptide and interacting with the antigen receptor on T cells (TCR) (Stern *et al.*, 1994). In particular, the lysine at position 71 contributes a positive charge to the P4 specificity pocket. *In vitro* binding studies have defined properties characterizing peptides that are able to bind to RA-associated HLA-DR molecules (Hammer *et al.*, 1994; Sinigaglia & Hammer, 1994; Woulfe *et al.*, 1995). Such distinctions have allowed prediction of potential autoantigenic peptides, which include type II collagen (Fugger, Rothbard & Sonderstrup-McDevitt, 1996) and the 65 kDA heat shock protein (Hammer *et al.*, 1995).

The significance of the P4 specificity pocket is underlined further in pemphigus vulgaris. In addition to HLA-DQβ, susceptibility to this disease is also associated with DRB1*0402, a rare subtype of HLA-DR4. This differs from the RA-associated DRB1*0404 at only three residues (DRβ 67, 70 and 71), introducing a negative charge into the P4 pocket. Analysis of the self-peptide related to pemphigus vulgaris from the desmoglein 3 autoantigen (residues 190–204) reveals a complementary positive charge at position 4, appropriate for occupying the P4 pocket. Site-directed mutagenesis of DRB1*0402 confirmed that binding of desmoglein 3 (190–204) was indeed via the negatively charged residues of the P4 pocket (DRβ 70 and 71) (Wucherpfennig *et al.*, 1995), highlighting the importance of the charge in the P4 pocket for binding of appropriate disease-specific peptides to HLA-DR4.

Disease-associated MHC class II alleles may also contribute to the development of autoimmunity by mechanisms other than the presentation of pathogenic peptides to T cells. For example, such molecules may *fail* to present some peptide(s) that is important in *preventing* development of disease. This would predict, for example, that non-RA-associated *DRB1* alleles would be protective, and T cell activation occurs with other MHC molecules. Such a hypothesis has indeed been suggested. *HLA-DQ8* has been proposed to confer susceptibility to collagen-induced arthritis in transgenic mice, while certain *DRB1* alleles are proposed to confer protection (Zanelli, Gonzalez-Gay & David, 1995). Other explanations for links between the shared epitope and RA include sequence homology with bacterial proteins (Zanelli *et al.*, 1995), and direct binding of an endogenous 73 kDa heat shock protein to the QKRAA motif (Albani *et al.*, 1995). The latter may impede surface expression of the class II MHC molecule or may alter peptide-binding capability (Auger *et al.*, 1996).

T cells in lesions

If T cells are the culprits, are they found at the scene of the crime? This is indeed the case. Dense T cell infiltrates are characteristically seen in inflammatory plaques of demyelination in multiple sclerosis (Hauser *et al.*, 1986), in islet beta cells in IDDM and in the synovium in RA. T cell infiltrates in RA synovial tissue differ from normal or peripheral blood T cells in RA patients in a number of respects. They show many histological similarities to paracortical areas of lymph nodes, with occasional germinal centres. In addition the presence of specialized high endothelial venules (HEV) (intimately associated with T cell migration into tissues) suggests extensive T cell activity (Kurosaka & Ziff, 1983) and T cell infiltrates may sometimes be observed in clinically normal knees of patients with RA (Soden *et al.*, 1989).

The detailed characterization of such infiltrates is now possible by immuno-histochemical staining and provides more clues as to what the T cells may be doing. In RA, the phenotype of synovial T cells differs significantly from that of the T cells in peripheral blood and in infiltrates in non-inflammatory joint lesions such as osteoarthrosis. The majority of infiltrating cells in the synovium express CD4, corresponding to the genetic MHC class II predisposition. They are highly differentiated, expressing the 'memory' CD45 RO+ marker in larger numbers than do peripheral blood cells from the same patients (reviewed in Salmon & Gaston, 1995). They also express markers of activation such as HLA-DR and the transferrin receptor (Smolen *et al.*, 1996). Other activation markers such as the IL-2 receptor (IL-2R) are lacking, or present on a smaller population of cells. However consideration of the dynamics of activation marker expression in response to mitogens *in vitro* (IL-2R, early and transient expression, HLA-DR later and prolonged expression), together with the expression of CD45 RO, suggests that they are in a stage of late activation.

Specificity of T cells

Detailed analysis of TCR usage has been performed in many conditions, but interpretation has been complicated by the fact that antigen-specific T cells represent only a small fraction of T cells in autoimmune lesions. A more convincing form of evidence for T cell-induced autoimmunity would be the characterization of self-proteins able to specifically activate T cells in patients. Furthermore, since autoreactive T cells may be isolated from normal individuals, autoaggressive T cells should occur with higher precursor frequency in patients. The search for candidate antigens for autoimmune responses started by focusing on proteins found in target organs, such as CNS myelin proteins in multiple sclerosis. Immunodominant myelin basic protein (MBP) peptide epitopes presented by disease-specific MHC molecules were characterized and T cells cloned. Such autoreactive MBP-specific T cells were found to be clonally expanded and persisted over time in patients with multiple sclerosis (Wucherpfenning *et al.*, 1994b). Other myelin components including proteolipid protein (PLP) were subsequently found to contain T cell epitopes. Similarly, T cells reactive to islet proteins such as glutamic acid decarboxylase (GAD 65) have been isolated in IDDM (Nepom, 1995), and to components of the acetylcholine receptor protein in myasthenia gravis (Newsom-Davis *et al.*, 1989).

Despite hard searching, no such autoantigen has yet been defined for RA, suggesting to some that T cells are not important in this disease. A number of candidates have, however, been proposed, including heat shock proteins, link protein and other proteoglycans. An important candidate is type II collagen (CII), expressed almost exclusively in synovial joints (Kuhn, 1987). An animal model, collagen-induced arthritis (CIA), has also been studied extensively. Here, an inflammatory erosive arthritis, with many similarities to RA, is induced by immunization with CII (Durie, Fava & Noelle, 1994) and mediated, at least in part, by CII-reactive T cells (Holmdahl *et al.*, 1989; Myers *et al.*, 1993). Reports of CII reactivity in humans, however, are limited to T cell lines, without characterization of peptide specificity. However, transgenic technology has lead to two recent reports describing T cell responses to CII restricted by HLA-DRI and HLA-DR4 in mice transgenic for human class II MHC and CD4 (Fugger *et al.*, 1996; Rosloniec *et al.*, 1997). In both cases, the immunodominant peptide, residues 259–271 of CII, was identical. The similarities in the peptide-binding site of these two MHC molecules support the hypothesis that presentation of a pathogenic 'arthritogenic' epitope to autoaggressive T cells is an important pathological mechanism.

Animal models

Many models for autoimmune disease exist in animals of many species, ranging from the tight-skinned chicken (systemic sclerosis) to the non-obese diabetic mouse (IDDM). These animal models have helped to define basic mechanisms of autoimmunity, although their relevance to the human diseases is not yet known. The major susceptibility factor in many of these models also lies within the MHC. The non-obese diabetic (NOD) mouse, for example, is spontaneously prone to develop an autoimmune insulitis, with an islet T cell infiltrate specific for islet proteins such as GAD 65 (Haskins & Wegmann, 1996). Susceptibility in NOD mice maps to the murine MHC class II molecule I-A^{g7} and appears to be T cell mediated. Similarly, experimental allergic encephalomyelitis (EAE) in mice and rats is associated with a specific T cell response to CNS proteins including MBP, PLP and myelin oligodendrocyte glycoprotein (MOG). Myelin-specific T cell lines and clones have been produced, and specific peptides defined. T cell clones can transfer disease, even in the absence of antibodies or B lymphocytes (Steinman, 1996).

Collagen-induced arthritis is one of a number of animal models for RA, including adjuvant- and pristane-induced arthritis. It is characterized by an inflammatory polyarthritis sharing many features with RA. Disease develops in susceptible mouse or rat strains after immunization with CII and is characterized by specific T and B cell responses to CII (Staines & Wooley, 1994). It is interesting to note, however, that mice transgenic for a TCR reactive against a systemically expressed antigen were serendipitously observed to develop a localized joint disease

(Kouskoff *et al.*, 1996). This suggests that the mechanisms underlying T cell autoimmunity may be considerably more complex than previously believed.

Clinical observations

The basic idea that pathological T cells cause autoimmune diseases is supported by clinical observations from different groups. An open pilot study of the use of IFN-γ therapy in multiple sclerosis was terminated soon after starting, because of an increased early relapse rate. This was associated with a high rate of spontaneous proliferation of peripheral blood lymphocytes and an increase in the specific response to MBP (Panitch *et al.*, 1987).

In RA, a variety of procedures designed to reduce T cell numbers or affect function have been used with some success. These include thoracic duct drainage (Vaughan *et al.*, 1984), total lymphoid irradiation (Helfgott, 1989), lymphapheresis (Wilder, Yarboro & Decker, 1982), and treatment with cyclosporin A (Forre, 1995). Recent clinical trials using a depleting anti-CD4+ monoclonal antibody did not produce clinical benefit, despite significant reduction in peripheral CD4+ cells (Weinblatt *et al.*, 1995). This has been cited as evidence against a significant role for T cells. However, measurement of peripheral cells may not accurately reflect an effect on T cells within the joint. Indeed, a different humanized *non-depleting* anti-CD4 monoclonal antibody appears to induce some clinical benefit (Panayi *et al.*, 1996).

What triggers autoreactivity in T cells?

The incomplete deletion of all potentially autoreactive T cells in the thymus may occur for a number of reasons. For example, not all self-proteins may be accessible to the thymus for presentation to maturing T cells. The resultant 'resting' autoreactive T cells in peripheral blood are considered a normal part of the immune repertoire and do not normally induce disease. Peripheral mechanisms hold these potentially pathogenic T cells in check. The key event in the induction of T cell-mediated autoimmunity would, therefore, need to overcome this and allow activation of autoreactive T cells. This is supported by data from animal models such as EAE, where disease can be adoptively transferred only with activated and not resting T cells (Zamvil & Steinman, 1990). In conditions such as multiple sclerosis and the murine model EAE, activation must occur outside the CNS and with a different protein, since the target proteins are not expressed outside the blood–brain barrier. A number of hypotheses have been proposed to explain this. The two major hypotheses currently are T cell activation by superantigen, and molecular mimicry.

Both of these hypotheses implicate microbial pathogens. This is supported by both clinical and epidemiological evidence for potential infectious triggers of autoimmunity. For example, common viral infections such as measles and rubella may occasionally result in inflammatory CNS disease. In these conditions, there has been T cell reactivity to MBP, with no evidence of virus in the CNS (Johnson *et al.*, 1984). Viral infections have been reported to precede the development of IDDM and autoimmune myocarditis, and infection with a variety of pathogens has been thought for a long time to trigger RA. The complex epidemiology of all human autoimmune diseases indicates that a number of pathogens may be involved.

The potential role of superantigens in the triggering of autoreactive T cells

Superantigens are small proteins that are able to activate T cells by a mechanism bypassing the normal requirement for antigen processing (Marrack & Kappler, 1990). They bind to class II MHC molecules at conserved regions outside the peptide binding cleft and to TCR Vβ sequences away from the highly polymorphic CDR3 loops. Such an interaction with TCR is specific to particular Vβ families and, as such, superantigens are able to activate a large proportion of T cells. Indeed the term superantigen arose because of their potent T cell stimulatory capacity (in concentrations down to 10^{-13} M), leading to a marked skewing of the TCR Vβ repertoire. Many superantigens have been identified, including staphylococcal and streptococcal enterotoxins, a soluble mitogen from *Mycoplasma arthritidis* (MAM) and endogenous retroviral gene products.

Initially, superantigens were found to induce severe clinical conditions charactized by a massive secretion of cytokines, such as toxic shock syndrome (Jupin *et al.*, 1988). However, it soon became apparent that the binding of superantigen to MHC class II molecules and selected TCR Vβ gene products, coupled with their potency as T cell mitogens, could result in the activation of quiescent circulating T cells with a TCR specificity for self-protein. After clearance of the superantigen, most activated T cells would return to a resting state or be deleted. A small subset, however, of autoreactive T cells may home in to the site of expression of autoantigen and mediate disease (Fig. 2.1).

In the murine EAE model, MBP-specific I-A^u-restricted T cells using the Vβ8.2 gene segment induce disease. The bacterial superantigen staphylococcal enterotoxin B (SEB) activates T cells expressing Vβ8 and is able to induce clinical relapse or exacerbation in mice previously immunized with the MBP peptide (Brocke *et al.*, 1993). The murine Vβ8 gene family is also utilized by pathogenic T cells in several other experimental models, including collagen-induced

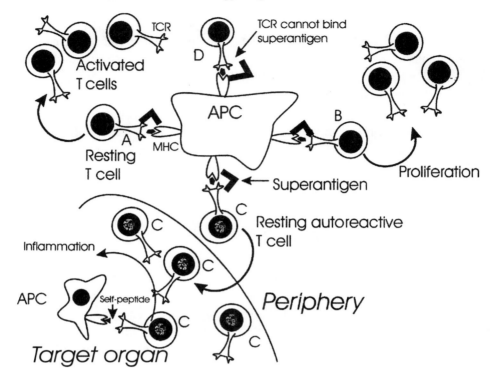

Fig. 2.1. Superantigen-mediated activation of autoreactive T cells APC, antigen-presenting cell.

arthritis. Injection of MAM, a potent superantigen for cells with such TCRs, caused an exacerbation of arthritis in mice recovering from collagen-induced arthritis. Such a result is intriguing, as the organism from which MAM is derived is known itself to induce a chronic inflammatory erosive arthritis in rodents. Furthermore, while not a human pathogen, the major MAM-responsive human Vβ gene family is Vβ17, reported to be overrepresented in synovial T cells in patients with RA (Zagon *et al.*, 1994). These observations suggest that super-antigens could be significantly involved in the pathogenesis of chronic auto-immune disease, perhaps by inducing exacerbations and relapses. To test this hypothesis further, it will be important to compare the functional properties and fine specificity of, for example, Vβ17-positive T cells in the blood and synovial fluid of RA patients. Such an involvement of superantigen in auto-immune disease would not only provide a link to infection – long postulated to be involved in the triggering of these disorders – but also offer the potential for novel therapy.

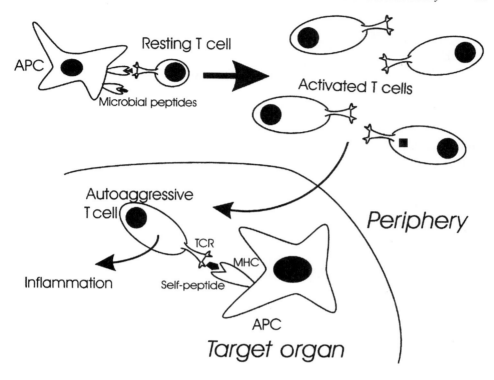

Fig. 2.2. Molecular mimicry. APC, antigen-presenting cell.

Molecular mimicry as trigger for autoreactive T cells

In many ways, the concept of mimicry, which depends upon a structural homology between self and foreign antigens, is intuitive. It would result in a cross-reactive T cell response if there were sufficient similarities between the two peptide epitopes. Microbial and host determinants would need to be similar enough to induce a cross-reacting immune response, yet different enough to break immunological tolerance (Fig. 2.2).

Molecular mimicry between microbes and antibodies that induce autoimmunity is well established. One of the earliest and best known is between group A streptococcal M antigens and myocardial and glomerular tissues, which occurs in rheumatic fever (Robinson & Kehoe, 1992). If such a phenomenon exists for T cells, it should be possible to demonstrate TCR cross-reactivity for self-peptides and foreign peptides presented by appropriate (disease-associated) MHC molecules. Many workers have searched for this in vain, hampered by the far greater complexity of antigen recognition for T cells compared with antibodies. A cross-reactive T cell epitope must retain its ability to bind not only MHC but also a clonally distributed TCR. Another problem has been the equally complex biochemical identification of cross-reactive T cell epitopes from pathogens, requiring extensive biochemical fractionation before testing on T cell clones. In order to overcome these problems, many authors have used computer-based sequence homology searches to align linear sequences of similarity between self-proteins and foreign proteins. Predicted peptide epitopes were then synthesized and tested with specific T cell clones. Fujinami and Oldstone (1985) used this approach to immunize rabbits with a hepatitis B virus polymerase peptide, successfully inducing cross-reactive autoantibodies to MBP and hepatitis B virus polymerase peptide. Some cross-reactive T cells could be found, together with CNS perivascular infiltrates characteristic of EAE in four out of eleven rabbits. However, while EAE was induced normally by the MBP peptide, it was not possible to induce disease by immunization with the hepatitis B virus polymerase peptide.

This study demonstrated that immune-mediated injury may occur *after* the triggering immunogen had been cleared, a 'hit and run' event. It also made it much harder to link infection with autoimmunity clinically because the inducing agent was likely to have been cleared before the onset of autoimmune symptoms. If this time lag were a matter of years, it would be extremely difficult to prove an association between a common pathogen and autoimmune disease by epidemiological methods. Similar studies in animal models such as experimental autoimmune uveitis (hepatitis B virus DNA polymerase and S-antigen photoreceptor protein) (Singh *et al.*, 1990) and adjuvant arthritis (mycobacterial 65 kDa heat shock protein and joint proteoglycan) (van Eolen *et al.*, 1988) confirmed that different pathogens could induce autoimmune disease. While replicating infectious agents were not required to trigger molecular mimicry in those models, the triggering epitopes were derived from pathogens that did not normally affect the animal in question.

An early criticism of the T cell molecular mimicry hypothesis was that it appeared to counter the commonly held view that the TCR is exquisitely specific for a particular peptide–MHC complex. Unless the self and foreign sequences were identical (up to a 1 in 20^6 chance), there would be no significant recognition. Over the last few years, however, it has become apparent that TCR recognition is more degenerate, and cross-reactivity at the T cell level may be more common than previously appreciated. In the mouse, a number of T cells clones have been reported that, while specific for MBP (Ac 1–9), were also able to recognize a dissimilar peptide presented by the same MHC class II molecule, I-A^u. As the two peptides had no obvious sequence similarity, the term 'space mimicry' was coined (Bhardwaj *et al.*, 1993).

Bearing in mind the evolving concept of degeneracy in TCR recognition, a different strategy to investigate potential molecular mimicry in human auto-immune disease has been devised. Specific T cell clones reactive to human MBP were generated from patients with multiple sclerosis and used to characterize the structural requirements for recognition of the immunodominant MBP(85–99) peptide (Wucherpfennig *et al.*, 1994a) in terms of MHC binding and TCR recognition. A series of amino acid substitutions were then selectively introduced at each critical position and the effects on T cell recognition analysed to define the sets of amino acids permitted at each critical residue. These structural data, together with the knowledge that amino acids side-chains required for binding to MHC molecules are degenerate, were used to search a protein sequence data-base of human pathogens. Candidate peptides were synthesized and tested for recognition by MBP-reactive human T cell clones derived from the peripheral blood of patients with multiple sclerosis. Seven viral and one bacterial peptide, from the 129 synthesized, were able to stimulate MBP-specific T cell clones efficiently, mimicking the immunodominant MBP(85–99) peptide (Wucherpfennig & Strominger, 1995a). Because of the degenerate MHC-binding motif, the viral/bacterial peptides had no obvious sequence homology with the MBP peptide. This indicated that some TCRs recognize not just a single peptide but rather a set of structurally related peptides derived from different antigens. A recent study that used combinatorial peptide libraries for definition of the T cell recognition motif has also detected cross-reactivity between dissimilar viral peptides and self-peptides for recognition by a MBP-specific T cell clone (Hemmer *et al.*, 1997). The diverse nature of the viral peptides able to stimulate MBP-specific T cell clones in these data would suggest that more than one single pathogen is able to trigger autoimmunity. This may explain why it has been so difficult to link conclusively the pathogenesis of individual autoimmune diseases to particular pathogens, in the face of considerable evidence for association of disease with infection in general. Rather, it may be that a group of common microbial pathogens could be involved in the pathogenesis of autoimmune processes.

How do pathological T cells cause disease?

There is much evidence implicating T cells in the autoimmune process in humans. Moreover, T cells are able to transfer disease directly in animals. However, one basic problem remains. Many target cells, such as pancreatic beta cells and oligodendrocytes, do not express class II MHC. How, therefore, can CD4+ T cells mediate the damage? A number of mechanisms may explain this. Firstly, T cells secrete cytokines. Some induce expression of class II MHC, allowing T cell-induced damage to occur. Others recruit immune system cells, which damage target organs. Secondly, CD4+ T cells may kill target cells directly, particularly utilizing the Fas/FasL pathway. These mechanisms will now be discussed in more detail.

Cytokine release

One consequence of CD4+ T cell activation is secretion of cytokines, in particular TNFα and TNFβ, IFN-γ, and IL-2. These potent mediators have a variety of biological effects, potentially contributing to the autoimmune disease processes in several different ways (Cavallo, Pozzilli & Thorpe, 1994). IFN-γ is a significant contributor to inflammation. It is able to recruit and activate a variety of inflammatory leukocytes, including macrophages. It also promotes upregulation of MHC class II molecules on antigen-presenting cells and induces their expression on non-professional antigen-presenting cells. Such a dysregulated expression of class II MHC molecules on target cells may amplify or facilitate an autoimmune response (Bottazzo *et al.*, 1983) (Fig. 2.3). Indeed the aberrant expression of MHC class II molecules by non-immune cells has been described in a variety of conditions, such as thyrocytes in autoimmune thyroiditis (Hanafusa *et al.*, 1983) and pancreatic cells in IDDM patients (Bottazzo *et al.*, 1985; Foulis, Farquharson & Hardman, 1987). In both cases this would allow presentation of autoantigen to T cells. Cytokines that directly influence the immune system, such as IL-2, would have an obvious impact on an autoimmune response. Originally described as a T cell growth factor, IL-2 plays a critical role in the proliferation and differentiation of numerous classes of lymphocyte. Indeed, monoclonal anti-IL-2 antibodies may inhibit disease in animal models. Conversely, agents that stimulate the secretion of IL-2, such as IFN-α and IL-12, potentiate disease.

T helper cells (T_H1 cells) secreting IL-2, IFN-γ and TNF can trigger EAE in rodent models and diabetes in the NOD mouse. TNF is one of the cytokines found in high concentration in rheumatoid joints. There is little doubt that this cytokine plays an important role in the pathophysiology of joint inflammation and destruction in both animals and humans (Feldmann, 1996; Feldmann, Brennan & Maini, 1996; Szekanecz, Szegedi & Koch, 1996). The biological effects include apoptosis, macrophage and polymorphonuclear leukocyte activation, B and T cell proliferation, secretion of proinflammatory cytokines (in a variety of cells), enhancement of fibroblast proliferation, nitric oxide release, secretion of collagenase and prostaglandin E_2 (PGE_2) by fibroblasts, and the resorption of bone and cartilage (Arend & Dayer, 1995; Lotz, 1996). Not surprisingly, there has been a considerable effort to modulate this cytokine as therapy for RA. Indeed, monoclonal anti-TNF antibody therapy induces dramatic early remissions in patients with RA (Elliott *et al.*, 1993; 1994), but, as yet, the effect is

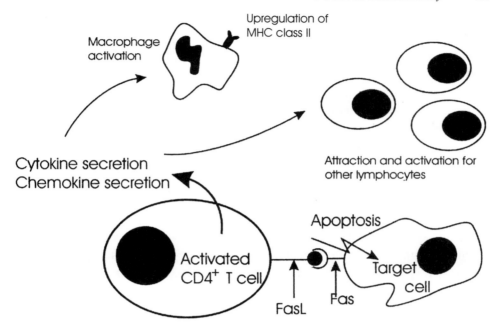

Fig. 2.3. Effector mechanisms.

not long-lasting. Despite this, the full cytokine profile of synovial tissue and fluid is still being elucidated.

Fas–FasL interaction

Fas (APO-1, CD95) is a cell-surface receptor of the TNF receptor superfamily; it is able to induce apoptotic cell death when ligated by an appropriate antibody, or Fas ligand (FasL) (Nagata & Golstein, 1995). Indeed, membrane-bound TNF on T cells is also able to perform this and may synergize with the Fas/FasL pathway (Cleveland & Ihie, 1995). Although Fas signalling induces apoptosis, Fas ligation has also been shown to trigger cellular proliferation (Aggarwal *et al.*, 1995). FasL was originally identified on CD8+ T cells and can function as an effective perforin-independent mechanism whereby cytotoxic T cells (CTL) can induce target cell cytolysis (Lowin *et al.*, 1994). Subsequently, expression of Fas and FasL has been found to be highly regulated in T cells. Expression of FasL is observed on activated T cells, CD45 RO+ cells expressing very little until stimulated. Fas expression, in contrast, is generally found on peripheral blood T cells. The potential role for this molecule in regulating normal immune responses and maintaining self-tolerance became evident with the description of lymphoproliferative diseases in *lpr/lpr* and *gld/gld* mice, with defects in the genes encoding

Fas and FasL, respectively (reviewed in Lynch, Ramsdell & Alderson, 1995). These observations, together with the discovery that previously activated T cells expressing Fas may apoptose when stimulated through the TCR–CD3 complex (activation-induced cell death), suggested an intimate role for the Fas–FasL interactions in autoimmune disease (Kabelitz, Pohl & Pechhold, 1993; Crichfield *et al.*, 1994). Fas–FasL interaction occurring between T cells and other cells appear to result in clonal 'downsizing' of immune responses. If there was a dysfunction in this mechanism, then disordered immune responses and autoimmunity may result (Lynch *et al.*, 1995).

Recently, other observations have implicated an additional important role for Fas–FasL interactions: the direct killing of target cells by autoreactive CD4[+] T cells. D'Souza *et al.* (1996) reported that CNS lesions in patients with multiple sclerosis demonstrated elevated levels of expression of Fas on oligodendrocytes, compared with tissue from normal subjects. In these lesions, microglia and infiltrating lymphocytes displayed an intense immunoreactivity for FasL. Rapid cell death in Fas-expressing oligodendrocytes could be induced by ligation with specific anti-Fas antibody or FasL, but, interestingly, apoptosis (as indicated by DNA fragmentation) did not occur.

Fas-mediated cell death appears to be a final common pathway in several T cell-mediated autoimmune diseases. The mechanism of beta cell loss in diabetes was investigated by crossing a transgenic mouse carrying a beta cell-specific TCR onto the NOD.scid background. These mice produced CD4[+] T cells bearing transgenic TCR but were devoid of B cells or CD8[+] cells. The mice developed an accelerated insulitis and overt disease. Pancreatic beta cell destruction was mediated by Fas-induced apoptosis (Chervonsky *et al.*, 1997; Kurrer *et al.*, 1997). Similarly, in a study by Giordano *et al.* (1997), thyrocytes from thyroid glands of patients with Hashimoto's thyroiditis, but not from non-autoimmune thyroids, expressed Fas. *In vitro* Fas expression was induced by IL-1β, which is abundantly produced in the thyroid in Hashimoto's glands thyroiditis. Massive thyrocyte apoptosis was observed on cross-linking of Fas. Thyrocyte suicide or fratricide resulted because FasL was constitutively expressed both in normal and thyroiditis thyrocytes. Activated T cells that express FasL may also induce cross-linking of Fas.

Potential relevance to therapy

The goal behind so much of the work on T cell immunology in autoimmune disease has been to identify potential strategies for therapeutic intervention. The recent developments in the molecular and cellular immunology of T cells, discussed here, can now be used to develop alternative approaches to conventional

Table 2.1. *Potential targets for treatment of autoimmune diseases*

Process	Target
Antigen processing	Blockade of DM-mediated CLIP removal
	Selective inhibition of key proteases
Interference with target organ localization of T cells	Blockade of adhesion molecules/homing receptors
	Blockade of chemokines/chemoattractants
Blockade of T cell effector functions	Inhibition of T cell produced cytokines
	Inhibition of Fas–FasL interactions
Deletion/inactivation of autoaggressive T cells	Monoclonal antibody
	Mucosal or systemic administration of autoantigen/peptide

immunosuppression for the treatment of autoimmune diseases (Table 2.1). An ideal therapy would reverse established disease, or at least prevent further progression, by selectively inhibiting autoreactive cells while leaving the rest of the immune system intact.

As yet there appears to be a number of potential pitfalls with some of these approaches. A specific means of treating autoimmune disease would be to induce tolerance to key autoantigens. Perhaps the best (and oldest) known means of achieving this is by the administration of protein (or preferably peptide). It has long been realised that systemic or mucosal administration of protein or peptide in high doses can induce tolerance to the same protein. In animal models, these strategies have proved effective. Unfortunately their great potential has yet to be realised in humans. Early trials of oral MBP and CII in multiple sclerosis (Weiner *et al.*, 1993) and RA (Trentham *et al.*, 1993) have not provided any clinical benefit when subjected to larger formal study. However, systemic administration of specific peptides, or targeting to the mucosal immune system (such as with cholera toxin B subunit (Sun *et al.*, 1996)), may improve the efficiency of tolerance induction and allow this to be of use in human disease. While we still rely on non-specific drug therapy at present, the developments in understanding autoimmune disease discussed here suggest that there is considerable potential for major new developments.

References

Aggarwal, B.B., Singh, S., La Pushin, R. & Totpal, K. (1995). Fas antigen signals proliferation of normal human diploid fibroblast and its mechanism is different from tumor necrosis factor receptor. *FEBS Lett.* 364: 5–8.

Albani, S., Keystone, E.C., Nelson, J.L., Ollier, W.E., La, C.A., Montemayor, A.C., Weber, D.A., Montecucco, C., Martini, A. & Carson, D.A. (1995). Positive selection in autoimmunity: abnormal immune responses to a bacterial dnaJ antigenic determinant in patients with early rheumatoid arthritis. *Nature Med.* 1: 448–452.

Arend, W.P. & Dayer, J.M. (1995). Inhibition of the production and effects of inter-leukin-1 and tumor necrosis factor alpha in rheumatoid arthritis. *Arthritis Rheum.* 38: 151–160.

Auger, I., Escola, J.M., Gorvel, J.P. & Roudier, J. (1996). HLA-DR4 and HLA-DR10 motifs that carry susceptibility to rheumatoid arthritis bind 70-kD heat shock proteins. *Nature Med.* 2: 306–310.

Bhardwaj, V., Kumar, V., Geysen, H.M. & Sercarz, E.E. (1993). Degenerate recognition of a dissimilar antigenic peptide by myelin basic protein-reactive T cells. Implications for thymic education and autoimmunity. *J. Immunol.* 151: 5000–5010.

Bottazzo, G.F., Pujol-Borrell, R., Hanafusa, T. & Feldmann, M. (1983). Role of aberrant HLA-DR expression and antigen presentation in induction of endocrine autoimmunity. *Lancet* ii, 1115–1119.

Bottazzo, G.F., Dean, B.M., McNally, J.M., MacKay, E.H., Swift, P.G. & Gamble, D.R. (1985). In situ characterization of autoimmune phenomena and expression of HLA molecules in the pancreas in diabetic insulitis. *N. Eng. J. Med.* 313: 353–360.

Brocke, S., Gaur, A., Piercy, C., Gautam, A., Gijbels, K., Fathman, C.G. & Steinman, L. (1993). Induction of relapsing paralysis in experimental autoimmune encephalomyelitis by bacterial superantigen. *Nature* 365: 642–644.

Brown, J.H., Jardetzky, T.S., Gorga, J.C., Stern, L.J., Urban, R.G., Strominger, J.L. & Wiley, D.C. (1993). Three-dimensional structure of the human class II histocom-patibility antigen HLA-DR1. *Nature* 364: 33–39.

Cavallo, M.G., Pozzilli, P. & Thorpe, R. (1994). Cytokines and autoimmunity. *Clin. Exp. Immunol.* 96: 1–7.

Chervonsky, A.V., Wang, Y., Wong, F.S., Visintin, I., Flavell, R.A., Janeway, C.A., Jr & Matis, L.A. (1997). The role of Fas in autoimmune diabetes. *Cell* 89: 17–24.

Cleveland, J.L. & Ihle, J.N. (1995). Contenders in fasL/TNF death signalling. *Cell* 81: 479–482.

Crichfield, J.M., Racke, M.K., Zuniga-Pflucker, J.C., Canella, B., Raine, C.S., Goverman, J. & Lenardo, M.J. (1994). T cell deletion in high antigen dose therapy of autoimmune encephalomyelitis. *Science* 263: 1139–1143.

D'Souza, S.D., Bonetti, B., Balasingam, V., Cashman, N.R., Barker, P.A., Troutt, A.B., Raine, C.S. & Antel, J.P. (1996). Multiple sclerosis: fas signaling in oligodendrocyte cell death. *J. Exp. Med.* 184: 2361–2370.

Durie, F.H., Fava, R.A. & Noelle, R.J. (1994). Collagen-induced arthritis as a model of rheumatoid arthritis. *Clin. Immunol. Immunopathol.* 73: 11–18.

Elliott, M.J., Maini, R.N., Feldmann, M., Kalden, J.R., Antoni, C., Smolen, J.S., Leeb, B., Breedveld, F.C., Macfarlane, J.D. & Bijl, H. (1994). Randomised double-blind comparison of chimeric monoclonal antibody to tumour necrosis factor alpha (cA2) versus placebo in rheumatoid arthritis. *Lancet* 344: 1105–1110.

Elliott, M.J., Maini, R.N., Feldmann, M., Long-Fox, A., Charles, P., Katsikis, P., Brennan, F.M., Walker, J., Bijl, H. & Ghrayeb, J. (1993). Treatment of rheuma-toid arthritis with chimeric monoclonal antibodies to tumor necrosis factor alpha. *Arthritis Rheum.* 36: 1681–1690.

Feldmann, M. (1996). What is the mechanism of action of anti-tumour necrosis factor-alpha antibody in rheumatoid arthritis? *Int. Arch. Allergy Immunol.* 111: 362–365.

Feldmann, M., Brennan, F.M. & Maini, R.N. (1996). Role of cytokines in rheumatoid arthritis. *Annu. Rev. Immunol.* 14: 397–440.

Forre, O. (1995). Cyclosporine in rheumatoid arthritis: an overview. *Clin. Rheumatol.* 14 (Suppl. 2): 33–36.

Foulis, A.K., Farquharson, M.A. & Hardman, R. (1987). Aberrant expression of class II major histocompatibility complex molecules by B cells and hyperexpression of class I major histocompatibility complex molecules by insulin containing islets in type 1 (insulin-dependent) diabetes mellitus. *Diabetologia* 30: 333–343.

Fox, D.A. (1997). The role of T cells in the immunopathogenesis of rheumatoid arthritis. *Arthritis Rheum.* 40: 598–609.

Fugger, L., Rothbard, J.B. & Sonderstrup-McDevitt, G. (1996). Specificity of an HLA-DRB1*0401-restricted T cell response to type II collagen. *Eur. J. Immunol.* 26: 928–933.

Fujinami, R.S. & Oldstone, M.B. (1985). Amino acid homology between the encephalitogenic site of myelin basic protein and virus: mechanism for autoimmunity. *Science* 230: 1043–1045.

Giordano, C., Stassi, G., de Maria, R., Todaro, M., Richiusa, P., Papoff, G., Ruberti, G., Bagnasco, M., Testi, R. & Galluzzo, A. (1997). Potential involvement of Fas and its ligand in the pathogenesis of Hashimoto's thyroiditis. *Science* 275: 960–963.

Gough, A., Faint, J., Salmon, M., Hassell, A., Wordsworth, P., Pilling, D., Birley, A. & Emery, P. (1994). Genetic typing of patients with inflammatory arthritis at presentation can be used to predict outcome. *Arthritis Rheum.* 37: 1166–1170.

Gregersen, P.K., Silver, J. & Winchester, R.J. (1987). The shared epitope hypothesis. An approach to understanding the molecular genetics of susceptibility to rheumatoid arthritis. *Arthritis Rheum.* 30: 1205–1213.

Hammer, J., Bono, E., Gallazzi, F., Belunis, C., Nagy, Z. & Sinigaglia, F. (1994). Precise prediction of major histocompatibility complex class II-peptide interaction based on peptide side chain scanning. *J. Exp. Med.* 180: 2353–2358.

Hammer, J., Gallazzi, F., Bono, E., Karr, R.W., Guenot, J., Valsasnini, P., Nagy, Z.A. & Sinigaglia, F. (1995). Peptide binding specificity of HLA-DR4 molecules: correlation with rheumatoid arthritis association. *J. Exp. Med.* 181: 1847–1855.

Hanafusa, T., Pujol-Borrell, R., Chiovato, L., Russell, R.C., Doniach, D. & Bottazzo, G.F. (1983). Aberrant expression of HLA-DR antigen on thyrocytes in Graves' disease: relevance for autoimmunity. *Lancet* ii, 1111–1115.

Haskins, K. & Wegmann, D. (1996). Diabetogenic T-cell clones. *Diabetes* 45: 1299–1305.

Hauser, S.L., Bhan, A.K., Gilles, F., Kemp, M., Kerr, C. & Weiner, H.L. (1986). Immunohistochemical analysis of the cellular infiltrate in multiple sclerosis lesions. *Ann. Neurol.* 19: 578–587.

Helfgott, S.M. (1989). Total lymphoid irradiation. *Rheum. Dis. Clin. N. Am.* 15: 577–582.

Hemmer, B., Fleckenstein, B.T., Vergelli, M., Jung, G., McFarland, H.F., Martin, R. & Wiesmuller, K.-H. (1997). Identification of high potency microbial and self ligands for a human autoreactive class II-restricted T cell clone. *J. Exp. Med.* 185: 1651–1659.

Holmdahl, R., Karlsson, M., Andersson, M.E., Rask, L. & Andersson, L. (1989). Localization of a critical restriction site on the I-Ab chain that determines susceptibility to collagen-induced arthritis in mice. *Proc. Natl. Acad. Sci., USA* 86: 9475–9479.

Johnson, R.T., Griffin, D.E., Hirsch, J.S., Wolinsky, J.S., Rodenbeck, S., Lindo de Soriano, I. & Vaisberg, A. (1984). Measles encephalomyelitis: clinical and immunological studies. *N. Eng. J. Med.* 310: 137–141.

Jupin, C., Anderson, S., Damais, C., Alouf, J.E. & Parant, M. (1988). Toxic shock syndrome toxin 1 as an inducer of human tumor necrosis factors and gamma interferon. *J. Exp. Med.* 167, 752–761.

Kabelitz, D., Pohl, T. & Pechhold, K. (1993). Activation-induced cell death (apoptosis) of mature peripheral T lymphocytes. *Immunol. Today* 14: 338–339.

Kouskoff, V., Korganow, A.S., Duchatelle, V., Degott, C., Benoist, C. & Mathis, D. (1996). Organ-specific disease provoked by systemic autoimmunity. *Cell* 87, 811–822.

Kuhn, K. (1987). The classical collagens: types I, II, and III. In *Structure and Function of Collagen Types*, ed. R. Mayne & R.E. Burgeson, pp. 1–43. Orlando, FL: Academic Press.

Kurosaka, M. & Ziff, M. (1983). Immunoelectron microscopic study of the distribution of T cell subsets in rheumatoid synovium. *J. Exp. Med.* 158: 1191–1210.

Kurrer, M.O., Pakala, S.V., Hanson, H.L. & Katz, J.D. (1997). β Cell apoptosis in T cell-mediated autoimmune diabetes. *Proc. Nat. Acad. Sci., USA* 94: 213–218.

Lotz, M. (1996). Cytokines and their receptors. In *Arthritis and Allied Conditions: a Textbook of Rheumatology*, ed. W.J. Koopman, Baltimore, MD: Williams and Wilkins. pp. 439–479.

Lowin, B., Hahne, M., Mattmann, C. & Tschopp, J. (1994). Cytolytic T-cell cytotoxicity is mediated through perforin and Fas lytic pathways. *Nature* 370: 650–652.

Lynch, D.H., Ramsdell, F. & Alderson, M.R. (1995). Fas and FasL in the homeostatic regulation of the immune responses. *Immunol. Today* 16: 569–574.

Marrack, P. & Kappler, J. (1990). The staphylococcal enterotoxins and their relatives. *Science* 248: 1066.

Morel, P.A., Dorman, J.S., Todd, J.A., McDevitt, H.O. & Trucco, M. (1988). Aspartic acid at position 57 of the HLA-DQ beta chain protects against type I diabetes: a family study. *Proc. Natl. Acad. Sci., USA* 85: 8111–8115.

Myers, L.K., Seyer, J.M., Stuart, J.M., Terato, K., David, C.S. & Kang, A.H. (1993). T cell epitopes of type II collagen that regulate murine collagen-induced arthritis. *J. Immunol.* 151: 500–505.

Nagata, S. & Golstein, P. (1995). The Fas death factor. *Science* 267: 1449–1456.

Nepom, G.T. (1995). Glutamic acid decarboxylase and other autoantigens in IDDM. *Curr. Opin. Immunol.* 7: 825–830.

Nepom, G.T. & Erlich, H. (1991). MHC class-II molecules and autoimmunity. *Annu. Rev. Immunol.* 9: 493–525.

Newsom-Davis, J., Harcourt, G., Sommer, N., Beeson, D., Willcox, N. & Rothbard, J.B. (1989). T-cell reactivity in myasthenia gravis. *J. Autoimmun.* 2 (Suppl.), 101–108.

Panayi, G.S., Choy, E.H.S., Connolly, D.J.A., Manna, V.K., Regan, T., Rapson, N., Kingsley, G.H. & Johnston, J.M. (1996). T-cell hypothesis in rheumatoid-arthritis (RA) tested by humanized non-depleting anti-CD4 monoclonal-antibody (mAb) treatment .1. Suppression of disease-activity and acute-phase response. *Immunology* 89: OG379–OG379.

Panitch, H.S., Hirsch, R.L., Schindler, J. & Johnson, K.P. (1987). Treatment of multiple sclerosis with gamma interferon: exacerbations associated with activation of the immune system. *Neurology* 37: 1097–1102.

Robinson, J.H. & Kehoe, M.A. (1992). Group A streptococcal M proteins: virulence factors and protective anitgens. *Immunol. Today* 13: 362–367.

Rosloniec, E.F., Brand, D.D., Myers, L.K., Whittington, K.B., Gumanovskaya, M., Zaller, D.M., Woods, A., Altmann, D.M., Stuart, J.M. & Kang, A.H. (1997). An HLA-DR1 transgene confers susceptibility to collagen-induced arthritis elicited with human type II collagen. *J. Exp. Med.* 185: 1113–1122.

Salmon, M. & Gaston, J.S. (1995) The role of T-lymphocytes in rheumatoid arthritis. *Br. Med. Bull.* 51: 332–345.

Salmon, M., Wordsworth, P., Emery, P., Tunn, E., Bacon, P.A. & Bell, J.I. (1993). The association of HLA DR beta alleles with self-limiting and persistent forms of early symmetrical polyarthritis. *Br. J. Rheumatol.* 32, 628–630.

Scharf, S.J., Freidmann, A., Steinman, L., Brautbar, C. & Erlich, H.A. (1989). Specific HLA-DQB and HLA-DRB1 alleles confer susceptibility to pemphigus vulgaris. *Proc. Natl. Acad. Sci., USA* 86, 6215–6219.

Singh, V.K., Kalra, H.K., Yamaki, K., Abe, T., Donoso, L.A. & Shinohara, T. (1990). Molecular mimicry between a uveitopathogenic site of S-antigen and viral peptides. Induction of experimental autoimmune uveitis in Lewis rats. *J. Immunol.* 144, 1282–1287.

Sinigaglia, F. & Hammer, J. (1994). Defining rules for the peptide-MHC class II interaction. *Curr. Opin. Immunol.* 6, 52–56.

Smolen, J.S., Tohidast-Akrad, M., Gal, A., Kunaver, M., Eberl, G., Zenz, P., Falus, A. & Steiner, G. (1996). The role of T-lymphocytes and cytokines in rheumatoid arthritis. *Scand. J. Rheumatol.* 25, 1–4.

Soden, M., Rooney, M., Cullen, A., Whelan, A., Feighery, C. & Bresnihan, B. (1989). Immunohistological features in the synovium obtained from clinically uninvolved knee joints of patients with rheumatoid arthritis. *Br. J. Rheumatol.* 28, 287–292.

Staines, N.A. & Wooley, P.H. (1994). Collagen arthritis – that can it teach us. *Br J. Rheumatol.* 33, 798–807.

Steinman, L. (1996). Multiple sclerosis: a coordinated immunological attack against myelin in the central nervous system. *Cell* 85, 299–302.

Stern, L.J., Brown, J.H., Jardetzky, T.S., Gorga, J.C., Urban, R.G., Strominger, J.L. & Wiley, D.C. (1994). Crystal structure of the human class II MHC protein HLA-DR1 complexed with an influenza virus peptide. *Nature* 368, 215–221.

Sun, J.-B., Rask, C., Olsson, T., Holmgren, J. & Czerkinsky, C. (1996). Treatment of experimental autoimmune encephalomyelitis by feeding myelin basic protein conjugated to cholera toxin B subunit. *Proc. Natl. Acad. Sci., USA* 93, 7196–7201.

Szekanecz, Z., Szegedi, G. & Koch, A.E. (1996). Cellular adhesion molecules in rheumatoid arthritis: regulation by cytokines and possible clinical importance. *J. Invest. Med.* 44, 124–135.

Theofilopoulos, A.N. (1995). The basis of autoimmunity: Part I. Mechanisms of aberrant self-recognition. *Immunol. Today* 16, 90–98.

Todd, J.A., Bell, J.I. & McDevitt, H.O. (1987). HLA-DQ beta gene contributes to susceptibility and resistance to insulin-dependent diabetes mellitus. *Nature* 329, 599–604.

Trentham, D.E., Dynesius-Trentham, R.A., Orav, E.J., Combitchi, D., Lorenzo, C., Sewell, K.L., Hafler, D.A. & Weiner, H.L. (1993). Effects of oral administration of type II collagen on rheumatoid arthritis. *Science* 261, 1727–1730.

Trowsdale, J. (1993). Genomic structure and function in the MHC. *Trends Genet.* 9, 117–22.

van Eolen, W., Thole, J.E., van der Zee, R., Noordzij, A., van Embden, J.D., Hensen, E.J., Cohen, I.R. (1988). Cloning of the mycobacterial epitope recognized by T lymphocytes in adjuvant arthritis. *Nature* 331: 171–173.

Vaughan, J.H., Fox, R.I., Abresch, R.J., Tsoukas, C.D., Curd, J.G. & Carson, D.A. (1984). Thoracic duct drainage in rheumatoid arthritis. *Clin. Exp. Immunol.* 58: 645–653.

Weinblatt, M.E., Maddison, P.J., Bulpitt, K.J., Hazleman, B.L., Urowitz, M.B., Sturrock, R.D., Coblyn, J.S., Maier, A.L., Spreen, W.R. & Manna, V.K. (1995). CAMPATH-1H, a humanized monoclonal antibody, in refractory rheumatoid arthritis. An intravenous dose-escalation study. *Arthritis Rheum.* 38: 1589–1594.

Weiner, H.L., Mackin, G.A., Matsui, M., Orav, E.J., Khoury, S.J., Dawson, D.M. & Hafler, D.A. (1993). Double-blind pilot trial of oral tolerization with myelin antigens in multiple sclerosis. *Science* 259: 1321–1324.

Wilder, R.L., Yarboro, C.H. & Decker, J.L. (1982). The effects of repeated leukapheresis in patients with severe refractory rheumatoid arthritis. Prog. Clin. Biol. Res. 106: 49–59.

Woulfe, S.L., Bono, C.P., Zacheis, M.L., Kirschmann, D.A., Baudino, T.A., Swearingen, C,. Karr, R.W. & Schwartz, B.D. (1995). Negatively charged residues interacting with the p4 pocket confer binding specificity to DRB1*0401. *Arthritis Rheum.* 38: 1744–1753.

Wucherpfennig, K.W. & Strominger, J.L. (1995a). Molecular mimicry in T cell-mediated autoimmunity: viral peptides activate human T cell clones specific for myelin basic protein. *Cell* 80: 695–705.

Wucherpfennig, K.W. & Strominger, J.L. (1995b). Selective binding of self-peptides to disease-associated major histocompatibility complex (MHC) molecules: a mechanism for MHC-linked susceptibility to human autoimmune diseases. *J. Exp. Med.* 181: 1597–1601.

Wucherpfennig, K.W., Sette, A., Southwood, S., Oseroff, C., Matsui, M., Strominger, J.L. & Hafler, D.A. (1994a). Structural requirements for binding of an immunodominant myelin basic protein peptide to DR2 isotypes and for its recognition by human T cell clones. *J. Exp. Med.* 179: 279–290.

Wucherpfennig, K.W., Zhang, J., Witek, C., Matsui, M., Modabber, Y., Ota, K. & Hafler, D.A. (1994b). Clonal expansion and persistence of human T cells specific for an immunodominant myelin basic protein peptide. *J. Immunol.* 152: 5581–92.

Wucherpfennig, K.W., Yu, B., Bhol, K., Monos, D.S., Argyris, E., Karr, R.W., Ahmed, A.R. & Strominger, J.L. (1995). Structural basis for major histocompatibility complex (MHC)-linked susceptibility to autoimmunity: charged residues of a single MHC binding pocket confer selective presentation of self-peptides in pemphigus vulgaris. *Proc. Natl. Acad. Sci., USA* 92, 11 935–11 939.

Zagon, G., Tumang, J.R., Li, Y., Friedman, S.M. & Crow, M.K. (1994). Increased frequency of Vβ17-positive T cells in patients with rheumatoid arthritis. Arthritis Rheum. 37: 1431–1440.

Zamvil, S.S. & Steinman, L. (1990). The T lymphocyte in experimental allergic encephalomyelitis. *Annu. Rev. Immunol.* 8: 579–621.

Zanelli, E., Gonzalez-Gay, M.A. & David, C.S. (1995). Could HLA-DRB1 be the protective locus in rheumatoid arthritis? *Immunol. Today* 16: 274–278.

3

The role of MHC antigens in autoimmunity

J. HOYT BUCKNER and G. T. NEPOM

Introduction

The immunological basis for autoimmune disease is complex, and autoimmune diseases themselves are diverse in character. The pathogenesis of specific autoimmune diseases may well be different, involving both genetic and environmental factors. However, many autoimmune diseases share an association with the HLA locus and, more specifically, the highly polymorphic class I and class II alleles found in this region. Recent advances in the understanding of the structure and function of HLA class I and class II molecules have made it possible to begin to decipher mechanisms by which these genes may be contributing to the development of autoimmunity. In this chapter, we will address the evidence that the HLA locus is associated with autoimmunity, the possible mechanisms by which HLA genes could contribute to disease, and the implication that this information will have on future assessment and treatment of patients with autoimmune diseases.

The HLA locus

The HLA locus is a cluster of genes found on chromosome 6 (6p21.3). This region includes the genes encoding HLA class I and class II proteins, complement and other factors important in the generation of the immune response. Figure 3.1 demonstrates the distribution of genes across this region. The HLA class I genes are located at the telomeric end of the human MHC. The *HLA-A*, *HLA-B* and *HLA-C* loci are referred to as class I genes and encode the principle transplantation antigens, which are expressed in all nucleated cells. The class I genes each encode a single polypeptide, the HLA class I heavy chain. The class I heavy chain forms a complex with β_2-microglobulin, a protein encoded outside of the MHC region, to form the functional HLA class I molecule. The HLA class II complex is also shown in Fig. 3.1. Each class II haplotype may contain up to 14

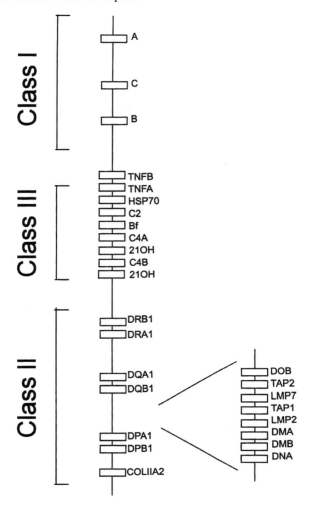

Fig. 3.1. A representation of the HLA locus on chromosome 6 emphasizing the genes discussed in the text.

different class II loci, clustered into three subregions, termed *HLA-DR, HLA-DQ* and *HLA-DP*. Each subregion contains at least one functional beta (B) locus and one functional alpha (A) locus. The *HLA-DRA* and *HLA-DRB1* loci encode the α and β chains, respectively, which together form a mature class II HLA-DR molecule. Similarly, the products of the *HLA-DQA1* and *HLA-DQB1* loci form the DQ molecule, and the *HLA-DPA1* and *HLA-DPB1* loci encode the DP molecule. A second DR molecule is encoded on most HLA haplotypes by the *HLA-DRA* and *HLA-DRB3, HLA-DRB4* or *HLA-DRB5* loci. Thus, most HLA haplotypes encode four distinct expressed class II molecules. The HLA class I and class II molecules produced by this genetically complex system are highly polymorphic in the population, leading to a source of interindividual differences (Dupont, 1989).

The class I and class II genes mentioned above represent only about half of the known genes lying within the HLA region (Ragoussis *et al.*, 1991; Kelly & Trowsdale, 1994). Among the remaining genes, several have interesting immunological functions that could be important in pathogenic events relating to HLA-associated autoimmune disease. One such region is the HLA class III region, a cluster of genes between the class I and class II complexes (Fig. 3.1). This region includes the genes for 21-hydroxylase and complement components C2, C4 and Bf (Carroll *et al.*, 1984; White, 1989). Within the class II complex between the *DQ* and *DP* clusters lies a group of genes involved in antigen processing. The genes for a transporter, TAP, and for low molecular weight protein (LMP) are within this region. These polypeptides are implicated in HLA class I antigen processing and peptide transport (Spies *et al.*, 1989; 1990; Deverson *et al.*, 1990; Trowsdale *et al.*, 1990). The *DMA* and *DMB* genes found in this region have a similar involvement in the class II antigen-processing pathway (Mellins *et al.*, 1990). Other genes of particular interest include a collagen gene centromeric of the class II region, an *hsp 70* gene found near the HLA class I complex and the cytokine genes for lymphotoxin, TNFβ and TNFα, centromeric of the *HLA-B* locus (Carroll *et al.*, 1987; Hanson *et al.*, 1989; Sargent *et al.*, 1989; Trowsdale, Ragoussis & Campbell, 1991).

The HLA region is, therefore, densely packed with genes important in the immune response. The polymorphic nature of these genes may contribute to differences in the immune response between individuals, and probably accounts for the HLA genetic linkage to a predisposition to autoimmunity. The structure and function of the proteins that these genes encode have been elucidated by crystallography and cellular biology. This information has deepened our understanding of how the HLA locus is associated with autoimmunity and the possible mechanisms by which this region contributes to the development of autoimmunity.

The structure of HLA molecules and the trimolecular complex

The crystal structure of both class I and class II molecules has been solved, allowing us a look at the structure of these HLA proteins. Both molecules are heterodimers with a peptide-binding site defined by an eight-stranded β sheet and two α helices. For class I, a constant chain β_2-microglobulin combines with either HLA-A, HLA-B, or HLA-C heavy chain to form a binding pocket in which peptides of only 8–10 amino acid residues in length are able to bind (Fig. 3.2*a*) (Madden *et al.*, 1991; Madden, Garboczi & Wiley, 1993). The class II proteins

(a)   (b)

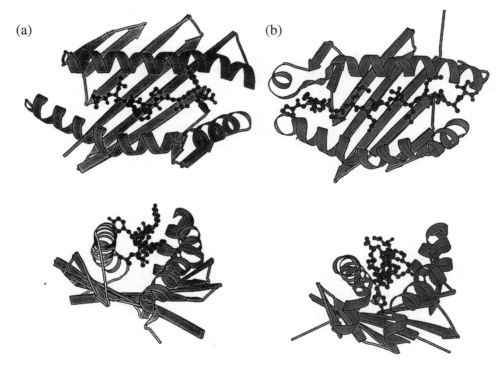

Fig. 3.2. Computer-generated models of HLA molecules based on known crystal structures (Kraulis, 1991). (*a*) A model of the HLA class I heavy chain molecule. Two views of the HLA-A*0201/TAX peptide complex are shown (Garboczi *et al.*, 1996). The top view has the α_2 helix on the bottom and the α_1 helix on the top with peptide amino terminus on the left end of the binding pocket. The bottom view includes the α_2 helix on the right and the α_1 helix on the left, with the peptide amino terminus coming out of the page. (*b*) A model of HLA class II molecule. Two views of the DR1/HA peptide are shown (Stern *et al.*, 1994). In the top view, the DR α chain forms the top α helix, and the DR β chain forms the bottom α helix; the peptide is bound with the amino terminus on the left. In the bottom view, the DR α chain is shown on the left, the DR β chain on the right and the peptide amino terminus is coming out of the page. The peptide extends beyond the groove, unlike the class I molecule.

include α and β chains, which combine to form a more open binding groove, allowing peptides of greater length to bind in the groove (Fig. 3.2*b*) (Stern *et al.*, 1994). The crystal structure of class I and class II molecules has also demonstrated that within the binding groove there are pockets which act as anchors for the peptide; these pockets favour interactions with specific amino acids based on size and polarity. Interestingly, those pockets that are essential for peptide-binding specificity are the regions where the most polymorphic residues are found.

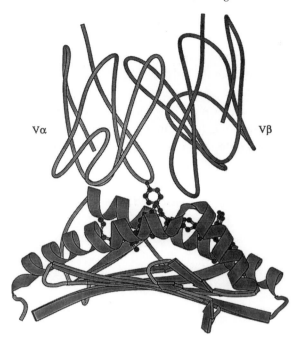

Vα   Vβ

Fig. 3.3. Model of the trimolecular complex based on the crystal structure of HLA-A2–TAX–TCR A6 (Garboczi *et al.*, 1996). This model demonstrates the interaction of the TCR with both the polymorphic regions of the HLA molecule and the peptide.

The HLA class I and class II molecules are found on the surface of cells and interact with CD8[+] and CD4[+] T cells, respectively, via the T cell receptor (TCR). The complex formed in this interaction – HLA molecule, bound peptide in the groove and the TCR – is referred to as the trimolecular complex. Here the crystal structure is enlightening as well. The crystal structure of the class I molecule HLA-A2 has been solved with a peptide TAX and the TCR A6 (Garboczi *et al.*, 1996). This structure demonstrates that the TCR has a relatively flat surface that interacts with the class I molecule and peptide in such a way as to contact both peptide and HLA molecule (Fig. 3.3). Of importance is the finding that half of the contact sites are with peptide residues, while the other contact sites are with the class I molecule and include polymorphic residues. This demonstrates that a TCR is not only peptide specific but is also specific for self-MHC. Indeed, the peptide may be altered as long as the residues that contact the TCR are not altered, allowing for the possibility of several different peptides being able to interact with the TCR in the context of one HLA molecule.

These studies of the structure of HLA class I and class II molecules demonstrate that the polymorphisms found in these genes encode the region important for T cell contact and for the peptide bound in the groove, leading to a unique surface appearance to the TCR for each HLA allele. At the level of the gene, the importance of these polymorphisms is demonstrated by the fact that the HLA class II genes share sequence over large regions, intermixed with regions of polymorphism, that correlate with T cell contact or with the binding pockets. These regions of polymorphism seem to be like 'cassettes' that are shuffled between alleles. An example of this concept can be found in the *DRB* locus, as shown in Fig. 3.4. Not only are these cassettes found among the *DRB* loci of humans, but they can be seen in other primates, suggesting that they play an important role in the immune response and have been conserved through evolution (Erlich & Gyllensten, 1991; Gaur *et al.*, 1997). Of further significance is the fact that these cassettes have been linked to disease susceptibility (see below).

Function of class I and class II genes

The function of the HLA class I and class II alleles are similar. Both molecules form heterodimers on the cell surface with peptide bound in the binding groove which forms a recognition signal for the TCR. Binding and activation of an antigen-specific T cell requires both HLA molecule and bound peptide. Class I and class II molecules differ in several ways. The HLA class I molecule contains a binding site for recognition by the T cell co-receptor known as CD8 (Rosenstein *et al.*, 1989) and the class II molecule contains a binding site preferential for the T-cell differentiation antigen CD4 (Mittler *et al.*, 1989). Binding of CD8 to the class I molecule achieves at least two things: it increases the affinity of interaction between T cell and antigen-presenting cell, which facilitates activation, and it provides for specificity by focusing the attention of CD8[+] T cells on antigens presented via the class I pathway (Garcia *et al.*, 1996; Gao *et al.*, 1997). The binding of the CD4 molecule to the class II molecule acts in a similar manner by increasing the affinity of interaction between T cell and the class II–peptide complex and it facilitates activation (Mittler *et al.*, 1989). Therefore, the engagement of the HLA–peptide complex with the TCR leads to the formation of the trimolecular complex and to the generation of the T cell response. The specificity of this interaction is dependent on the recognition of the self-HLA molecule and a specific peptide bound in the cleft.

The primary function of HLA molecules in the immune activation pathway is to bind antigenic peptides for presentation to a T cell. Therefore, the ability of an antigenic peptide to be bound by an HLA molecule is a primary determinant of whether or not an immune response to that peptide can be generated. The question of whether or not a peptide will satisfactorily bind to an HLA molecule is

HLA DRB1*	60	61	62	63	64	65	66	67	68	69	70	71	72	73	74	75	76	77	78
0101	Y	W	N	S	Q	K	D	L	L	E	Q	R	R	A	A	V	D	T	Y
0401												K							
0404																			
0405																			
1402																			
0402								I			D	E							
1301								I			D	E							
0801								F			D				L				
1101								F			D								
0701	S							I			D		G	Q					
0301	S											K	G	Q			N		
1501								I				A							

Fig. 3.4. The single letter amino acid code for residues 60–78 is given for several *HLA-DRB1* alleles. The shaded region is the third hypervariable region of the class II molecule. Those alleles producing similar sequences are grouped together. Notably these patterns fall into groups; the sequence shared by *0101, *0401, *0404, *0405 and *1402 is found only in alleles associated with RA and is referred to as 'the shared epitope'.

determined by the amino acid residues on the peptide in combination with the amino acid residues of the binding pockets of the HLA molecule (Buus, Sette & Grey, 1987; Krieger *et al.*, 1991). This structural interaction between an antigenic peptide and the HLA peptide-binding groove is one of the key ways in which HLA genes control the immune response. Only a few peptides have the potential to be immunogenic, by virtue of their ability to bind to an HLA molecule. The genetic control in this system is achieved by allelic variation. The principle polymorphic regions of HLA molecules include residues in the peptide-binding groove. Therefore, individual variation in the HLA molecule caused by genetic polymorphism determine which peptides are antigenic in one individual but are not in another individual.

The structural interaction between a peptide and the HLA peptide-binding groove determines which peptides are allowed to bind but it does not determine which peptides are actually available to bind. This aspect of peptide binding is determined by the intracellular events of antigen processing. Antigen processing takes place within a series of specialized compartments in the cell. Within this compartmentalized pathway, HLA molecules assemble, bind peptide and move to the cell surface where interactions with selected T cells occur (reviewed in Braciale & Braciale (1991) and Neefjes & Ploegh (1992)). Peptide comes to be bound by class I or II molecules via distinct processing pathways.

After synthesis, the class I heavy chain is transported to the endoplasmic reticulum (ER). In the ER, class I heavy chain forms a heterodimer with β_2-microglobulin and binds peptides derived from cytosolic proteins. These proteins have been partially degraded by proteasomes (which utilize the MHC-encoded *LMP* gene products) and make their way as proteolytically cleaved peptides into the ER in a form suitable for binding to class I molecules (Belich & Trowsdale, 1995). This movement of peptides into the ER is accomplished by a transporter molecule, TAP, which is itself encoded by genes within the MHC complex (Spies & de Mars, 1991). The interaction of the class I heavy chain and peptide in the ER results in transport of the class I–peptide complex into the Golgi and post-Golgi compartments on the way to the plasma membrane. In general, as a result of these features of the class I pathway, the peptides bound by class I molecules predominantly derive from self-peptides, viral or other endogenously synthesized proteins.

MHC class II molecules are synthesized in the ER, where the invariant (Ii) chain then aids in the assembly and transport of the nascent class II into the lysosome-like MIIC compartment and other endosomal compartments (Peters *et al.*, 1991). During this process the Ii is cleaved, leaving a peptide, CLIP, in the binding cleft. Proteins enter the cell via pinocytosis or receptor-mediated endocytosis. They then enter the acidic environment of the endosomes where proteases digest them into peptides. These peptides and the class II heterodimers both localize to the MIIC where CLIP is replaced by exogenous peptide in the MHC class II binding groove (Pieters, 1997). The non-classical class II molecule DM is thought to facilitate the removal of CLIP and the binding of peptides in this compartment (Sanderson *et al.*, 1994; Kropshofer *et al.*, 1997). The newly formed HLA–peptide complex then moves to the cell surface, possibly via endosomal fusion, where it becomes a mediator of T cell activation. As a result of these features of class II antigen processing, exogenous peptides are bound by class II molecules, although it has been demonstrated that class II molecules do present endogenous peptides as well (Nuchtern *et al.*, 1990; Chicz *et al.*, 1992).

Epidemiology of disease association

The association of HLA with several of the rheumatic diseases has been well recognized for some time (Tiwari & Terasaki, 1985a). This evidence has come from family, twin and population studies. Initially this work correlated serological specificities associated with HLA polymorphisms with patients and with con-

Table 3.1. *Some autoimmune diseases which have HLA associations and the* ￼
risk conferred by the associated HLA gene

Disease	HLA-associated allele	Race	Relative risk	Referen￼
Ankylosing spondylitis	B27		90	Khan and Kellner (1992)
Reiter's syndrome	B27		41	Khan and Kellner (1992)
Inflammatory bowel disease	B27		10	Khan and Kellner (1992)
Psoriatic arthritis	B27		10	Khan and Kellner (1992)
Rheumatoid arthritis	DRB1*0101	Israeli Jews	6	Gao *et al.* (1991)
	DRB1*0401	Caucasians	6	Nepom *et al.* (1989)
	DRB1*0404	Caucasians	5	
	DRB1*0405	Japanese	3.5	Ohta *et al.* (1982);
	DRB1*1402	Yakima Indians	3.3	Willkens *et al.* (1991)
Systemic lupus	DR2	Caucasians	3	Arnett and Reveille
	DR3		3	(1992)
Sjögren's syndrome	DR3		6	Arnett *et al.* (1989)
Pauciarticular juvenile rheumatoid arthritis	DR8		5	Nepom (1991)
	DR5		4.5	
	DP2.1		4	
Polyarticular juvenile rheumatoid arthritis	DRB1*0401 DRB1*0404		7	Nepom *et al.* (1984)
Juvenile dermatomyositis	DR3		6	–

trols. More recent studies have used molecular techniques to identify specific haplotypes and, in some cases, specific genes that account for these associations. Table 3.1 lists the best characterized examples of rheumatic disorders associated with HLA genes. The strength of the association of HLA and disease is reflected in the term 'relative risk', which is an odds ratio representing the risk of disease in an individual carrying a particular genetic marker compared with the risk in individuals in that population without that marker.

In many rheumatic diseases there is an increased frequency of the disease found among family members of affected individuals, suggesting a genetic link. This has been seen in SLE, where a patient with SLE has a 10-fold increased likelihood of having a first-degree relative with SLE (Arnett & Reveille, 1992); similar results are seen in RA (Deighton & Walker, 1991) and multiple sclerosis (Ebers *et al.*, 1986). Studies of monozygotic and dizygotic twins also support a strong genetic component to these diseases. The concordance rate for monozygotic twins in SLE is 24–69% compared with dizygotic twins, where the rate is 2–9% (Deapen *et al.*, 1992). In RA, twin studies have shown that 30–50% of identical twin pairs will be concordant for RA, compared with fraternal twins, which have 3–5% concordance rate (Winchester, 1981). These findings confirm a strong genetic basis for these diseases and suggest that the genetic contribution to these diseases is polygenic in nature, and not a simple single gene trait. However, a lack of complete penetrance in the genetically identical siblings also implicates other factors (Winchester *et al.*, 1992). These factors could include environmental exposures, both infectious and chemical, and stochastic events. The 30–50% concordance rate in identical twins is found in many autoimmune diseases. This finding may occur because, although identical twins have identical germ-line genes, they do not have identical immune systems since much of the immune system is developed along stochastic lines. Therefore, recombination events such as the formation of the TCR and immunoglobulins may be implicated as factors in the development of autoimmunity.

Population studies have been a further source for evaluation of the link between the HLA locus and autoimmunity. These studies have involved HLA typing patients with disease and controls taken from the population. When an allele is found to be more frequent in the disease population it is thought to be associated with the disease. Population studies allow the study of large groups of individuals and have broad applicability of findings. However, interpretation of findings may differ between ethnic groups. The strength of an association may differ based on the disease frequency and the baseline frequency of the susceptibility allele in the population.

An example of this is the *HLA-DR4* association with RA. In Caucasians, there is a frequency of disease that reaches 1%, and the presence of *DR4* in the general population is 23%. Of those affected by RA in this population 70% are *DR4*, thus demonstrating a clear association (Nepom & Nepom, 1992). However, in the African American population of the USA, the frequency of RA is similar to whites, but the presence of *DR4* in this population is lower, at 14%. In this population, *DR4* is found in 45% of patients with RA. This is considerably lower than the number of *DR4*-positive Caucasian RA patients; however, when the low overall frequency of *DR4* in the population is taken into account the association between disease and *DR4* is still present (Karr *et al.*, 1980).

Interpretation of the epidemiological data is complicated by several phenomenon that may lead to a demonstrable HLA association but also lead to differing interpretations of the data. These include variation in ethnic groups (as discussed above), allelic differences, linkage disequilibrium and *trans* complementing dimers.

Most HLA alleles within a single locus are highly related. Therefore, when a disease is associated with a specific allele within a single locus, differences between alleles may be quite small, as little as one nucleotide difference leading to an alteration in one amino acid residue on the entire molecule. As was discussed above, these polymorphisms play an important part in the structure at the site of T cell interaction and peptide binding. Therefore, it is important to identify differences between alleles because they have direct implications for the structure and function of the HLA molecules. An example of this is the association of both RA and pemphigus vulgaris with *HLA-DR4*. *DR4* is marker for a family of alleles that are quite similar; however, if the association of *DR4* with these two diseases is looked at at the allelic level important differences are found. RA is associated with *DRB1**alleles *0401, 0404, 0405* and *0408* (Nepom & Nepom, 1992), whereas pemphigus is found to be associated with *DRB1*0402* (Ahmed *et al.*, 1990; Scharf *et al.*, 1988a; Scharf, Long & Erlich, 1988b). Table 3.2 demonstrates the significant polymorphism between these alleles. The RA-associated alleles share a strong similarity at the β67, β70, β71 residues, which differ in size and charge on *DRB1*0402*. The aspartic acid and glutamic acid at positions 70 and 71, respectively, both carry a negative charge, unlike those positions in the RA-associated allelic products, which include a glutamine at β70 and a positive residue at β71, either a lysine or an arginine. These polymorphisms are structurally and functionally significant and link the genetic variability with disease-specific properties.

Genetic association must also be interpreted with the understanding that HLA genes are physically linked to one another. A high degree of linkage disequilibrium found among HLA loci means that different alleles at the different HLA loci do not randomly assort in each generation but rather exist on haplotypes that are relatively fixed in the population. Therefore, inheritance of a specific allele at one locus is often accompanied by the inheritance of a specific allele at a nearby linked locus. This means that when a polymorphic HLA marker is noted to be associated with a particular disease, the actual susceptibility gene may correspond to a linked gene elsewhere on the haplotype.

This may be the case with the HLA association of multiple sclerosis. Multiple sclerosis has been associated with the *DR2* haplotype in Caucasians (Tiwari & Terasaki, 1985b). This haplotype includes *DRB1*1501*, *DRB5*0101*, *DQA1*0102* and *DQB1*0602*. These genes are usually found as linked alleles in patients with multiple sclerosis (Allen *et al.*, 1994). Therefore, the high degree of linkage disequilibrium does not allow a distinction to be made between the contribution of individual genes in the *DRB1* and that of the *DQB1* region to the risk for multiple sclerosis.

Table 3.2. *Comparison of amino acid residues produced by DR4 alleles*

DRB1* alleles	Residue position				
	57	67	70	71	86
0401	D	L	Q	K	G
0402	D	I	D	E	V
0404	D	L	Q	R	V
0405	S	L	Q	R	G
0408	D	L	Q	R	G

Another phenomenon that must be taken into consideration is that of *trans*-complementary dimers. Most individuals in the population are heterozygotes, and, therefore, an individual's HLA phenotype is determined by two HLA haplotypes. Most individuals express six class I molecules and at least eight class II molecules. A further source of diversity in individuals heterozygous for class II haplotypes is provided by *trans*-complementation. *Trans*-complementation occurs when the HLA class II molecule α–β heterodimer is formed from an α chain encoded on one haplotype and a β chain encoded on the other haplotype, creating novel dimers in heterozygotes. For example, an individual heterozygous for the *DQA1*0501* and *DQB1*0201* genes on one haplotype, and the *DQA1*0301* and *DQB1*0302* genes on the other haplotype, will actually express four, not two, different DQ heterodimers resulting from the combinatorial association of each of the α and β chains. *Trans*-complementing dimers cannot occur with all combinations of α and β chains in the class II complex, so the extent of the additional diversity provided by this mechanism depends on the specific haplotypes in each individual (Kwok *et al.*, 1988).

One such example is coeliac disease. This disease has been associated with *HLA-DR3* and to a lesser extent with *HLA-DR7* (Kagnoff *et al.*, 1989). The *DR3* haplotype is relatively fixed as *DQB1*0201 DQA1*0501 DRB1*0301*, while the *DR7* haplotype shares the *DQB1*0201* allele (in common with *DR3*) but not the *DQA1*0501* allele. However, a high frequency of patients who are not *DR3* carry both *DR7* and *DR5*. The *DR5* haplotype includes *DQ1*0301* and *DQA1*0501*; as a result when the *DR7* haplotype is also present a *trans*-complementing DQ heterodimer DQA1*0501 DQB1*0201 can be formed in *DR5/DR7* heterozygotes (Sollid *et al.*, 1989). When population studies are evaluated in this light, 90% of patients with coeliac disease have DOA1*0501 DOB1*0201, demonstrating a clear association (Fig. 3.5).

When these factors are considered, many clear associations with the HLA locus

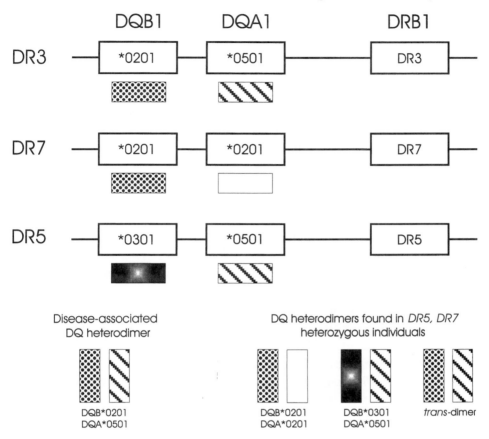

Fig. 3.5. *Trans*-complementing dimers in the susceptibility to coeliac disease. The DQ heterodimer DQB*0201 DQA*0501 is associated with coeliac disease. In individuals heterozygous for *DR7* and *DR5*, three combinations of *DQB* and *DQA* alleles are possible through *trans*-complementation, one of which is the heterodimer DQB*0201 DQA*0501.

and in some cases specific genes can be shown. With this knowledge the mechanisms by which these genes confer increased risk can be investigated.

Mechanisms by which HLA may contribute to autoimmunity

Genetic associations with autoimmunity can be applied to clinical use for prediction and prognostic purposes and can also be used as a means to define the mechanism by which these genes lead to autoimmunity. The structure of the HLA molecule and its role in the formation of the trimolecular complex give us clues to follow. In the remaining part of this chapter we will discuss the hypotheses that have been generated based on this information and summarize data that support these hypotheses.

Disease-associated alleles give rise to unique peptide binding

As discussed above, the function of HLA class I and class II heterodimers is to bind peptides in their binding groove and interact with the TCR. This then leads to signalling within the T cell and activation of the immune response. Since this is the primary immunological function of these molecules, it is reasonable to consider the ability of specific allelic products to present a pathogenic peptide as the basis by which they contribute to autoimmunity. This hypothesis would require evidence that allelic differences in HLA molecules lead to differences in the peptides which are bound, and the identification of pathogenic peptides.

The ability of a peptide to be bound in the groove of an HLA molecule is determined by the residues lining the pockets of the binding groove (as demonstrated by the crystal structure). These pockets determine a 'motif' for the amino acid residues needed or tolerated within the groove. Allelic polymorphisms occur at these sites and, therefore, alter the binding pockets and the binding motifs. Investigation into binding motifs has been carried out for many of the class I and class II alleles (Rammensee, Friede & Stevanoviic, 1995). These studies have shown that allelic differences do alter the peptide-binding motifs. An example of these differences can be demonstrated with the motif produced by the *DR4* alleles *0401, 0402* and *0404*. As described above, these *DR4* molecules are similar except at several residues located on the β chain (Table 3.2 above). These differences are most profound at residues 70 and 71, where 0401 and 0404 both have a glutamine at 70 and a positive residue at position 71. These residues line pocket 4, and motif studies have demonstrated that pocket 4 in these alleles favours a negatively charged residue. In contrast, the 0402 molecule carries a negative charge at both position 70 and 71, leading to an alteration in motif, with a preference for a positive charge at pocket 4 (Table 3.3). In this way, these alleles favour binding of different peptides and, therefore, generate different antigen-specific responses. In this instance, the allelic polymorphism, which is disease-associated, demonstrates a functional difference which can be associated with disease (Wucherpfennig & Strominger, 1995).

If disease is caused by the binding of a pathogenic peptide, then understanding of these motifs, in theory, could lead to the definition of important autoantigens. In diseases with known HLA associations, suspect autoantigens can be screened for peptides compatible with the motif of disease-associated allelic products.

This type of work has been done in the setting of pemphigus vulgaris and the

Table 3.3. *Binding motifs formed by DR4 alleles*

DRB1*	DRb71	Pocket 1 binding preference	Pocket 4 binding preference	Pocket 6 binding preference	Disease association
0401	K (positive)	V, L, I, M, F	D, E, (negative)	S, T, N, V	Rheumatoid arthritis
0402	E (negative)	V, L, I, M, F	K, R (positive)	S, T, N, V	Pemphigus vulgaris
0404	R (positive)	V, L, I, M, F	D, E, (negative)	S, T, N, V	Rheumatoid arthritis

*DRB1*0402* allele. Pemphigus is an immune-mediated, blistering disease of the skin. Patients with phemphigus vulgaris frequently carry the *DRB1*0402* allele. These patients have a specific antibody response to desmoglian, a skin protein, and this antibody response is directly implicated in the pathogenesis of the disease (Merlob *et al.*, 1986). Using the predicted binding motif of 0402 to scan the protein desmoglian for a peptide that could bind 0402, a peptide from this protein was identified that had the predicted binding motif for 0402, and in four patients T cells responsive to this peptide have been demonstrated. This finding suggests that an immune response to this self-peptide may be a component of the autoimmune phenomenon leading to disease, and that this occurs in 0402 individuals (Wucherpfennig *et al.*, 1995).

As described above, the motif is important in determining what peptides are allowed to bind, but which peptides are actually available to bind is determined by antigen processing. The mechanisms by which antigens are processed are being elucidated and at this time are not completely understood. However, it is clear that antigen processing may be important in determining the peptides available for binding, particularly since aspects of these processes may have allelic specificity. Interestingly, many of the proteins involved in processing are encoded by genes on the HLA locus. Several factors important in processing have been shown to be allele specific, including the effect of different intracellular environments such as pH, affinity for the chaperone CLIP, and the stability of the heterodimer. A specific example of this type has been suggested by Auger and Roudier. They have shown that a member of the heat shock protein family HSP73 binds DR4 molecules and may act as a molecular chaperone. This may lead to an alteration in the processing pathway for DR4 molecules with changes in the set of peptides accessible to this group of alleles (Auger *et al.*, 1996).

These concepts also suggest another method by which differences between alleles in the ability to bind a peptide may influence autoimmunity. In these scenarios instead of a pathogenic peptide being bound in the disease-associated allele, a protective epitope may be bound and presented in other alleles, leaving individuals without the protective allele at risk.

Unique MHC–TCR interactions

The crystal structure of the trimolecular complex discussed above demonstrates that the surface of the HLA molecule–peptide complex seen by the TCR is relatively flat. Contact with the TCR occurs via both the residues of the peptide and the components of the α helix of the HLA molecule. Therefore, class I and class II molecules may influence the immune response via direct contact between the TCR and HLA residues. One such mechanism would require direct interaction between the polymorphic residues on the HLA molecule with the TCR, leading to selection and activation of autoreactive T cells. The crystal structure of TCR–peptide–class I demonstrates interaction between the polymorphic sites on the class I protein and the TCR, and although a ternary complex has not yet been crystallized for class II it is likely from what is known of the structure that polymorphic residues will be in contact with the TCR in this setting as well. This has been demonstrated with alloclones, which specifically 'see' polymorphic residues on DRB1*0404, this recognition is lost on DRB1 mutant proteins, which differ only by one residue (Hiraiwa *et al.*, 1990; Penzotti *et al.*, 1996).

Another mechanism by which a direct interaction between the TCR and HLA molecule might occur is in the presence of a bacterial superantigen. Superantigens are molecules that are able to interact with the MHC and the TCR outside of the peptide-binding groove, usually using a common structural component from the TCR Vβ region (Dellabona *et al.*, 1990). These molecules then lead to an immune response that is not antigen specific. If a superantigen was specific for a class I or class II allele, it could lead to an amplification of autoreactive T cells in those patients with the disease-associated HLA type and initiation of autoimmunity. Such a mechanism might help explain the link between the genetic and environmental influences in autoimmunity.

Yet another hypothesis to be considered when thinking of HLA–TCR interactions is the ability of two closely related alleles to produce proteins that interact with the same TCR. Many HLA alleles are closely related and their products may be able to bind the same peptides. The surface of these molecules may be similar enough to be recognized by a TCR yet include polymorphisms on the HLA molecule that could subtly alter the interaction, leading to differences in signalling and possibly the immune outcome of the response (Madrenas & Germain, 1996). This type of mechanism could come into play in individuals who are heterozygous for two closely related HLA alleles, such as *0401* and

0404. A T cell may be positively selected in the thymus on 0401, but recognition of 0404 with a self-peptide may lead to activation and an autoimmune response. In this model, heterozygosity is important, as has been demonstrated in RA where most severe disease is found in individuals who are *DRB1*0401/DRB1*0404* (Weyand *et al.*, 1992).

Molecular mimicry

A model referred to as molecular mimicry has been suggested to explain the association of HLA with some autoimmune diseases. This model suggests that the contribution to the disease-associated region of the HLA complex is not functioning as a class I or class II molecule but is itself presented as a peptide on class II. In the example of RA, this would mean that the *HLA-DR*-encoded 'shared epitope' would be the peptide bound by other class II molecules and would lead to recognition by an autoreactive T cell. Although direct evidence of this phenomenon has not been demonstrated in disease, several lines of evidence suggest that it may be possible. Elution of peptides from HLA class II molecules have revealed that, although an important role of HLA class II is to present exogenous peptides to CD4+ T cells, the majority of peptides found bound to class II are derived from (membrane-bound) endogenous proteins, and some of these peptides are from the polymorphic regions of the MHC molecules (Chicz *et al.*, 1993; Rammensee *et al.*, 1995).

Evidence that self-peptides derived from the polymorphic regions of HLA molecules generate an immune response in humans has been demonstrated (Liu *et al.*, 1992; Salva *et al.*, 1994). These endogenous peptides may well play a role in the immune response, either at the level of T cell repertoire selection or later in immune modulation. In these cases, of course, studies would show linkage or association with the MHC. One trigger for mimicry could be an infection. Searches for infectious agents that have proteins homologous to these regions have been done. In the case of HLA B27, several proteins derived from *Klebsiella pneumoniae* and a *Shigella* sp. plasmid have been described (Schwimmbeck, Yu & Oldstone, 1987; Stieglitz, Fosmire & Lipsky, 1989) and the 'shared epitope' of RA has been shown to be present both in an Epstein–Barr virus protein and in a protein found in *Escherichia coli* (La Cava *et al.*, 1995). In this setting, a patient's ability to continue presenting a peptide similar to that of the infectious agent may lead to persistence of inflammation. These data raise the possibility that the polymorphic regions of self-proteins may act as peptides that are a factor in the protection from, or the initiation and propagation of, autoimmunity.

HLA genes other than those for class I and II may contribute to disease association

Other genes on the MHC certainly may contribute to autoimmunity. As discussed above, only half of the known genes found within the HLA locus encode HLA class I and II. Several of these other genes are important in immunological function, such as the cytokine genes for TNFβ and TNFα, genes involved in processing and genes of the class II region, which includes the complement components. In these cases, an HLA association may result from linkage with nearby non-HLA genes. Some forms of SLE may represent this type of disease association (Arnett *et al.*, 1984). Both *HLA-DR2* and *HLA-DR3* haplotypes are associated with SLE in Caucasians, and the predominant *HLA-DR3+* haplotype in Caucasians has very tight linkage with other genes within the MHC, notably *A1*, *B8*, *Cw7* and *C4A*. This last gene, a structural gene for the C4 complement component, is a silent allele on this *DR3* haplotype. The *C4A* 'null' alleles are significantly increased in patients with SLE, even on non-*DR3* haplotypes, and particularly when the patient is also *HLA-DR2+* (Fielder *et al.*, 1983; Christiansen *et al.*, 1991). This relationship may indicate that it is the presence of a *C4A* silent allele, rather than the expression of any particular class II gene, which is the primary predisposing genetic element in these patients.

Case studies in rheumatological disease

To demonstrate the concepts discussed above, we will discuss two rheumatic diseases with well known HLA associations. The possible mechanisms of disease can be explored for each of these diseases, although the relationship to HLA is different for each.

HLA-B27 and spondyloarthropathies

The association of HLA-B27 with the spondyloarthropathies is well established. Initial population studies in patients with ankylosing spondylitis demonstrated a marked predominance of HLA-B27 in the population with disease (90%) compared with the control population (10% Caucasians) (Benjamin & Parham, 1990). This association has been confirmed in different racial and ethnic groups (Khan & Kellner, 1992). To further establish the importance of the gene in development of this disease, a transgenic animal model has been developed in which the HLA-B27 molecule is expressed in the rat (Hammer *et al.*, 1990). In this model, the rats which express HLA-B27 develop a disease that bears striking similarity to spondyloarthropathies, directly validating the role of HLA-B27 in development of disease.

Another finding in the rat model confirms data found in humans. This is the finding that disease develops only in the rats that are exposed to infections (Taurog *et al.*, 1994), similar to reactive arthritis in humans (a form of spondylo-arthropathy), which has been clearly associated with preceding infectious diarrhoea (Hahn, 1993). These findings support the concept that both an environmental agent and HLA are important in this disease. However, the pathogenic mechanism by which B27 triggers disease is not yet known. Possible mechanisms include (i) the binding of a pathogenic peptide to HLA-B27, which leads to a CD8+ CTL response that causes joint inflammation; (ii) molecular mimicry, in which a bacterial peptide similar to a peptide found on the HLA-B27 heavy chain drives an immune response that persists after infection because of the persistent presence of the peptide from the HLA-B27 molecule itself; and (iii) HLA-B27 having a unique immunological role that is not yet defined.

Evidence to support the idea that the HLA-B27 molecule can bind a unique pathogenic peptide is supported by the finding that several subtypes of HLA-B27 exist (Khan & Kellner, 1992). These subtypes are all quite similar and all are associated with disease. These class I alleles share strong similarity in their peptide-binding pockets, particularly P2 (arginine site) (Khan & Kellner, 1992). An exception to this is the allele *B*2703*, which is found in West Africans and African Americans. Spondyloarthropathies are rare among these groups and this rarity may result from the differences found on the *HLA-B*2703* allele, which differs from the most common allele *B*2705* in giving a single residue change at position 59 (tyrosine to histidine) (Hill *et al.*, 1991). Molecular mimicry models for HLA-B27 are supported by the finding that several pathogens share similar amino acid sequences with HLA-B27 AA71–77. A more novel mechanism involving a less well-defined function of the HLA B27 heavy chain is suggested by the finding that *HLA-B27* transgenic mice, which do not express the β_2-microglobulin chain, still develop disease (Khare *et al.*, 1995). The mice are unable to form stable HLA-B27 heterodimers on the cell surface yet still get disease, suggesting a role that may not require the β_2-microglobulin chain for this molecule, such as HLA-B27 acting as a port of entry into the cell for pathogens or as a unique receptor on the cell surface.

RA and the shared epitope

Unlike the spondyloarthropathies, RA is a disease in which the HLA association has been mapped not to one allele but to a specific amino acid sequence found in several DR allelic forms. This sequence is referred to as the shared epitope. Population studies have demonstrated an association with *DRB1*0401* and *DRB1*0404* in the Caucasian population. Studies in several ethnic groups that have a low prevalence of *DR4* have shown other *DR* associations includ-ing: *DRB1*0101* in Israel, *DRB1*0405* among Japanese and *DRB1*1402* in the people of the Yakima Nation (Willkens *et al.*, 1991; Ollier & Thomson, 1992). Remarkably, each of these HLA alleles have in common the β67–74 region. As shown in Fig. 3.4, this region is not found on any other haplotype and although all these RA-associated alleles carry the same shared epitope, they differ in other regions of the HLA molecule. Therefore, it appears that it is the shared epitope itself, rather than any specific single HLA allele, that is the principle determi-nant of the genetic susceptibility for RA.

As discussed for HLA-B27, similar theories for the role of the associated HLA molecules in RA have been proposed: the ability of these molecules to bind a unique arthritogenic peptide, the shared epitope presenting itself as a peptide, leading to molecular mimicry, and a unique immunological interaction with the T cell by the disease-associated molecules. However, in RA these ideas need to be viewed differently. In RA, the idea that a unique peptide is bound in the RA-associated alleles can be supported by some similarities in the binding motifs of the molecules in pocket 4 (Woulfe *et al.*, 1995). However, unlike the *HLA-B27* alleles, the similarity between the associated molecules is not over the entire binding groove but is in one region of the class II β chain only (Fig. 3.6). This region includes the α helix. Other regions of the binding groove are not conserved between the associated alleles; therefore differences in binding motif occur in the disease-associated alleles. The molecular mimicry hypothesis, as in HLA-B27, is supported by the finding that there are bacterial sequences which are similar to the amino acid sequence found in the region of the shared epitope. The position of the shared epitope on the α helix also suggests that it may lead to unique interactions with the T cell, as dis-cussed above. Hopefully, as our understanding of the importance of allelic dif-ferences on the immune response broadens, we can clarify the underlying mechanisms involved with the HLA molecule and diseases such as RA and the spondyloarthropathies.

Future directions in research and therapy

Understanding the association of HLA and autoimmune disease has led to new areas of investigation into the pathogenesis of these diseases. It has also had an impact on clinical practice. The use of these genetic markers to identify mem-bers of the general population at risk is not feasible, since these HLA types are found in many more unaffected individuals than those affected by autoimmunity. However, use of these genetic markers is already helpful in assessing patients with arthritis. In the case of a patient presenting with signs and symptoms that

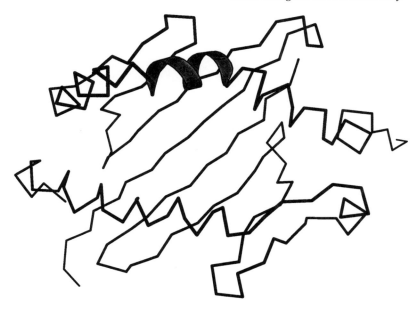

Fig. 3.6. Location of the shared epitope. The backbone trace of the DR1 variable domain is shown with the amino acid residues 67–74 highlighted as a ribbon. This region is the location of the shared epitope on DR molecules.

may be consistent with spondyloarthropathy, information regarding the presence of *HLA-B27* can help determine the likelihood of the diagnosis of spondyloarthropathy. This must always be done with the knowledge of the prevalence of the allele in the general population. In RA, the role of HLA typing is not helpful for diagnosis but may be useful for prognostic purposes and therapeutic decisions. It has been suggested that the presence of the shared epitope is associated with severity of disease, particularly having both the *0401* and *0404* alleles (Weyand *et al.*, 1992). Knowledge that the patient may expect more severe disease, particularly joint destruction, may lead to more aggressive early treatment. Response to therapy may also be influenced by a patient's HLA type. In a study comparing the response to methotrexate or combination therapy, patients carrying the shared epitope did better on combination therapy (O'Dell *et al.*, 1998). In this setting, knowledge of a patient's HLA type may help in the choice of initial therapies. Several new therapies are being developed to take advantage of our understanding of the structure and function of class II alleles; peptide-based therapies are being studied in multiple sclerosis and RA with the hope of interfering in the abnormal immune response to self by altering the peptides presented via the HLA molecules. Understanding the specific genes and the mechanisms by which they predispose to disease, and the environmental factors that influence disease, will allow us to target diagnostics and therapeutics more specifically in the future.

Acknowledgement

The structural models for the figures in this chapter were constructed using molecular homology modelling techniques, by Julie Penzotti, Virginia Mason Research Center and Dept of Bioengineering, University of Washington School of Medicine.

References

Ahmed, A.R., Yunis, E.J., Khatri, K., Wagner, R., Notani, G., Awdeh, Z. & Alper, C.A. (1990). Major histocompatibility complex haplotype studies in Ashkenazi Jewish patients with pemphigus vulgaris. *Proc. Natl. Acad. Sci., USA* 87: 7658–7662.

Allen, M., Sandberg-Wollheim, M., Sjogren, K., Erlich, H.A., Petterson, U. & Gyllensten, U. (1994). Association of susceptibility to multiple sclerosis in Sweden with HLA class II DRB1 and DQB1 alleles. *Human Immunol.* 39: 41–48.

Arnett, F. & Reveille, J.D. (1992). Genetics of systemic lupus erythematosus. In *Rheumatic Disease Clinics of North America*, ed. G.T. Nepom, p. 865. Philadelphia, PA: Saunders.

Arnett, F.C., Reveille, J.D., Wilson, R.W., Provost, T.T. & Bias, W.B. (1984). Systemic lupus erythematosus: current state of the genetic hypothesis. *Semin. Arthritis Rheum.* 14: 24–35.

Arnett, F.C., Bias, W.B. & Reveille, J.D. (1989). Genetic studies in Sjogren's syndrome and systemic lupus erythematosus. *J. Autoimmun.* 2: 403–413.

Auger, I., Escola, J.M., Gorvel, J.P. & Roudier, J. (1996). HLA-DR4 and HLA-DR10 motifs that carry susceptibility to rheumatoid arthritis bind 70-kD heat shock proteins. *Nature Med.* 2: 306–310.

Belich, M.P. & Trowsdale, J. (1995). Proteasome and class I antigen processing and presentation. (Review) *Mol. Biol. Rep.* 21: 53–56.

Benjamin, R. & Parham, P. (1990). Guilt by association: HLA-B27 and ankylosing spondylitis. *Immunol. Today* 11: 137–142.

Braciale, T.J. & Braciale, V.L. (1991). Antigen presentation: structural themes and functional variations. (Review) *Immunol. Today* 12: 124–129.

Buus, S., Sette, A. & Grey, H. (1987). The interaction between protein-derived immunogenic peptides and Ia. *Immunol. Rev.* 98: 115–141.

Carroll, M.C., Campbell, R.D., Bentley, D.R. & Porter, R.R. (1984). A molecular map of the human major histocompatibility complex class III region linking complement genes C4, C2, and factor B. *Nature* 307: 237–241.

Carroll, M.C., Katzman, P., Alicot, E.M., Koller, B.H., Geraghty, D.E., Orr, H.T., Strominger, J.L. & Spies, T. (1987). Linkage map of the human major histocompatibility complex including the tumor necrosis factor genes. *Proc. Natl. Acad. Sci., USA* 84: 8535–8539.

Chicz, R.M., Urban, R.G., Lane, W.S., Gorga, J.C., Stern, L.J., Vignali, D.A. & Strominger, J.L. (1992). Predominant naturally processed peptides bound to HLA-

DR1 are derived from MHC-related molecules and are heterogeneous in size. *Nature* 358: 764–768.

Chicz, R.M., Urban, R.G., Gorga, J.C., Vignali, D.A., Lane, W.S. & Strominger, J.L. (1993). Specificity and promiscuity among naturally processed peptides bound to HLA-DR alleles. *J. Exp. Med.* 178: 27–47.

Christiansen, F.T., Zhang, W.J., Griffiths, M., Mallal, S.A. & Dawkins, R.L. (1991). Major histocompatibility complex (MHC) complement deficiency, ancestral haplotypes and systemic lupus erythematosus (SLE): C4 deficiency explains some but not all the influence of the MHC. *J. Rheumatol.* 18: 1350–1358.

Deapen, D., Escalante, A., Weinrib, L., Horwitz, D., Bachman, B., Roy-Burman, P., Walker, A. & Mack, T.M. (1992). A revised estimate of twin concordance in systemic lupus erythematosus. *Arthritis Rheum.* 35: 311–318.

Deighton, C.M. & Walker, D.J. (1991). The familial nature of rheumatoid arthritis. (Review) *Ann Rheum. Dis.* 50: 62–65.

Dellabona, P., Peccoud, J., Kappler, J., Marrack, P., Benoist, C. & Mathis, D. (1990). Superantigens interact with MHC class II molecules outside of the antigen groove. *Cell* 62: 1115–1121.

Deverson, E.V., Gow, I.R., Coadwell, W.J., Monaco, J.J., Butcher, G.W. & Howard, J.C. (1990). MHC class II region encoding proteins related to multidrug resistance family of transmembrane transporters. *Nature* 348: 738.

Dupont, B. (1989). *Immunobiology of HLA*. New York: Springer-Verlag.

Ebers, C.G., Bulman, D.E., Sadovnick, A.D., Paty, D.W., Warren, S., Hader, W., Murray, T.J., Seland, T.P., Duquette, P. & Grey, T. (1986). A population-based study of multiple sclerosis in twins. *N. Engl. J. Med.* 315: 1638–1642.

Erlich, H.A. & Gyllensten, U.B. (1991). Shared epitopes among HLA class II alleles: gene conversion, common ancestry and balancing selection. (Review) *Immunol. Today* 12: 411–414.

Fielder, A.H., Walport, M.J., Batchelor, J.R. & Rynes, R.I. (1983). Family study of the major histocompatibility complex in patients with systemic lupus erythematosus: importance of null alleles of C4A and C4B in determining disease susceptibility. *Br. Med. J.* 286: 425–428.

Gao, G.F., Tormo, J., Gerth, U.C., Wyer, J.R., McMichael, A.J., Stuart, D.I., Bell, J.I., Jones, E.Y. & Jakobsen, B.K. (1997). Crystal structure of the complex between human CD8αα and HLA-A2. *Nature* 387: 630–634.

Gao, X., Gazit, E., Livneh, A. & Stastny, P. (1991). Rheumatoid arthritis in Israeli Jews: shared sequences in the third hypervariable region of DRB1 alleles are associated with susceptibility. *J. Rheumatol.* 18: 801–803.

Garboczi, D.N., Ghosh, P., Utz, U., Fan, Q.R., Biddison, W.E. & Wiley, D.C. (1996). Structure of the complex between human T-cell receptor, viral peptide and HLA-A2. *Nature* 384: 134–141.

Garcia, K.C., Scott, C.A., Brunmark, A., Carbone, F.R., Peterson, P.A., Wilson, I.A. & Teyton, L. (1996). CD8 enhances formation of stable T-cell receptor/MHC class I molecule complexes. *Nature* 384: 577–581.

Gaur, L.K., Nepom, G.T., Snyder, K.E., Anderson, J., Pradarpurkar, M., Yadock, W. & Heise, E.R. (1997). MHC-DRB allelic sequences incorporate distinct intragenic *trans*-specific segments. *Tissue Antigens* 49: 342–355.

Hahn, B.H. (1993). Management of systemic lupus erythematosus. In *Textbook of Rheumatology*, ed. W.N. Kelley, E.D. Harris, S. Ruddy & C.B. Sledge, p. 1043. Philadelphia, PA: Saunders.

Hammer, R.E., Maika, S.D., Richardson, J.A., Tang, J.-P. & Taurog, J.D. (1990). Spontaneous inflammatory disease in transgenic rats expressing HLA-B27 and human β₂m: an animal model of HLA-B27-associated human disorders. *Cell* 63: 1099–1112.

Hanson, I.M., Gorman, P., Lui, V.C.H., Cheah, K.S.E., Solomon, E. & Trowsdale, J. (1989). The human α₂(XI) collagen gene (COL11A2) maps to the centromeric border of the major histocompatibility complex on chromosome 6. *Genomics* 5: 925–931.

Hill, A.V.S., Allsopp, C.E.M., Kwiatowski, D., Anstey, N.M., Greenwood, B.M. & McMichael, A.J. (1991). HLA class I typing by PCR: HLA-B27 and an African B27 subtype. *Lancet* 337: 640–642.

Hiraiwa, A., Yamanaka, K., Kwok, W.W., Mickelson, E.M., Masewicz, S., Hansen, J.A., Radka, S.F. & Nepom, G.T. (1990). Structural requirements for recognition of the HLA-Dw14 class II epitope: a key HLA determinant associated with rheumatoid arthritis. *Proc. Natl. Acad. Sci., USA* 87: 8051–8055.

Kagnoff, M.F., Harwood, J.I., Bugawan, T.L. & Erlich, H.A. (1989). Structural analysis of the HLA-DR, -DQ, and -DP alleles on the celiac disease-associated HLA-DR3 (DRw17) haplotype. *Proc. Natl. Acad. Sci., USA* 86: 6274–6278.

Karr, R.W., Rodey, G.E., Lee, T. & Schwartz, B.D. (1980). Association of HLA-DRw4 with rheumatoid arthritis in black and white patients. *Arthritis Rheum.* 23: 1241–1245.

Kelly, A. & Trowsdale, J. (1994). Novel genes in the human major histocompatibility complex class II region. *Int. Arch. Allergy Immunol.* 103: 11–15.

Khan, M.A. & Kellner, H. (1992). Immunogenetics of spondyloarthropathies. In *Rheumatic Disease Clinics of North America*, ed. G.T. Nepom, p. 837. Philadelphia, PA: Saunders.

Khare, S.D., Luthra, H.S. & David, C.S. (1995). Spontaneous inflammatory arthritis in HLA-B27 transgenic mice lacking beta 2-microglobulin: a model of human spondyloarthropathies. *J. Exp. Med.* 182: 1153–1158.

Kraulis, P.J. (1991). MOLSCRIPT: a program to produce both detailed and schematic plots of protein structures. *J. Appl. Crystallogr.* 24: 946-950.

Krieger, J.I., Karr, R.W., Grey, H.M., Yu, W.-Y., O'Sullivan, D., Batovsky, L., Zheng, Z.-L., Colón, S.M., Gaeta, F.C.A., Sidney, J., Albertson, M., del Guercio, M.-F., Chesnut, R.W. & Sette, A. (1991). Single amino acid changes in DR and antigen define residues critical for peptide-MHC binding and T cell recognition. *J. Immunol.* 146: 2331–2340.

Kropshofer, H., Hammerling, G.J. & Vogt, A.B. (1997). How HLA-DM edits the MHC class II peptide repertoire: survival of the fittest? *Immunol. Today* 18: 77–82.

Kwok, W.W., Schwarz, D., Nepom, B.S., Thurtle, P.S., Hock, R.A. & Nepom, G.T. (1988). HLA-DQ molecules form α–β heterodimers of mixed allotype. *J. Immunol.* 141: 3123–3127.

La Cava, A., Nelson, J.L., Ollier, W.E., Keystone, E.C., Carson, D.A. & Albani, S. (1995). The OKRAA susceptibility sequence to rheumatoid arthritis (RA) is an immunological cassette expressed by microorganisms related to RA etiopathogenesis. *Arthritis Rheum.* 38: S371.

Liu, Z., Sun, Y.-K., Xi, Y.-P., Harris, P. & Suciu-Foca, N. (1992). T cell recognition of self-human histocompatibility leukocyte antigens (HLA)-DR peptides in context of syngeneic HLA-DR molecules. *J. Exp. Med.* 175: 1663–1668.

Madden, D.R., Gorga, J.C., Strominger, J.L. & Wiley, D.C. (1991). The structure of HLA-B27 reveals nonamer self-peptides bound in an extended conformation. *Nature* 353: 321–325.

Madden, D.R., Garboczi, D.N. & Wiley, D.C. (1993). The antigenic identity of peptide-MHC complexes: a comparison of the conformations of five viral peptides presented by HLA-A2 [published erratum appears in *Cell* 1994, 76(2): following 410]. *Cell* 75: 693–708.

Madrenas, J. & Germain, R.N. (1996). Variant TCR ligands: new insights into the molecular basis of antigen-dependent signal transduction and T-cell activation. (Review) *Semin. Immunol.* 8: 83–101.

Mellins, E., Smith, L., Arp, B., Cotner, T., Celis, E. & Pious, D. (1990). Defective processing and presentation of exogenous antigens in mutants with normal HLA class II genes. *Nature* 343: 71–74.

Merlob, P., Metzker, A., Hazaz, B., Rogovin. H. & Reisner, S.H. (1986). Neonatal pemphigus vulgaris. *Pediatrics* 78: 1102–1105.

Mittler, R.S., Goldman, S.J., Spitalny, G.L. & Burakoff, S.J. (1989). T-cell receptor–CD4 physical association in a murine T-cell hybridoma: induction by antigen receptor ligation. *Proc. Natl. Acad. Sci., USA* 86: 8531–8535.

Neefjes, J.J. & Ploegh, H.L. (1992). Intracellular transport of MHC class II molecules. *Immunol. Today* 13: 179–184.

Nepom, B.S. (1991). The immunogenetics of juvenile rheumatoid arthritis. In *Rheumatic Disease Clinics of North America*, ed. B.H. Athreya, p. 825. Philadelphia, PA: Saunders.

Nepom, B., Nepom, G.T., Schaller, J., Mickelson, E. & Antonelli P. (1984). Characterization of specific HLA-DR4-associated histocompatiblity molecules in patients with juvenile rheumatoid arthritis. *J. Clin. Invest.* 74: 287–291.

Nepom, G.T. & Nepom, B.S. (1992). Prediction of susceptibility to rheumatoid arthritis by human leukocyte antigen genotyping. In *Rheumatic Disease Clinics of North America*, ed. G.T. Nepom, p. 785. Philadelphia, PA: Saunders.

Nepom, G.T., Byers, P., Seyfried, C., Healey, L.A., Wilske, K.R., Stage, D. & Nepom, B.S. (1989) HLA genes associated with rheumatoid arthritis. *Arthritis Rheum.* 32: 15–21.

Nuchtern, J.G., Biddison, W.E. & Klausner, R.D. (1990). Class II MHC molecules can use the endogenous pathway of antigen presentation. *Nature* 343: 74–76.

O'Dell, J.R., Nepom, B.S., Haire, C., Gersuk, V.H., Gaur, L., Moore, G.F., Drymalski, W., Palmer, W., Eckhoff, P.J., Klassen, L.W., Wees, S., Thiele, G., & Nepom, G.T. (1998). HLA-DRB1 typing in rheumatoid arthritis: predicting response to specific treatments. *Ann. Rheum. Dis.* 57: 209–213.

Ohta, N., Nishimura, Y.K., Tanimoto, K., Horiuchi, Y., Abe, C., Shiokawa, Y., Abe, T., Katagiri, M., Yoshiki, T. & Sasazuki, T. (1982). Association between HLA and Japanese patients with rheumatoid arthritis. *Human Immunol.* 5: 123–132.

Ollier, W. & Thomson, W. (1992). Population genetics of rheumatoid arthritis. In *Rheumatic Disease Clinics of North America*, ed. G.T. Nepom, p. 741. Philadelphia, PA: Saunders.

Penzotti, J.E., Doherty, D., Lybrand, T.P. & Nepom, G.T. (1996). A structural model for TCR recognition of the HLA class II shared epitope sequence implicated in susceptibility to rheumatoid arthritis. *J. Autoimmun.* 9: 287–293.

Peters, P.J., Neefjes, J.J., Oorschot, V., Ploegh, H.L. & Geuze, H.J. (1991). Segregation of MHC class II molecules from MHC class I molecules in the Golgi complex for transport to lysosomal compartments. *Nature* 349: 669.

Pieters, J. (1997). MHC class II restricted antigen presentation. *Curr. Opin. Immunol.* 9: 89–96.

Ragoussis, J., Monaco, A., Mockridge, I., Kendall, E., Campbell, R.D. & Trowsdale, J. (1991). Cloning of the HLA class II region in yeast artificial chromosomes. *Proc. Natl. Acad. Sci., USA* 88: 3753–3757.

Rammensee, H.G., Friede, T. & Stevanoviic, S. (1995). MHC ligands and peptide motifs: first listing. *Immunogenetics* 41: 178–228.

Rosenstein, Y., Ratnofsky, S., Burakoff, S.J. & Hermann, S.H. (1989). Direct evidence for binding of CD8 to HLA class I antigens. *J. Exp. Med.* 169: 149–160.

Salva, S., Auger, I., Rochelle, L., Begovich, A., Geburher, L., Sette, A. & Roudier, J. (1994). Tolerance to a self-peptide from the third hypervariable region of HLA DRB1*0401 in rheumatoid arthritis patients and normal subjects. *J. Immunol.* 153: 5321–5329.

Sanderson, F., Kleijmeer, M.J., Kelly, A., Verwoerd, D., Tulp, A., Neefjes, J.J., Geuze, H.J. & Trowsdale, J. (1994). Accumulation of HLA-DM, a regulator of antigen presentation, in MHC class II compartments. *Science* 266: 1566–1573.

Sargent, C.A., Dunham, I., Trowsdale, J. & Campbell, R.D. (1989). Human major histocompatibility complex contains genes for the major heat shock protein HSP70. *Proc. Natl. Acad. Sci., USA* 86: 1968–1972.

Scharf, S.J., Friedman, A., Brautbar, C., Szafer, F., Steinman, L., Horn, G., Gyllensten, U. & Erlich, H.A. (1988a). HLA class II allelic variation and susceptibility to pemphigus vulgaris. *Proc. Natl. Acad. Sci., USA* 85: 3504–3508.

Scharf, S.J., Long, C.M. & Erlich, H.A. (1988b). Sequence analysis of the HLA-DRb and HLA-DQb loci from three pemphigus vulgaris patients. *Human Immunol.* 22: 61–69.

Schwimmbeck, P.L., Yu, D.T.Y. & Oldstone, M.B.A. (1987). Autoantibodies to HLA B27 in the sera of HLA B27 patients with ankylosing spondylitis and Reiter's syndrome. *J. Exp. Med.* 166: 173–181.

Sollid, L.M., Markussen, G., Ek, J., Gjerde, H., Vartdal, F. & Thorsby, E. (1989). Evidence for a primary association of celiac disease to a particular HLA-DQ α/β heterodimer. *J. Exp. Med.* 169: 345–350.

Spies, T. & de Mars, R. (1991). Restored expression of major histocompatibility class I molecules by gene transfer of a putative peptide transporter. *Nature* 351: 323–324.

Spies, T., Blanck, G., Bresnahan, M., Sands, J. & Strominger, J.L. (1989). A new cluster of genes within the human major histocompatibility complex. *Science* 243: 214–217.

Spies, T., Bresnahan, M., Bahram, S., Arnold, D., Blanck, G., Mellins, E., Pious, D. & de Mars, R. (1990). A gene in the human major histocompatibility complex class II region controlling the class I antigen presentation pathway. *Nature* 348: 744.

Stern, L.J., Brown, J.H., Jardetzky, T.S., Gorga, J.C., Urban, R.G., Strominger, J.L. & Wiley, D.C. (1994). Crystal structure of the human class II MHC protein HLA-DR1 complexed with an influenza virus peptide. *Nature* 368: 215–221.

Stieglitz, H., Fosmire, S. & Lipsky, P. (1989). Identification of a 2-Md plasmid from *Shigella flexneri* associated with reactive arthritis. *Arthritis Rheum.* 32: 937–946.

Taurog, J.D., Richardson, J.A., Croft, J.T., Simmons, W.A., Zhou, M., Fernández-Sueiro, J.L., Balish, E. & Hammer, R.E. (1994). The germfree state prevents development of gut and joint inflammatory disease in HLA-B27 transgenic rats. *J. Exp. Med.* 180: 2359–2364.

Tiwari, J. & Terasaki, P. (1985a). *HLA and Disease Associations*. New York: Springer-Verlag.

Tiwari, J.L. & Terasaki, P.I. (1985b). Neurology. In *HLA and Disease Associations*, p. 152. New York: Springer-Verlag.

Trowsdale, J., Hanson, I., Mockridge, I., Beck, S., Townsend, A. & Kelly, A. (1990). Sequences encoded in the class II region of the MHC related to the 'ABC' superfamily of transporters. *Nature* 348: 741–744.

Trowsdale, J., Ragoussis, J. & Campbell, R.D. (1991). Map of the human MHC. *Immunol. Today* 12: 443–446.

Weyand, C.M., Hicok, K.C., Conn, D.L. & Goronzy, J.J. (1992). The influence of HLA-DRB1 genes on disease severity in rheumatoid arthritis. *Ann. Intern. Med.* 117: 801–806.

White, P.C. (1989). Molecular genetics of the class III region of the HLA complex. In *Immunobiology of HLA. Immunogenetics and Histocompatibility*, ed. B. Dupont, p. 62. New York: Springer-Verlag.

Willkens, R.F., Nepom, G.T., Marks, C.R., Nettles, J.W. & Nepom, B.S. (1991). The association of HLA-Dw16 with rheumatoid arthritis in Yakima Indians: further evidence for the 'shared epitope' hypothesis. *Arthritis Rheum.* 34: 43–47.

Winchester, R.J. (1981). Genetic aspects of rheumatoid arthritis. *Springer Semin. Immunopath.* 4: 89–102.

Winchester, R., Dwyer, E. & Rose, S. (1992). The genetic basis of rheumatoid arthritis: the shared epitope hypothesis. In *Rheumatic Disease Clinics of North America*, ed. G.T. Nepom, p. 761. Philadelphia, PA: Saunders.

Woulfe, S.L., Bono, C.P., Zacheis, M.L., Kirschmann, D.A., Baudino, T.A., Swearingen, C., Karr, R.W. & Schwartz, B.D. (1995). Negatively charged residues interacting with the p4 pocket confer binding specificity to DRB1*0401. *Arthritis Rheum.* 38: 1744–1753.

Wucherpfennig, K.W. & Strominger, J.L. (1995). Selective binding of self peptides to disease-associated major histocompatibility complex (MHC) molecules: a mechanism for MHC-linked susceptibility to human autoimmune diseases. *J. Exp. Med.* 181: 1597–1601.

Wucherpfennig, K.W., Yu, B., Bhol, K., Monos, D.S., Argyris, E., Karr, R.W., Ahmed, A.R. & Strominger, J.L. (1995). Structural basis for major histocompatibility complex (MHC)-linked susceptibility to autoimmunity: charged residues of a single MHC binding pocket confer selective presentation of self-peptides in pemphigus vulgaris. *Proc. Natl. Acad. Sci., USA* 92: 11 935–11 939.

4

B cells: formation and structure of autoantibodies

A. RAHMAN, F. K. STEVENSON and D. A. ISENBERG

Introduction

Many autoimmune diseases are characterized by production of autoantibodies, and detection and measurement of these antibodies in patients' sera is used in diagnosis and monitoring of disease. For some autoantibodies, such as antibodies to double-stranded DNA (dsDNA) in SLE, or anti-acetylcholine receptor antibodies in myasthenia gravis, the autoantibodies appear to be involved in pathogenesis. Until recently, investigation in patients has been restricted largely to the mixed antibody populations in serum. However, using hybridoma and molecular biological technology, it is now possible to dissect out the individual antibodies from patients' sera and analyse specificity and molecular structure. By combining cloned and sequenced antibodies with the increasingly defined autoantigens, we are gaining insight into the features of autoantibodies that are responsible for pathogenicity. This review will describe our current understanding of antibody structure and the immunoglobulin (Ig) genes that encode the binding sites of autoantibodies. Knowledge at the genetic level may offer therapeutic opportunities based on rational design in order to block pathogenic interactions.

Variable region genes

V *gene recombination*

The events occurring in immunoglobulin genes during maturation of a B cell from a pro-B cell to a fully differentiated plasma cell are shown in Fig. 4.1. The genes encoding the heavy chains of immunoglobulin are highly unusual in having three separate genetic elements that must be combined prior to transcription (Tonegawa, 1983). Recombination takes place in two steps and is initiated by the lymphoid-specific RAG1 and RAG2 proteins (Gellert, 1992). Patients with

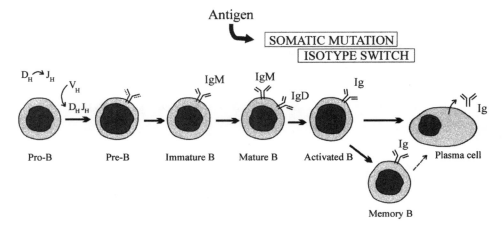

Fig 4.1. Changes in immunoglobulin occurring during normal B cell development. As B cells mature from the pluripotential stem cell to the fully differentiated plasma cell, immunoglobulin genes are recombined and modified. Following recombination, the pre-B cell expresses immunoglobulin μ chains with a surrogate light chain. Subsequently, light chains recombine and naive B cells express both IgM and IgD. Binding of antigen may then initiate further processes of somatic mutation and isotype switching, leading to plasma cells and memory cells.

certain rare forms of severe combined immunodeficiency (SCID) have defects in these proteins and consequently fail to generate immunoglobulin or T cell receptors (Kamachi *et al.*, 1993). Recombination begins at the pro-B cell level with the joining of a D_H segment gene to one of the six potentially functional J_H genes. Only a limited level of transcription occurs at this point until one of the available V_H genes combines to generate V_H–D_H–J_H. Transcription is then activated by the proximity of the promoter upstream of V_H to the immunoglobulin enhancer sequence, and the cell at this pre-B stage can synthesize μ heavy chains. As maturation proceeds, a similar recombination event takes place for the light chain to create V_L–J_L, and IgM is expressed (Fig. 4.1) at the immature B cell stage. Subsequent events following recognition of antigen are described below.

One feature of the joining process is that it may be imprecise, with gain or loss of nucleotides at the junctions, and in V_H the D segment gene may be read in different reading frames. Complexity at this site may be increased by D–D gene fusion or inversion, leading to a virtually unique sequence in the third complementarity-determining region (CDR3), which becomes the 'clonal signature' of a B cell. This sequence is maintained when a B cell clone undergoes expansion or neoplastic transformation and is proving useful in tracking tumour cells in patients after therapy (Steward, Potter & Oakhill, 1992). For normal B cells, the consequence of this potentially hazardous rearrangement of DNA is generation of a wide range of sequences, with CDR3 positioned at the centre of the antibody combining site (Kirkham & Schroeder, 1994). In some cases, the rearrangement will produce non-functional sequences, and if the second chance provided by the allelic chromosome also fails, the cell will die.

V_H gene usage

The choice of V_H gene for recombination is from a repertoire of approximately 51 potentially functional genes available in unrearranged germ-line DNA (Cook & Tomlinson, 1995). These genes can be divided into seven families, V_H1-V_H7, with members of each family having >80% sequence similarity (Table 4.1). Size of family varies from a single gene segment (V_H6) to 22 gene segments (V_H3) (Cook & Tomlinson, 1995). The V κ and λ light chains have a similar family structure, with 32 (Schable & Zachau, 1993) and 24 (Williams & Winter, 1993) potentially functional genes identified, respectively. The nature of the V gene segment dictates the basic sequence of V_H and V_L, although further diversification of sequence can occur by somatic hypermutation (see below). However, the sequence of the framework regions (FWs) tends to be conserved, and replaced amino acids often cluster in the CDRs, which are the known contact points for antigen (Fig. 4.2).

It has been difficult to estimate the relative use of different V_H genes by the normal expressed antibody repertoire, partly because of possible perturbation of gene usage by encounter with environmental antigens. In fact, studies using complementary DNA (cDNA) libraries (Logtenberg *et al.*, 1992), or *in situ* hybridization (Guigou *et al.*, 1990), have demonstrated that the expression of each V_H family is approximately equivalent to that expected from the available repertoire. However, recent analysis of single B cells from the blood of two normal subjects has shown that use of individual V_H genes varies, with the V_{3-23} gene (DP-47) being apparently overrepresented (Brezinschek *et al.*, 1997). One explanation may be that this gene is duplicated in certain haplotypes (Sasso, Buckner & Suzuki, 1995). Increased usage of particular V_H genes also occurs as a result of stimulation by B cell superantigens (Goodglick & Braun, 1994). Examples of B cell superantigens are found among common pathogens, such as staphylococcal protein A, which binds to immunoglobulin encoded by genes from the V_H3 family (Goodglick & Braun, 1994). Superantigen binding is to the FWs of the V_H sequence, rather than to the conventional sites in CDR1, CDR2 and CDR3 (Fig. 4.2). By this means, superantigens can stimulate a wide range of B cells, perhaps generating an early low-affinity IgM antibody response against invading pathogens.

Table 4.1. V_H *content of the functional locus on chromosome* $14_q32.3$

V_H family	Number of gene segments
V_H1	11
V_H2	3
V_H3	22
V_H4	11
V_H5	2
V_H6	1
V_H7	1
Total	51

Cook & Tomlinson, 1995

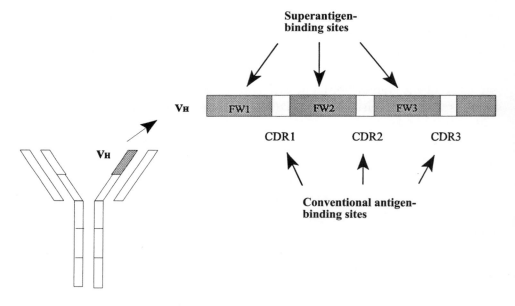

Fig. 4.2. Expanded view of the immunoglobulin heavy chain variable region (V_H) indicating the complementarity-determining regions (CDRs), known to be involved in high-affinity binding to conventional antigen. Also shown are the framework (FW) regions, which provide structural support for V_H, but which also may bind to certain 'superantigens'.

Somatic hypermutation

The naive mature IgM+ IgD+ B cell repertoire may undergo negative selection in the bone marrow environment, with removal of cells expressing immunoglobulin recognizing local autoantigens (Ghia *et al.*, 1995). This could be a crucial step in avoiding subsequent production of autoantibodies. Circulating B cells then can encounter antigen and enter the germinal centre of the lymphoid tissue (Fig. 4.1). In this site, the available range of *V* region sequence is extended by somatic hypermutation, which introduces mutations across V_H and V_L (Berek & Milstein, 1987). If the mutations generate replacement amino acids, they can be selected by limiting antigen, leading to a concentration of optimal amino acids in the contact points in the CDRs (Berek & Milstein, 1987). If mutations are deleterious, or if the cells are not selected, they will die by apoptosis (Liu *et al.*, 1989). Antigen-selected B cells will proliferate and, in the presence of CD4+ T cells and appropriate cytokines, undergo isotype switching (Berek & Milstein, 1987). Memory B cells and plasma cells are the final products of this maturation process.

Clearly, at this stage, where a new repertoire is being developed, there is a possibility of producing autoantibodies, some of which could be of high affinity. To avoid this, a second process of negative selection must operate. One of the mechanisms could be counter-selection against sequences containing mutations in CDRs that confer increased affinity for autoantigen. Intriguingly, this appears to occur in rheumatoid factors produced by normal individuals, but not in patients with RA (Borretzen *et al.*, 1994). Studies in transgenic mouse models have shown that there are several alternative mechanisms that can operate to suppress auto-antibody production, including inactivation or deletion of B cells (Shokat & Goodnow, 1995). At the levels of *V* genes, a further process, termed 'receptor editing', has been described, whereby a transgenic heavy and light chain pair from an autoanti-DNA antibody is rendered non-reactive by substitution of a rearranged endogenous V_L sequence (Tiegs, Russell & Nemazee, 1993). Finally, high levels of soluble protein antigen can induce apoptosis in specific B cells (Shokat & Goodnow, 1995). Evidently there are many potential checks and balances to prevent autoimmunity, and these shape the B cell repertoire. However, the normal shaped repertoire includes B cells capable of secreting IgM auto-antibodies. These B cells can produce significant levels of these antibodies under certain conditions, such as following infection with Epstein–Barr virus (EBV) (Chapman *et al.*, 1993). One possible check point is at isotype switch, since these B cells may either fail to undergo isotype switch or lose autoantibody activity in the switched variant.

Isotype switching

The process of isotype switching is likely to take place close to the site of somatic mutation in the germinal centre. Isotype switching results from a deletional DNA recombination event in which the *Cμ* constant region, initially located downstream of the *VDJ* region, is replaced by a *Cγ*, *Cα* or *Cε* constant region

(Coffman, Lebman & Rothman, 1993). The deletional endpoints are within or close to repetitive switch region sequences situated upstream of each constant region gene (Coffman et al., 1993). DNA between the switch sites is excised and can form a released 'switch circle'. Switching is influenced by cytokines, with IL-4, IFN-γ, and TGFβ being particularly important. Patients with X-linked hyper-IgM syndrome, who lack CD40 ligand (CD40L) normally expressed by T cells in the germinal centre, make IgM but fail to produce germinal centres and to generate significant amounts of IgG and IgA. They also show minimal levels of somatic mutations, implicating CD40L+ T cells in both somatic mutation and isotype switching events (Di Santo et al., 1993).

It appears that a considerable amount of somatic mutation can occur prior to isotype switch, and mutated IgM+ B cells can enter the blood (Klein, Kuppers & Rajewsky, 1994). However, there may be further accumulation of mutations after switching, and the change in the Fc region of the protein will influence the pathogenicity of autoantibodies. In fact, in autoimmune diseases such as SLE, pathogenic high-affinity antibodies tend to be of the IgG isotype. This points to a major role for CD4+ T cells in autoimmune disease, and there has been immense effort in investigating the T cell populations in various autoimmune diseases. In SLE, CD4+ T cell clones have been isolated that appear to recognize peptides from nucleosomes, and these clones are able to help B cells to produce anti-DNA antibodies (Mao et al., 1994).

Autoantibodies in rheumatic diseases

The knowledge of B cell biology described in the first part of this chapter can be applied to the study of potentially pathogenic autoantibodies found in rheumatic disorders. In this section, we will discuss this with reference to two examples, anti-dsDNA and anti-phospholipid (aPL) antibodies.

Anti-dsDNA antibodies in SLE

Although many different autoantibodies can be found in the serum of patients with SLE, those binding to dsDNA are most closely linked with tissue damage, particularly glomerulonephritis (reviewed in Isenberg et al., 1997). There is a considerable body of evidence to support this statement. While anti-dsDNA antibodies are found in approximately 75% of patients with SLE (Cervera et al. 1993), they are almost never seen in those with other diseases or in healthy individuals, including the normal relatives of patients with lupus (Christian & Elkon 1980; Isenberg et al., 1985). The levels of these antibodies tend to be high when the disease is at its most active (Ter Borg et al., 1990; Cervera et al., 1993) and they are deposited in the inflamed glomeruli of patients with lupus nephritis (Koffler, Schur & Kunkel, 1967).

In a number of animal models, it has been shown that monoclonal mouse or human anti-dsDNA antibodies can deposit in glomeruli to give proteinuria and nephritis (Madaio *et al.*, 1987; Raz *et al.*, 1989; Ehrenstein *et al.*, 1995). However, it is important to note that not all anti-dsDNA antibodies are equally pathogenic in such models. This correlates with the clinical data showing that a subset of human anti-dsDNA is particularly closely involved in renal damage in lupus. This subset consists primarily of IgG antibodies that bind specifically to dsDNA with high affinity. Okamura *et al.* (1993) demonstrated that in 40 patients with untreated lupus nephritis the degree of renal damage was related to the serum level of IgG anti-dsDNA but not to that of IgM anti-dsDNA or to anti-single stranded (ss)DNA of either isotype.

It is important to recognize that the high-affinity antibodies associated with tissue damage in a single patient arise from a number of different B cell clones, and that the study of any single clone will not necessarily give a true picture of the whole disease process. However, in order to draw conclusions about antibody sequence, genetic origin and fine structure, it is usually necessary to study monoclonal antibodies. These can be produced from peripheral blood lymphocytes or spleen cells by making hybridomas or by EBV transformation of cells.

Attempts have been made to define pathogenically important antibodies by means of idiotypes. An idiotype is a determinant in the variable region of an antibody molecule that is definable by a polyclonal antiserum. An idiotope is a variable region determinant defined by a monoclonal antibody. Some idiotypes are present on antibodies of several different specificities. These *public* idiotypes are generally believed to be encoded by elements in the FWs. Other idiotypes are more restricted and such *private* idiotypes are encoded primarily by the CDRs. Where it can be shown that the level of a particular idiotype is high in patients with SLE and that antibodies carrying it are detectable in damaged tissues (Isenberg & Collins, 1985; Kalunian *et al.*, 1989), it suggests that monoclonal anti-dsDNA antibodies carrying the same idiotype may be representative of the pathogenetically important clones in such patients.

In rare cases, it has been possible to localize an idiotope accurately. For example the idiotope 9G4 is encoded by the amino acid residues AVY at positions 23–25 in FW1 of the germ-line gene V_{4-34} (Potter *et al.*, 1993) and, therefore, serves as a marker for antibodies where the heavy chain is encoded by this gene. More recently, it has been shown that the idiotope actually comprises an interaction between these three amino acids and a tryptophan at position 7 in FW1 (Mockridge *et al.*, 1996). It has been estimated that 45% of patients with SLE may possess raised levels of 9G4 idiotope-positive antibodies in their serum and that in 3 out of 11 patients these antibodies were deposited in the kidneys (Isenberg *et al.*, 1993). Studies of monoclonal anti-dsDNA antibodies encoded by V_{4-34} may, therefore, be relevant to the pathogenesis of lupus nephritis.

Evidence from sequence analysis of monoclonal anti-dsDNA antibodies

By cloning and sequencing cDNA encoding the V_H and V_L regions of a monoclonal antibody, it is possible to discover a great deal about the history of the B cell clone which produced it. Firstly, the identities of the *V* and *J* genes that have been rearranged functionally to produce the heavy and light chains of this antibody can be deduced. It may be possible to identify the *D* genes, though this is more difficult because of the complexity of recombination in this area. The cDNA sequence can then be compared with the sequence of the corresponding germline gene, ideally by sequencing non-rearranged genomic DNA from the individual from whose cells the monoclonal antibody was derived. Differences between the two sequences are likely to result from somatic mutation.

Many monoclonal anti-dsDNA antibodies have been derived from mouse models of SLE. Certain genes seem to be used preferentially to encode such antibodies. For example, antibodies from three different mouse models all use the same V_H genes, which are members of the J558 gene family (Krishnan & Marion, 1993). The relevance of mouse autoantibody data to human disease is not entirely clear, however. The mouse V_H gene repertoire has not been fully sequenced and is more complicated than that of humans. Estimates of the number of functional mouse V_H genes vary from 100 to 1000 (Kofler *et al.*, 1992), compared with 51 in humans. In addition, expressed mouse *V* genes show a generally lower degree of complexity in CDR3 sequences, and of somatic mutation, than human *V* genes. These facts suggest that choice of V_H gene may play a more important role in generation of antibody diversity in the mouse than in humans. Nevertheless, certain features, such as the role of basic amino acids in binding to DNA, seem to be common to both species (see below).

In humans, cold agglutinins (which bind to the I/i antigen on the surface of erythrocytes) all use the V_{4-34} gene. Although this shows that gene preference can be involved in determining antigen specificity in humans, the available evidence from human monoclonal anti-dsDNA antibodies shows no definite preference for any particular family or for particular *V* genes (Isenberg *et al.*, 1997). However, the numbers of antibodies studied are small, especially those of IgG isotype. This conclusion must 'therefore' be guarded.

By studying IgM and IgG cDNA libraries from unstimulated human peripheral blood lymphocytes, Huang and Stollar (1993) demonstrated that IgG generally tend to carry more somatic mutations. This is also true of human monoclonal anti-dsDNA antibodies. IgM monoclonal antibodies with relatively low affinity and low specificity for DNA have been isolated from healthy subjects as well as from patients with SLE. These antibodies have often shown cDNA sequences almost identical to those of the germ-line genes (reviewed in Isenberg *et al.*, 1994), although some mutated IgM have been reported (Rioux *et al.*, 1995). In contrast, it has proved very difficult to produce human IgG monoclonal anti-dsDNA antibodies, even from patients with active disease. The few IgG molecules that have been reported tend to have numerous somatic mutations, particularly in the V_H regions (van Es *et al.*, 1991; Winkler, Fehr & Kalden, 1992; Stevenson *et al.*, 1993; Ehrenstein *et al.*, 1994). The replacement mutations are not evenly distributed, being clustered in the CDRs. This is often expressed in the form of the ratio of replacement to silent mutations (R:S) in each region of the sequence. Where R:S is higher in the CDRs than the FWs, this finding suggests that the B cell clone producing the monoclonal antibody has been subject to antigen-driven clonal expansion. This observation can be expressed statistically by using the binomial theorem to calculate the probability that a particular distribution of R and S mutations could have arisen by chance without requiring antigen-mediated selection (Chang & Casali, 1994).

Antigen promotes accumulation of sequence motifs associated with high-affinity binding

The theory that a particular clone of antibody-producing cells is stimulated to expand by antigen and that later generations of cells accumulate R mutations in the CDRs predicts that it should be possible to produce distinct but clonally related hybridomas from an individual patient with SLE. Such clonally related hybridomas have been reported in studies of both rheumatoid factors (Schlomchik *et al.*, 1987) and anti-DNA antibodies (Schlomchik *et al.*, 1990) in mice. The clonal relationship is deduced from the fact that the antibodies share the same 'clonal signature' in V_H CDR3. Dersimonian *et al.* (1987) reported three IgM monoclonal anti-DNA antibodies derived from a single patient that showed very few differences from the germ-line V_H26 (now called V_{3-23}). Two of these showed exactly the same V_H sequence, including the clonal signature. Therefore, even where extensive mutation has not occurred, clonal expansion may contribute to the production of anti-DNA antibodies.

In patients with SLE and in murine models of the disease, therefore, certain clones of autoreactive B cells seem to escape the normal control mechanisms. Under the influence of appropriate cytokines, antigen drives these clones to expand and to produce high-affinity 'pathogenic' antibodies. As noted above, this may be associated temporally with isotype switching. By comparing the sequences of many such antibodies, it has been possible to suggest which particular mutations contribute most to this high affinity. Much of this work has been done in mice, simply because of the large number of monoclonal antibodies available. The most striking feature is that the number of basic or positively charged amino acids in the sequence is often increased in high-affinity anti-dsDNA antibodies, especially in V_H CDR3, where they may arise from junctional diversity or N base addition as well as from mutation (Krishnan & Marion, 1993). It has been postulated that these changes enhance binding to negatively charged DNA. Computer programs can use the variable region sequence of such an antibody to construct a three-dimensional model of the antibody–DNA complex. In an extensive review of murine anti-DNA antibodies, Radic and Weigert (1994) showed that such models often demonstrate an important role for basic amino acids such as arginine (R), asparagine (N) and lysine (K) at the site of binding to the DNA double helix. These amino acids could be situated in any of a number of different CDRs, particularly V_H CDR1, V_H CDR2, V_H CDR3 and V_L CDR1.

In human IgG anti-DNA antibodies, similar patterns have been found. As in mice, basic or positively charged residues are prominent especially, but not exclusively, in V_H CDR3 (Winkler *et al.*, 1992; Ehrenstein *et al.*, 1994). The mere presence of such residues is not sufficient to confer high affinity for dsDNA. Some aPL, for example, have basic CDRs but no DNA-binding activity (Rahman *et al.*, 1996). This may be because of the different spatial arrangement of charged groups in DNA and in anionic phospholipids, which are the main targets of these aPL. The repeating double helical structure of DNA can provide a regular array of negative charge whereas this is not true of phospholipids.

Nevertheless, studies of anti-DNA antibodies encoded by V_{4-34} support the importance of basic residues in V_H CDR3. D5 and RT 79 are monoclonal anti-DNA antibodies produced in the same laboratory, that both use this V_H gene. Their heavy chain sequences have many basic residues in V_H CDR3, a feature not seen in monoclonal cold agglutinins encoded by V_{4-34} that do not bind to DNA (Stevenson *et al.*, 1993). Conversely, some groups have described sequence motifs that occur commonly in anti-dsDNA antibodies but do not contain positive residues. An example is the tetrapeptide YYGS, which has been reported to occur in several such antibodies and to be derived from the germ-line D segment DXP'1 (Cairns *et al.*, 1989).

There is, therefore, no simple relationship between the absolute number of basic amino acids in the CDRs of a monoclonal antibody and its affinity for dsDNA. It is the actual position of these residues that is critical. It is possible to use computer-generated models of the type mentioned above to hypothesize that particular residues are crucial in the binding site (Radic *et al.*, 1993; Kalsi *et al.*, 1996). To test such a hypothesis, it is necessary to compare the binding properties of the original antibody with those of a slightly modified molecule that differs only at the residues in question. Whereas such modifications can be readily achieved by site-directed mutagenesis, it is more problematic to develop systems for expressing the mutant and wild-type anti-DNA antibodies.

Use of expression systems to investigate autoantibody function

To be useful scientifically, the expressed product must possess a complete antigen-binding site, and expression of both V_H and V_L cDNA in the same cell is, therefore, required. Some workers have sought to express the cloned V_H and V_L genes of previously characterized monoclonal antibodies for which the binding properties are known. This has been achieved in a number of ways: as whole antibodies in mammalian cells (Radic *et al.*, 1993; Pewzner-Jung, Simon & Eilat, 1996), as single chain Fv fragments (Polymenis & Stollar, 1994) or as phage-bound Fab fragments (Mockridge *et al.*, 1996). Phage-bound Fab can also be used in a different way by creating heavy and light chain cDNA libraries, allowing a large number of different heavy and light chain combinations to be expressed on the surface of phage molecules and testing for DNA-binding affinity (Barbas *et al.*, 1995). In general, the results of experiments using all these techniques have tended to confirm the predictions of sequencing and modelling studies. For example, Radic *et al.* (1993) showed that removal of arginine residues from sites believed to be important in the heavy chain of the murine monoclonal antibody 3H9 did result in reduced DNA-binding affinity. The sequential addition of arginine residues increased affinity, but not in a linear fashion, and some sites appeared more critical than others. Using a similar method, Katz, Limpanasithikul & Diamond (1994) found that DNA-binding affinity could be perceptibly altered by single amino acid residue changes in the V_H sequence of another murine antibody, R4A. However, some changes that increased positive charge actually reduced affinity for DNA, and when the mutant antibodies were introduced into SCID mice, the ability to cause glomerulonephritis did not always vary in parallel with the ability to bind dsDNA.

Much less work has involved mutagenesis of human monoclonal anti-dsDNA. However, in a recent study of the V_{4-34}-encoded antibody D5, Mockridge *et al.* (1996) demonstrated that basic residues in V_H CDR3 were important in binding dsDNA, as were changes caused by somatic mutations in the light chain but not the heavy chain. Intriguingly, binding to the 9G4 idiotope carried on this antibody was independent of changes in V_H CDR3 but completely abolished by specific mutations in the gene for V_H FW1. This framework region is also known to be important for the binding of the red cell antigen I/i, so that in V_{4-34}-encoded antibodies, it seems clear that sites for two different antigens can be encoded by different parts of the V_H sequence. As noted previously, binding to the framework regions is characteristic of B cell superantigens (Fig. 4.2), and the fact that the red cell binding site is in FW1 may result from molecular mimicry between the I/i antigen and such a superantigen.

Overall, the method of reasoning described above can show how high-affinity anti-dsDNA antibodies might develop and can help to build up a picture of the antibody–DNA interaction. It does not tell us the identity of the stimulating antigen, or exactly how the antibodies cause tissue damage. Although there are small amounts of DNA present in the bloodstream, mammalian DNA is a poor immunogen and it seems likely that a low-affinity autoantibody response is initially stimulated by a DNA – protein complex such as the nucleosome (Rumore & Steinman, 1990). Antibodies more specific for dsDNA might then develop after clonal expansion, antigen-driven mutation and isotype switching. A number of different mechanisms have been suggested to explain how these antibodies could cause glomerulonephritis. For example, they may cross-react with cell surface proteins (Raz et al., 1993) or antibody – DNA – histone complexes might interact with heparan sulphate in the glomerular basement membrane (Brinkman et al., 1990). The more it becomes possible to distinguish the fine structure of those antibodies which do cause such clinical effects from those which do not, the closer we will be to resolving these issues.

Anti-phospholipid antibodies

Antibodies to phospholipid occur in 1.5 to 5% of the population (Harris & Spinnato, 1991) but are present at much higher frequency (up to 25–40%) in patients with SLE (Harris, Gharavi & Hughes, 1985). These antibodies bind to a variety of neutral or negatively charged phospholipids. aPL can occur in patients with a variety of infectious or neoplastic conditions but under these circumstances they appear to bind cardiolipin without the need for a cofactor and are not associated with an increased risk of thrombosis (Hunt et al., 1992). aPL found in patients with autoimmune disorders appear to recognize the antigen in association with a serum cofactor known as β_2-glycoprotein I (β_2-GPI) and are, in some cases, associated with increased risk of thrombosis, leading to the clinical features of the anti-phospholipid antibody syndrome (APS) (Hunt et al., 1992). These features include venous thromboses, increased prevalence of stroke, skin rash, thrombocytopenia and recurrent spontaneous miscarriages (Asherson et al., 1989). As in the case of anti-dsDNA antibodies described above, it has been found that high-affinity aPL of the IgG isotype are more closely associated with the presence of disease features than IgM antibodies of lower affinity and specificity (Alarçon-Segovia *et al.*, 1989).

As has been described, the methods of molecular biology and immunology have been used extensively to study the origin and properties of anti-dsDNA antibodies. It is becoming clear that very similar reasoning can be applied to the study of other potentially pathogenic antibodies. aPL antibodies provide a good example as they share many characteristics with anti-DNA antibodies. A number of low-affinity monoclonal IgM antibodies bind both these antigens, and it has been known since the early 1980s that a single replacement mutation in a murine antibody can be enough to convert it from an anti-DNA into an aPL antibody (Diamond & Scharff, 1984).

Just as for anti-DNA antibodies, human IgG monoclonal aPL antibodies are commonly more mutated than IgM and bind with higher affinity and specificity (van Es *et al.*, 1992; Menon *et al.*, 1997). This suggests a role for antigen-driven clonal expansion in the development of pathogenic, high-affinity IgG aPL. Further evidence supporting this is the isolation of two clonally related monoclonal aPL antibodies from a single patient with features of APS (Menon *et al.*, 1997). Attempts to identify sequence motifs conferring enhanced binding properties are not as far advanced as in anti-DNA antibodies. However, aPL antibodies found in patients with clinical features of APS bind primarily to negatively charged phospholipids. It is 'therefore' striking that monoclonal aPL antibodies that show specific binding or are derived from patients with active APS tend to have more basic residues in their CDRs than less-specific aPL antibodies from healthy volunteers (Rahman *et al.*, 1996). The next step will be to carry out modelling and mutagenesis experiments to investigate the antibody – phospholipid interface.

Summary

The complex processes whereby the immune system uses a relatively small number of gene segments to produce an antibody repertoire capable of defending the body against a vast number of potential antigenic targets have been described. A possible side effect of these mechanisms for generating antibody diversity is the production of dangerous autoantibodies. In some rheumatic diseases, clones producing such antibodies escape the normal regulatory systems and the autoantibodies produced can contribute to tissue damage. Knowledge of B cell biology can be used to study the sequence and properties of such antibodies so that we may eventually be able to prevent their formation or block their adverse effects.

Acknowledgements

The authors would like to thank the Arthritis Research Campaign for its support. Dr Rahman is supported by Wellcome Research Training Fellowship No. 040 366/Z/94/Z.

References

Alarçon-Segovia, D., Deleze, M., Oria, C.V. *et al.* (1989). Antiphospholipid antibodies and the antiphospholipid syndrome in systemic lupus erythematosus. *Medicine (Baltimore)* 68: 353–365.

Asherson, R.A., Khamashta, M.A., Ordi-Ros, J. *et al.* (1989). The 'primary' antiphospholipid syndrome: major clinical and serological features. *Medicine (Baltimore)* 68: 366–375.

Barbas, S.M., Ditzel, H.J., Salonen, E.M., Yang, W.P., Silverman, G.J. & Burton, D.R. (1995). Human autoantibody recognition of DNA. *Proc. Natl. Acad. Sci., USA* 92: 2529–2533.

Berek, C. & Milstein, C. (1987). Mutation drift and repertoire shift in the maturation of the immune response. *Immunol. Rev.* 96: 23–41.

Borretzen, M., Randen, I., Zdarsky, E., Forre, O., Natvig, J.B. & Thompson, K.M. (1994). Control of autoantibody affinity by selection against amino acid replacements in the complementarity determining regions. *Proc. Natl. Acad. Sci., USA* 91: 12 917–12 921.

Brezinschek, H.-P., Foster, S.J., Brezinschek, R.I., Dorner, T., Domiati-Saad, R. & Lipsky, P.E. (1997). Analysis of the human V_H gene repertoire. Differential effects of selection and somatic hypermutation on human peripheral CD5+/IgM+ and CD5-/IgM+ B cells. *J. Clin. Invest.* 99: 2488–2501.

Brinkman, K., Termaat, R.M., Berden, J.H.M. & Smeenk, R.J.T. (1990). Anti-DNA antibodies and lupus nephritis: the complexity of cross-reactivity. *Immunol. Today* 11: 232–234.

Cairns, E., Kwong, P.C., Misener, V.I.P. & Bell, D.A. (1989). Analysis of variable region genes encoding a human anti-DNA antibody of normal origin. *J. Immunol.* 143: 685–691.

Cervera, R., Khamashta, M.A., Font, J. *et al.* (1993). Systemic lupus erythematosus: clinical and immunologic patterns of disease expression in a cohort of 1000 patients. *Medicine (Baltimore)* 72: 113–124.

Chang, B. & Casali, P. (1994). The CDR1 sequences of a major proportion of human germline Ig V_H genes are inherently susceptible to amino acid replacement. *Immunol. Today* 15: 367–373.

Chapman, C.J., Spellerberg, M.B., Smith, G.A., Carter, S.J., Hamblin, T.J. & Stevenson, F.K. (1993). Autoanti-red cell antibodies synthesized by patients with infectious mononucleosis utilize the V_H4–21 gene segment. *J. Immunol.* 151: 1051–1061.

Christian, C.L. & Elkon, K.B. (1980). Antibodies to intracellular proteins: clinical and biological significance. *Am. J. Med.* 80: 53–61.

Coffman, R.L., Lebman, D.A. & Rothman, P. (1993). The mechanism and regulation of immunoglobulin isotype switching. *Adv. Immunol.* 54: 229–270.

Cook, G.P. & Tomlinson, I.M. (1995). The human immunoglobulin V_H repertoire. *Immunol. Today* 16: 237–242.

Dersimonian, H., Schwartz, R.S., Barrett, K.J. & Stollar, B.D. (1987). Relationship of human variable region heavy chain germline genes to genes encoding anti-DNA autoantibodies. *J. Immunol.* 139: 2496–2501.

Diamond, B. & Scharff, M.D. (1984). Somatic mutation of T15 heavy chain gives rise to an antibody with autoantibody specificity. *Proc. Natl. Acad. Sci., USA* 81: 5841–5844.

Di Santo, J.P., Bonnefoy, J.Y., Ganchat, J.F., Fischer, A. & de Saint Basile, G. (1993). CD40 ligand mutations in X-linked immunodeficiency with hyper-IgM. *Nature* 361: 541–543.

Ehrenstein, M.R., Longhurst, C.M., Latchman, D.S. & Isenberg, D.A. (1994). Serological and genetic characterization of a human monoclonal immunoglobulin G anti-DNA idiotype. *J. Clin. Invest.* 93: 1787–1797.

Ehrenstein, M.R., Katz, D.R., Griffiths, M.H., Papadaki, L., Winkler, T.H., Kalden, J.R. & Isenberg, D.A. (1995). Human IgG anti-DNA antibodies deposit in kidneys and induce proteinuria in SCID mice. *Kidney Int.* 48: 705–711.

Gellert, M. (1992). Molecular analysis of V(D)J recombination. *Annu. Rev. Genet.* 22: 425–446.

Ghia, P., Gratwohl, A., Signer, E., Winkler, T.H., Melchers, F. & Rolink, A.G. (1995). Immature B cells from human and mouse bone marrow can change their surface light chain expression. *Eur. J. Immunol.* 25: 3108–3114.

Goodglick, L. & Braun, J. (1994). Revenge of the microbes. Superantigens of the T and B cell lineage. *Am. J. Pathol.* 144: 623–636.

Guigou, V., Cuisinier, A.-M., Tonnelle, C., Moinier, D., Fougereau, M. & Fumoux, F. (1990). Human immunoglobulin V_H and V_κ repertoire revealed by *in situ* hybridization. *Mol. Immunol.* 27: 935–940.

Harris, E.N. & Spinnato, J.A. (1991). Should anticardiolipin tests be performed in otherwise healthy pregnant women? *Am. J. Obstet. Gynaecol.* 165: 1272–1277.

Harris, E.N., Gharavi, A.E. & Hughes, G.R.V. (1985). Antiphospholipid antibodies. *Clin. Rheumat. Dis.* 11: 591–596.

Huang, C. & Stollar, B.D. (1993). A majority of human IgH chain cDNA of normal human adult blood lymphocytes resembles cDNA for fetal Ig and natural autoantibodies. *J. Immunol.* 151: 5290–5300.

Hunt, J.E., McNeil, H.P., Morgan, G.J., Crameri, R.M. & Krillis, S.A. (1992). A phospholid-β_2-glycoprotein I complex is an antigen for anticardiolipin antibodies occurring in autoimmune disease but not with infection. *Lupus* 1: 75–81.

Isenberg, D.A. & Collins, C. (1985). Detection of cross-reactive anti-DNA antibody idiotypes on renal tissue-bound immunoglobulins from lupus patients. *J. Clin. Invest.* 76: 287–294.

Isenberg, D.A., Shoenfeld, Y., Walport, M. *et al.* (1985). Detection of cross-reactive anti-DNA idiotypes in the serum of systemic lupus erythematosus patients and of their relatives. *Arthritis Rheum.* 28: 999–1007.

Isenberg, D.A., Spellerberg, M., Williams, W., Griffiths, M. & Stevenson, F. (1993). Identification of a role for the 9G4 idiotope in systemic lupus erythematosus. *Br. J. Rheumatol.* 32: 876–882.

Isenberg, D.A., Ehrenstein, M.R., Longhurst, C. & Kalsi, J.K. (1994). The origin, sequence, structure, and consequences of developing anti-DNA antibodies: a human perspective. *Arthritis Rheum.* 37: 169–180.

Isenberg, D.A., Ravirajan, C.T., Rahman, A. & Kalsi, J. (1997). The role of antibodies to DNA in systemic lupus erythematosus. *Lupus* 6: 290–304.

Kalsi, J.K., Martin, A.C.R., Hirabayashi, Y. *et al.* (1996). Functional and modelling studies of the binding of human monoclonal anti-DNA antibodies to DNA. *Mol. Immunol.* 33: 471–482.

Kalunian, K.C., Panosian-Sahakian, N., Ebling, F.M., Cohen, A.H., Louie, J.S., Kaine, J. & Hahn, B.H. (1989). Idiotypic characteristics of immunoglobulins associated with systemic lupus erythematosus: studies of antibodies deposited in glomeruli of humans. *Arthritis Rheum.* 32: 513–522.

Kamachi, Y., Ichihara, Y., Tsuge, I., Abe, T., Torii, S., Kurosawa, Y. & Matsuoka, H. (1993). The gene loci for immunoglobulin heavy chains in precursor B cell lines from a patient with severe combined immunodeficiency appear able to participate in DNA rearrangement but have a germ-line configuration. *Eur. J. Immunol.* 23: 1401–1404.

Katz, J.B., Limpanasithikul, W. & Diamond, B. (1994). Mutational analysis of an autoantibody: differential binding and pathogenicity. *J. Exp. Med.* 180: 925–932.

Kirkham, P.M. & Schroeder, H.W. Jr (1994). Antibody structure and the evolution of immunoglobulin V gene segments. *Sem. Immunol.* 6: 347–360.

Klein, U., Kuppers, R. & Rajewsky, K. (1994). Variable region gene analysis of B cell subsets derived from a 4-year-old child: somatically mutated memory B cells accumulate in the peripheral blood already at a young age. *J. Exp. Med.* 180: 1383–1393.

Koffler, D., Schur, P.H. & Kunkel, H.G. (1967). Immunological studies concerning the nephritis of systemic lupus erythematosus. *J. Exp. Med.* 126: 607–624.

Kofler, R., Geley, S., Kofler, H. & Helmberg, A. (1992). Mouse variable region gene families: complexity, polymorphism and use in non-autoimmune responses. *Immunol. Rev.* 128: 5–21.

Krishnan, M.R. & Marion, T.N. (1993). Structural similarity of antibody variable regions from immune and autoimmune anti-DNA antibodies. *J. Immunol.* 150: 4948–4957.

Liu, Y.-J., Joshua, D.E., Williams, G.T., Smith, C.A., Gordon, J. & MacLennan, I.C.M. (1989). Mechanisms of antigen-driven selection in germinal centres. *Nature* 342: 929–931.

Logtenberg, T., Schutte, M.E.M., Ebeling, S.B., Gmelig-Meyling, F.H.J. & van Es, J.H. (1992). Molecular approaches to the study of human B cell and (auto)antibody repertoire generation and selection. *Immunol. Rev.* 128: 23–47.

Longhurst, C., Ehrenstein, M.R., Leaker, B. *et al.* (1996). Analysis of immunoglobulin variable genes of a human IgM anti-myeloperoxidase antibody derived from a patient with vasculitis. *Immunology* 87: 334–338.

Madaio, M.P., Carlson, J., Cataldo, J., Ucci, A., Migliorini, P. & Pankewycz, O. (1987). Murine monoclonal anti-DNA antibodies bind directly to glomerular antigens and form immune deposits. *J. Immunol.* 138: 2883–2889.

Mao, C., Osman, G.E., Adams, S. & Datta, S.K. (1994). T cell receptor alpha-chain repertoire of pathogenic autoantibody-inducing T cells in lupus mice. *J. Immunol.* 152: 1462–1470.

Menon, S., Rahman, M.A.A., Ravirajan, C.T. *et al.* (1997) The production, binding characteristics and sequence analysis of four human IgG monoclonal antiphospholipid antibodies. *J. Autoimmun.* 10: 43–57.

Mockridge, I., Chapman, C., Spellerberg, M., Isenberg, D.A. & Stevenson, F.K. (1996). Use of phage surface expression to analyze regions of a human V_{4-34} (V_H 4–21)-encoded IgG autoantibody required for recognition of DNA. *J. Immunol.* 157: 2449–2454.

Okamura, M., Kanayama, Y., Amastu, K., Negoro, N., Kohda, S., Takeda, T. & Inoue, T. (1993). Significance of enzyme linked immunosorbent assay (ELISA) for antibodies to double stranded and single stranded DNA in patients with lupus nephritis: correlation with severity of renal histology. *Ann. Rheum. Dis.* 52: 14–20.

Pewzner-Jung, Y., Simon, T. & Eilat, D. (1996). Structural elements controlling anti-DNA antibody affinity and their relationship to anti-phosphorylcholine affinity. *J. Immunol.* 156: 3065–3073.

Polymenis, M. & Stollar, B.D. (1994). Critical binding site amino acids of anti-Z DNA single chain Fv molecules: role of heavy and light chain CDR3 and relationship to autoantibody activity. *J. Immunol.* 152: 5318–5329.

Potter, K.N., Li, Y., Pascual, V. *et al.* (1993). Molecular characterization of a cross-reactive idiotope on human immunoglobulins using the V_H 4–21 gene segment. *J. Exp. Med.* 178: 1419–1428.

Radic, M.Z. & Weigert, M. (1994). Genetic and structural evidence for antigen selection of anti-DNA antibodies. *Annu. Rev. Immunol.* 12: 487–520.

Radic, M.Z., Mackle, J., Erikson, J., Mol, C., Anderson, W.F. & Weigert, M. (1993). Residues that mediate DNA binding of autoimmune antibodies. *J. Immunol.* 150: 4966–4977.

Rahman, A., Menon, S., Latchman, D.S. & Isenberg, D.A. (1996). Sequences of monoclonal antiphospholipid antibodies: variations on an anti-DNA antibody theme. *Sem. Arthritis Rheum.* 26: 515–525.

Raz, E., Brezis, M., Rosenmann, E. & Eilat, D. (1989). Anti-DNA antibodies bind directly to renal antigens and induce kidney dysfunction in the isolated perfused rat kidney. *J. Immunol.* 42: 3076–3082.

Raz, E., Ben-Bassat, H., Davidi, T., Shlomai, Z. & Eilat, D. (1993). Cross-reactions of anti-DNA antibodies with cell-surface proteins. *Eur. J. Immunol.* 23: 383–390.

Rioux, J.D., Zdarsky, E., Newkirk, M.M. & Rauch J. (1995). Anti-DNA and anti-platelet specificities of SLE-derived autoantibodies: evidence for CDR 2H mutations and CDR 3H motifs. *Mol. Immunol.* 32: 683–696.

Rumore, P.M. & Steinman, C.R. (1990). Endogenous circulating DNA in systemic lupus erythematosus. *J. Clin. Invest.* 86: 69–74.

Sasso, E.H., Buckner, J.H. & Suzuki, L.A. (1995). Ethnic differences in polymorphism of an immunoglobulin V_H3 gene. *J. Clin. Invest.* 96: 1591–1600.

Schable, K.F. & Zachau, H.-G. (1993). The variable genes of the human κ locus. *Biol. Chem. Hoppe-Seyler* 374: 1001–1022.

Schlomchik, M.J., Marshak-Rothstein, A., Wolfowicz, C.B., Rothstein, T.L. & Weigert, M.G. (1987). The role of clonal selection and somatic mutation in autoimmunity. *Nature* 328: 805–811.

Schlomchik, M.J., Mascelli, M., Shan, H. *et al.* (1990). Anti-DNA antibodies from autoimmune mice arise by clonal expansion and somatic mutation. *J. Exp. Med.* 171: 265–297.

Shokat, K.M. & Goodnow, C.C. (1995). Antigen-induced B-cell death and elimination during germinal-centre immune responses. *Nature* 375: 334–338.

Stevenson, F.K., Longhurst, C., Chapman, C.J. *et al.* (1993). Utilization of the V_H4–21 gene segment by anti-DNA antibodies from patients with SLE. *J. Autoimmun.* 6: 809–826.

Steward, C.G., Potter, M.N. & Oakhill, A. (1992). Third complementarity determining region (CDRIII) sequence analysis in childhood B-lineage acute lymphoblastic leukaemia: implications for the design of oligonucleotide probes for use in monitoring minimal residual disease. *Leukemia* 6: 1213–1219.

Ter Borg, E.J., Horst, G., Hummel, E.J., Limburg, P.L. & Kallenberg, C.G.M. (1990). Measurement of increases in anti-double-stranded DNA antibody levels as a predictor of disease exacerbation in systemic lupus erythematosus. *Arthritis Rheum.* 33: 634–643.

Tiegs, S.L., Russell, D.M. & Nemazee, D. (1993). Receptor editing in self-reactive bone marrow cells. *J. Exp. Med.* 177: 1009–1020.

Tonegawa, S. (1983). Somatic generation of antibody diversity. *Nature* 302: 575–581.

van Es, J.H., Gmelig-Meyling, F.H.J., van de Allker, A.R.F., Aanstoot, H., Derksen, R.H.W.M. & Logtenberg, T. (1991). Somatic mutations in the variable region of a human anti-dsDNA autoantibody suggest a role for antigen in the induction of systemic lupus erythematosus. *J. Exp. Med.* 173: 461–470.

van Es, J., Aanstoot, H., Gmelig-Meyling, F.H.J., Derksen, R.H.W.M. & Logtenberg, T. (1992). A human systemic lupus erythematosus-related anti-cardiolipin/single-stranded DNA autoantibody is encoded by a somatically mutated variant of the developmentally restricted 51P1 V_H gene. *J. Immunol.* 149: 2234–2240.

Williams, S.C. & Winter, G. (1993). Cloning and sequencing of human immunoglobulin Vλ gene segments. *Eur. J. Immunol.* 23: 1456–1461.

Winkler, T.H., Fehr, H. & Kalden, J.R. (1992). Analysis of immunoglobulin variable region genes from human IgG anti-DNA hybridomas. *Eur. J. Immunol.* 22: 1719–1728.

5

The role of CD40 in immune responses

P. LANE

Introduction

CD40 and its ligand (CD154: CD40L) play a central role in initiating and maintaining both T and B cell immune responses and are crucial in activating other effector cells such as macrophages. CD40 is far more widely expressed than previously thought, and recent data showing expression of this molecule on endothelium have implicated CD40 in the recruitment of cells at sites of inflammation. This review will focus on the experimental evidence in mouse and human that has contributed to our understanding of the normal function of this molecule *in vivo*. This will be viewed in the context of how CD40 contributes to disease processes, particularly autoimmune diseases, and how targeting of this model may offer new therapeutic possibilities for modifying disease activity. Although there is now some evidence for intracellular signalling pathways via CD40, these are covered elsewhere (Cheng *et al.*, 1995; Hanissian & Geha, 1997).

Structure of CD40 family members and their ligands

CD40 is a member of an ever increasing family of receptors for which the TNF receptor is the prototype (Smith, Farrah & Goodwin, 1994). The family includes the TNF receptors, CD30, CD27, OX40, the 4-1BB antigen, Fas, nerve growth factor receptor, several viral genome products and the newly described TRAIL molecule (Pan *et al.*, 1997). The extracellular portion of members of the TNF family share significant homology mainly because of conservation of the basic extracellular binding domain, which is composed of cysteine-rich pseudo-repeats, each containing about six cysteine motifs and 40 amino acid residues. Some molecules in the family encode soluble forms by alternative splicing. Intracellular domains, in contrast, vary considerably, indicating a likely diversity in intracellular signalling. CD40 has a cytoplasmic tail of 62 amino acid residues, which

79

is required for intracellular signalling. Mutation resulting in a change at position 234 of a threonine residue to serine abolishes intracellular signalling (Clark & Lane, 1991).

The ligands for the TNF family of receptors are type II membrane proteins, and their homology resides in the carboxyl terminal 150 residues. CD40L has a relatively long stretch of amino acids that link the carboxy terminal region to the 22 residue cytoplasmic tail. Like some of the receptors, there is potential for alternatively spliced forms of the ligands' which may be secreted as soluble factors. The ligand can certainly be shed from expressing cells after engagement of CD40, and there is some evidence that the molecule is downregulated after engagement (Yellin *et al.*, 1994).

The crystal structures of TNF and its receptor have given important insights into the mechanisms of action of the receptor/ligand family (Banner *et al.*, 1993). The ligands form trimeric structures that may dimerize or trimerize the receptors. Evidence from monoclonal antibody (mAb) binding studies suggests that dimerization is sufficient for activation. Conservation of the cytoplasmic domain of CD40L between mouse and humans indicates an important role, possibly related to the regulation of expression of the molecule or to regulation of the endocytosis that occurs following engagement of CD40 (Yellin *et al.*, 1994). Additionally, there is potential for signalling through the cytoplasmic domain in cells that express it, blurring the distinction between receptor and ligand (Smith *et al.*, 1994).

Expression of CD40 and its ligand

CD40 is expressed widely (Banchereau *et al.*, 1994). Virtually all cells of bone marrow origin express CD40; these include B cells from the earliest precursors until late plasmablasts (CD40 is lost on terminal differentiation to plasma cells), macrophages, monocytes and dendritic cells, CD34+ stem cell precursors and (most recently identified) T cells (Attrep *et al.*, 1996). Cells of other origins expressing CD40 include the basement layer of epithelial cells, many carcinoma cell lines (constitutively expressed), thymic epithelial cells in the cortex and medulla, and also endothelium. The function of the CD40 molecule in this other group of cell types is poorly defined.

Originally, the ligand for this molecule was found to be expressed on activated T cells (Armitage *et al.*, 1992; Lane *et al.*, 1992). Its expression has also been described at low levels on basophils and mast cells (Gauchat *et al.*, 1993) and also, surprisingly, on activated B cells (Grammer *et al.*, 1995). Initially there was some controversy with regard to the sites of expression of CD40L in lymphoid tissue (Foy *et al.*, 1994); now it is clear that activated T cells in the T cell areas and within germinal centres express CD40L (Casamayor-Palleja, Khan & MacLennan, 1995). It is not clear by immunohistology which, if any, B cells physiologically express the molecule. It is thought that CD40L expressed on mast cells may play a local role in switching B cells to IgE synthesis (Gauchat *et al.*, 1993).

Ontogeny of immune responses

Because CD40 plays such a pivotal role in both T and B cell immune responses, its function needs to be understood in the context of the normal sequence of events that leads to T and B cell priming.

Priming to T cells

T cell priming occurs in the T cell areas associated with specialized antigen-presenting cells called interdigitating dendritic cells (IDCs) (Inaba *et al.*, 1983). These cells are derived from Langerhans cells, which are phenotypically immature antigen-presenting cells that constitutively pick up soluble and particulate antigen via pinocytosis (Sallusto & Lanzavecchia, 1994). Subsequently, these cells migrate from the tissues via afferent lymphatics to lymph nodes, stop processing antigen and present peptide fragments derived from these proteins as they upregulate expression of class I and class II molecules as well as other co-stimulatory molecules. The migration of Langerhans cells from the tissue to central tissues probably occurs at a basal 'tickover' rate, but this is greatly augmented by inflammation and inflammatory cytokines like TNF (Austyn, 1996).

Resting T cells migrate from blood into lymphatic tissue via specialized post-capillary venules called high endothelial venules (HEV). Most evidence suggests that the T cells 'crawl' over antigen-presenting IDCs searching for antigen, which if encountered leads to T cell activation, proliferation and 'priming'. Primed antigen-specific T cells migrate to the outer T zone where they can interact with antigen-specific B cells. They also leave via efferent lymphatics. Activated T cells, through differential expression of adhesion receptors (Mackay, Marston & Dudler, 1991), can migrate out into inflamed tissues where they activate local inflammatory cells or are specifically cytotoxic against infected cells.

Primary B cell activation

By identifying antigen-specific B and T cells, it has been possible to study the primary interactions between B (Jacob, Kassir & Kelsoe, 1991; Liu *et al.*, 1991) and T cells (Gulbranson-Judge & MacLennan, 1996; Luther *et al.*, 1997).

Antigen-specific B cells carrying receptors that have been triggered by binding antigen get trapped in the T cell areas 'looking' for primed antigen-specific T cells (Cyster, Hartley & Goodnow, 1994). B cell presentation to unprimed T cells is poor (Lassila, Vainio & Matzinger, 1988; Fuchs *et al.*, 1992). There is an initial burst of B cell proliferation in the T cell areas. Many of these B cells differentiate locally to short-lived plasma cells in the red pulp of spleen, the medulla of lymph nodes and the lamina propria of the gut and respiratory mucosa.

Some B cells do not differentiate but migrate into follicles, where they proliferate and form germinal centres (MacLennan *et al.*, 1990); it appears that these B cells are clonally related to those B cells proliferating in the T cell areas (Jacob & Kelsoe, 1992). Germinal centres are sites where antigen-specific B cells are expanded, somatic mutation is switched on and mutants are selected. This environment allows affinity maturation to take place. B cell mutants that bind antigen better than other B cell clones are selected in germinal centres. Some progeny differentiate to produce plasma cells, which have most often switched to production of a different class of immunoglobulin, and memory B cells. Others continue the cycle of somatic mutation and selection.

Location of memory B cells and maintenance of antibody responses

Memory B cells that leave the germinal centre reaction enter the marginal zone in the spleen, where they exit the cell cycle (Liu, Oldfield & MacLennan, 1988). In lymph nodes, there is a comparable B cell area just underneath the capsule and adjacent to the lymphatics (Lagresle, Bella & Defrance, 1993). Both marginal zone and subepithelial B cells lie in antigen-traffic zones so are ideally situated to re-encounter antigen. Many of these memory B cells are long lived (MacLennan *et al.*, 1990), especially those that have switched to IgG production (Schittek & Rajewsky, 1990). Specific antibody responses are maintained by chronic activation of antigen-specific B cells within B cell follicles long after the germinal centre reaction has died down (MacLennan *et al.*, 1990).

Secondary B and T cell responses

Memory B cells activated through their antigen-specific receptors are rapidly recruited into immune responses and migrate again to the T cell areas. There is intense proliferation at this site, where the majority of proliferating cells differentiate to plasmablasts, which migrate to the bone marrow (Benner, Hijmans & Haaijman, 1981) and become long-lived plasma cells (Ho *et al.*, 1986). The observed cellular reaction is accompanied by elevated switched specific antibody responses in the sera.

Memory T cells are activated by antigen presented by IDCs, but they can also be restimulated by other antigen-presenting cells such as B cells because their stimulatory requirements are less stringent than those of unprimed cells.

Immunodeficiency resulting from CD40L and CD40 deficiency

The key insights into the function of CD40 and its ligand have come from studies in genetically deficient mice and humans. Deficient expression of CD40L was reported by several different groups more or less at the same time (reviewed in Callard *et al.*, 1993).

Humans

Deficiency of CD40L is associated in humans with the sex-linked hyper-IgM syndrome, where affected males have very low levels of IgG and IgA and often have elevated levels of IgM. The elevated levels of IgM are driven by infections, as IgM levels often return to normal with immunoglobulin replacement. In addition to their antibody defect, affected patients have problems dealing with infections with the intracellular fungal parasite *Pneumocystis carinii*. Variable neutropenia is also present.

Mice

Mice deficient in both CD40 and its ligand have been created using gene technology to make knock-out mice (Kawabe *et al.*, 1994; Xu *et al.*, 1994). The murine phenotype is similar to that seen in humans, indeed mice even get *P. carinii* infections. Normally they do not have elevated levels of IgM, but this probably reflects the fact that mice tend to be reared in specific pathogen-free conditions. Detailed analyses of these mice have contributed greatly to our understanding of the role of CD40 in T and B cell priming, although several questions remain unanswered. In general a few points need to be clarified.

Antibody responses that do not depend on T cells, so called thymus-independent responses to polysaccharide-based antigens, appear to be normal. Furthermore, B cells are able to switch to IgG_3, the IgG isotype associated with polysaccharide responses. It is not absolutely clear whether this is also true in humans where antibody responses may be partially dependent on T cells (Lane, 1996).

Primary antibody responses to conventional protein-based antigens occur but are restricted to the IgM isotype. This may partially reflect the relative T cell independence of B cells in primary immune responses.

Role of CD40 in primary immune responses

Effect on antigen-presenting cells: IDCs

The earliest event in T cell priming involves recognition of antigen presented by IDCs. It seems probable that antigen-specific triggering of T cells is sufficient to upregulate the expression of CD40L (Foy *et al.*, 1996), although others have found that expression is strongly upregulated by co-stimulation through CD28 (de Boer *et al.*, 1993; Klaus *et al.*, 1994). Whatever, the initial sequence of events, CD40 activation of IDCs leads to upregulation of the CD28 co-stimulatory B7 ligands (Chapter 6; Ranheim & Kipps, 1993) and HLA molecules and potently induces the expression of IL-12 (Cella *et al.*, 1996). This sequence of events clearly leads not only to more effective antigen presentation but also to co-stimulation of T cells.

T cell priming

The major influence of CD40 in T cell priming is probably through the effects of CD40L expressed by T cells on antigen presentation by IDCs. This conclusion is supported by observations of patients with CD40L deficiency, who have problems eradicating intracellular infections but are not profoundly T cell immunodeficient. Experimental studies in genetically deficient mice have given us a more detailed understanding of CD40's role. Using CD40L-deficient mice, Flavell's group have found T cell priming was impaired although not absent (Grewal, Xu & Flavell, 1995). In this system, CD40L-deficient T cells failed to proliferate *in vivo* in response to antigen. However, if IDCs were stimulated to upregulate B7 ligands by CD40-independent signals, then CD40L-deficient T cells were able to proliferate. This indicated that the dependence of T cell priming on CD40 was principally through upregulation of co-stimulation on antigen-presenting cells. Recently, this result has been repeated in a different way. CD40L-deficient mice cannot be primed to get encephalomyelitis, but priming can be restored by immunization with B7.1 expressing antigen-presenting cells, where upregulation of B7 ligands through CD40 has been bypassed (Grewal *et al.*, 1996).

The one caveat to the above experimental conclusions is that activated T cells can express CD40 (Attrep *et al.*, 1996) and CD40L will co-stimulate T cells directly (Armitage *et al.*, 1993; Fanslow *et al.*, 1994). Therefore, one might expect co-stimulatory effects between activated T cells mediated by CD40 to play some role in the expansion of T cell clones.

Role of CD40 in the effector phase of the immune response

Cytotoxic T cell priming

Humans with deficient CD40L expression do not, in general, have problems with viral infections. This is largely confirmed in mice. CD40-deficient mice make normal CD4+ T cell responses to infectious viruses (Oxenius *et al.*, 1996) although antibody responses are grossly impaired. Primary cytotoxic responses are also normal although memory responses are impaired, for reasons that are not clear (Borrow *et al.*, 1996).

Macrophage activation

Humans clearly have problems dealing with intracellular infections like that with *P. carinii*. CD40 activation of macrophages leads not only to IL-12 production but also to production of other proinflammatory cytokines like TNF and IFN-γ (reviewed in Grewal & Flavell (1996)). CD40L-negative mice are susceptible to leishmaniasis (Soong *et al.*, 1996), and the defect can be corrected by IL-12, which plays a key role in switching the T cell immune response to produce T_H1 cytokines (Trinchieri, 1995), which are instrumental in activating macrophages to kill intracellular organisms.

B cell priming

CD40L-deficient humans have impaired immunoglobulin class switching, no germinal centre formation and impaired affinity maturation of antibody responses because of a lack of somatic mutation. This phenotype is confirmed in CD40- (Kawabe *et al.*, 1994) and CD40L-deficient mice (Xu *et al.*, 1994).

Normal B cell responses depend on T cell priming and the appropriate helper signals, so it is appropriate to try to dissect the role of CD40 at different stages of this process. As stated above, T cell priming is impaired but not absent in mice deficient in CD40 signalling. Whether such T cells can efficiently deliver help for B cells is controversial. Two groups have taken T cells primed in the absence of CD40 and examined whether they can help normal B cells make antibody. Unfortunately, opposite answers were obtained: one group found T cells helped B cells (Oxenius *et al.*, 1996), the other did not (van Essen, Kikutani & Gray, 1995). The reasons for this discrepancy are not apparent and may be related to the degree of T cell priming.

B cell activation to plasma cells

B cell differentiation to plasma cells following cognate interactions between antigen-specific B and T cells in the T zones is relatively CD40 independent. Primary antibody responses are fairly normal and this is associated with the local differentiation of activated B cells to plasma cells. There is independent confirmation of this finding from *in vitro* studies: CD40L-deficient T cells will induce plasma cell differentiation in resting B cells (Lane *et al.*, 1995), and blocking CD40 induces plasma cell differentiation in activated B cells (Arpin *et al.*, 1995).

B cell proliferation

CD40 activation of B cells is a potent proliferation signal especially in conjunction with signals through the immunoglobulin receptor. Humans and mice deficient in this signalling pathway lack germinal centres in B cell follicles. Germinal centres are sites in the immune system that serve at least two functions.

1.   Clonal amplification of high-affinity B cells
2.   Somatic mutation and selection.

CD40 plays a clear role in B cell proliferation and selection (Liu *et al.*, 1989). Its role in somatic mutation is less clear because it is difficult to amplify and select somatic mutants and, therefore, they are difficult to detect. There is some published evidence that signalling through CD40 and surface immunoglobulin is important for maintaining somatic mutation in B cells *in vitro* (Källberg *et al.*, 1996), but this does not mean CD40 switches on mutation in B cells. There are some theoretical reasons to suppose that the mechanisms that regulate mutation and proliferation should be kept separate (Lane, 1997).

Class switching

Mice deficient in CD40 signalling have very low levels of IgA and IgG although levels of IgG_3, the isotype associated with thymus-independent responses, are normal. CD40 signalling induces sterile transcription of downstream IgG loci (Jumper *et al.*, 1994), indicating a significant contribution to successful class switching, although CD40 signalling alone seems to be insufficient.

Role of CD40 in B cell established immune responses

Because CD40 plays such a crucial role at so many different locations during immune responses, blocking CD40 interactions during established immune responses has profound immunosuppressive effects (Foy *et al.*, 1996). Its effect on established B cell immune responses where there is germinal centre formation is to cause dissolution of germinal centres and differentiation to plasma cells (Han *et al.*, 1995). This result is similar to that found *in vitro*, where CD40L-deficient T cell help leads to plasma cell formation (Arpin *et al.*, 1995; Lane *et al.*, 1995). The effects of blocking CD40 on long-term memory B cells are unknown.

Effects of CD40 in established T cell immune responses

Some effects of blocking CD40L are complicated by the fact that anti-CD40L antibodies may in some circumstances delete T cells expressing CD40L. In addition, it is very difficult to distinguish the role of CD40L-blocking events at distinct locations within the immune system because CD40 is so widely expressed. Nevertheless, its is clear that blocking CD40L *in vivo* exerts potent immunosuppressive effects. In mice prone to autoimmunity (Early, Zhao & Burns, 1996), anti-CD40L antibodies abrogate disease, as they do for graft-versus-host disease (Blazar *et al.*, 1997). Furthermore, in a transplantation model, antibodies to CD40L were potent enhancers of graft acceptance, especially in conjunction with blocking CD28 co-stimulation (Larsen *et al.*, 1996).

Tolerance induction

Although CD40L-deficient mice have relatively poor T cell priming (Grewal & Flavell, 1996), there is little evidence to suggest that T cells are tolerized by the lack of CD28 co-stimulation. Prior donor blood transfusion has been known for a long time to have a beneficial effect on the subsequent graft outcome, and it has been speculated that donor B cells induce tolerance to allogeneic antigens (Lassila *et al.*, 1988; Eynon & Parker, 1992; Fuchs *et al.*, 1992). Recent evidence suggests that CD40-deficient B cells are even more potent at inducing tolerance (Hollander *et al.*, 1996), and this is also true with blocking antibodies to CD40L (Buhlmann *et al.*, 1995). The exact mechanism by which B cells are tolerogenic is still not completely clear.

Summary

CD40 is widely expressed and plays a key role both in the afferent limb of the immune response in the priming of antigen-specific B and T cells and in the development of effector function, including macrophage activation, the development of effector T cells and in the clonal expansion and affinity maturation of B cells. Blocking CD40 with antagonists has the potential to block many different aspects of immune responses and exerts potent immunosuppressive effects that may be exploited in the treatment of autoimmune disease, transplant rejection and tolerance induction.

References

Armitage, R.J., Fanslow, W.C., Strockbine, O.L. *et al.* (1992), Molecular characterization of a murine ligand for CD40. *Nature.* 357: 80–82.

Armitage, R., Tough, T., Macduff, B. *et al.* (1993). CD40 ligand is a T cell growth factor. *Eur. J. Immunol.* 23: 2326–2331.

Arpin, C., Dechanet, J., van Kooten, C. *et al.* (1995). Generation of memory B cells and plasma cells in vitro. *Science* 268: 720–272.

Attrep, J., Brezinschek, H.P., Brezinschek, R.I. & Lipsky, P.F. (1996). Functional-activity of CD40 expressed by activated T-cells. *Arthritis Rheum.* 39: 1418.

Austyn, J.M. (1996). New insights into the mobilization and phagocytic-activity of dendritic cells. *J. Exp. Med.* 183: 1287–1292.

Bancherau, J., Bazan, F., Blanchard, D. *et al.* (1994). The CD40 antigen and its ligand. *Annu. Rev. Immunol.* 12: 881–922.

Banner, D.W., D'Arcy, A., Janes, W. *et al.* (1993). Crystal structure of the soluble human 55 kd TNF receptor-human TNF beta complex: implications for TNF receptor activation. *Cell* 73: 431–445.

Benner, R., Hijmans, W. & Haaijman, J.J. (1981). The bone marrow: the major source of immunoglobulins but still a neglected site of antibody formation. *Clin. Exp. Immunol.* 46: 1.

Blazar, B.R., Taylor, P.A., PanoskaltsisMortari, A. *et al.* (1997). Blockade of CD40ligand–CD40 interaction impairs CD4(+) T cell-mediated alloreactivity by inhibiting mature donor T cell expansion and function after bone marrow transplantation. *J. Immunol.* 158: 29–39.

Borrow, P., Tishon, A., Lee, S. *et al.* (1996). CD40I-deficient mice show deficits in antiviral immunity and have an impaired memory CD8(+) CTL response. *J. Exp. Med.* 183: 2129–2142.

Buhlmann, J.E., Foy, T.M., Aruffo, A. *et al.* (1995). In the absence of a CD40 signal B cells are tolerogenic. *Immunity* 2: 645–653.

Callard, R.E., Armitage, R.J., Fanslow, W.C. & Spriggs, M.K. (1993). CD40 ligand and its role in X-linked hyper-IgM syndrome. *Immunol. Today* 14: 559–564.

Casamayor-Palleja, M., Khan, M. & MacLennan, I.C.M. (1995). A subset of CD4+ memory T cells contain preformed CD40-ligand (gp39) that has rapid transient surface expression on activation via the T cell receptor complex. *J. Exp. Med.* 181: 1293–1301.

Cella, M., Scheidegger, D., Palmer-Lehman, K., Lane, P., Lanzavecchia, A. & Alber, G. (1996). Ligation of CD40 on dendritic cells triggers production of high levels of interleukin-12 and enhances T cell costimulatory capacity: T–T help via APC activation. *J. Exp. Med.* 184: 747–752.

Cheng, G.H., Cleary, A.M., Ye, Z.S., Hong, D.I., Lederman, S. & Baltimore, D. (1995). Involvement of CRAF1, a relative of TRAF, in CD40 signaling. *Science* 267: 1494–1498.

Clark, E.A. & Lane, P.J.L. (1991). Regulation of human B cell activation and adhesion. *Annu. Rev. Immunol.* 95: 97–127.

Cyster, J.G., Hartley, S.B. & Goodnow, C.C. (1994). Competition for follicular niches excludes self-reactive cells from the recirculating B-cell repertoire [see comments]. *Nature* 371: 389–395.

de Boer, M., Kasran, A., Kwekkeboom, J., Walter, H., Vandenberghe, P. & Ceuppens, J.L. (1993). Ligation of B7 with CD28/CTLA-4 on T cells results in CD40 ligand expression, interleukin-4 secretion and efficient help for antibody production by B cells. *Eur. J. Immunol.* 23: 3120–3125.

Early, G.S., Zhao, W.G. & Burns, C.M. (1996). Anti-CD40 ligand antibody treatment prevents the development of lupus-like nephritis in a subset of New-Zealand black x New-Zealand white mice – response correlates with the absence of an anti-antibody response. *J. Immunol.* 157: 3159–3164.

Eynon, E.E. & Parker, D.C. (1992). Small B cells as antigen-presenting cells in the induction of tolerance to soluble protein antigens. *J. Exp. Med.* 175: 131–138.

Fanslow, W., Clifford, K., Seaman, M. *et al.* (1994). Recombinant CD40 ligand exerts potent biologic effects on T cells. *J. Immunol.* 152: 4262–4269.

Foy, T.M., Laman, J.D., Ledbetter, J.A., Aruffo, A., Claassen, E. & Noelle, R.J. (1994). gp39–CD40 interactions are essential for germinal center formation and the development of B cell memory. *J. Exp. Med.* 180: 157–163.

Foy, T.M., Aruffo, A., Bajorath, J., Buhlmann, J.E. & Noelle, R.J. (1996). Immune regulation by CD40 and its ligand GP39. *Annu. Rev. Immunol.* 14: 591–617.

Fuchs, E.J., Matzinger, P., Eynon, E.E. & Parker, D.C. (1992). B cells turn off virgin but not memory T cells. *Science* 258: 1156–1159.

Gauchat, J.F., Henchoz, S., Mazzei, G. *et al.* (1993). Induction of human IgE synthesis in B-cells by mast-cells and basophils. *Nature* 365: 340–343.

Grammer, A.C., Bergman, M.C., Miura, Y., Fujita, K., Davis, L.S. & Lipsky, P.E. (1995). The CD40 ligand expressed by human B cells costimulates B cell responses. *J. Immunol.* 154: 4996–5010.

Grewal, I.S. & Flavell, R.A. (1996). A central role of CD40 ligand in the regulation of CD4(+) T-cell responses. *Immunol. Today* 17: 410–414.

Grewal, I.S., Xu, J. & Flavell, R.A. (1995). Impairment of antigen-specific T-cell priming in mice lacking CD40 ligand. *Nature* 378: 617–619.

Grewal, I.S., Foellmer, H.G., Grewal, K.D. *et al.* (1996). Requirement for CD40 ligand in costimulation induction, T cell activation, and experimental allergic encephalomyelitis. *Science* 273: 1864–1867.

Gulbranson-Judge, A. & MacLennan, I. (1996). Sequential antigen-specific growth of T cells in the T zones and follicles in response to pigeon cytochrome *c*. *Eur. J. Immunol.* 26: 1830–1837.

Han, S., Hathcock, K., Zheng, B., Kepler, T.B., Hodes, R. & Kelsoe, G. (1995). Cellular interaction in germinal centers. Roles of CD40 ligand and B7–2 in established germinal centers. *J. Immunol.* 155: 556–567.

Hanissian, S.H. & Geha, R.S. (1997). Jak3 is associated with CD40 and is critical for CD40 induction of gene expression in B cells. *Immunity* 6: 379–387.

Ho, F., Lortan, J., Khan, M. & MacLennan, I. (1986). Distinct short-lived and long-lived antibody-producing cell populations. *Eur. J. Immunol.* 16: 1297.

Hollander, G.A., Castigli, E., Kulbacki, R. *et al.* (1996). Induction of alloantigen-specific tolerance by B-cells from CD40-deficient mice. *Proc. Natl. Acad. Sci., USA* 93: 4994–4998.

Inaba, K., Steinman, R.M., Van Voorhis, W.C. & Muramatsu, S. (1983). Dendritic cells are critical accessory cells for thymus-dependent antibody responses in mouse and man. *Proc. Natl. Acad. Sci., USA* 80: 6041–6045.

Jacob, J. & Kelsoe, G. (1992). In situ studies of the primary immune response to

(4-hydroxy-3-nitrophenyl)acetyl. II. A common clonal origin for periarteriolar lymphoid sheath-associated foci and germinal centers. *J. Exp. Med.* 176: 679–687.

Jacob, J., Kassir, R. & Kelsoe, G. (1991). In situ studies of the primary immune response to (4-hydroxy-3-nitrophenyl)acetyl. I. The architecture and dynamics of responding cell populations. *J. Exp. Med.* 173: 1165–1176.

Jumper, M.D., Splawski, J.B., Lipsky, P.E. & Meek, K. (1994). Ligation of CD40 induces sterile transcripts of multiple Ig H chain isotypes in human B cells. *J. Immunol.* 152: 438–45.

Källberg, E., Jainandunsing, S., Gray, D. & Leanderson, T. (1996). Somatic mutation of immunoglobulin V genes *in vitro. Science* 271: 1285–1289.

Kawabe, T., Naka, T., Yoshida, K. *et al.* (1994). The immune response in CD40-deficient mice: impaired immunoglobulin class switching and germinal center formation. *Immunity* 1: 167–178.

Klaus, S.J., Pinchuk, L.M., Ochs, H.D. *et al.* (1994). Costimulation through CD28 enhances T cell-dependent B cell activation via CD40-CD40L interaction. *J. Immunol.* 152: 5643–5652.

Lagresle, C., Bella, C. & Defrance, T. (1993). Phenotypic and functional heterogeneity of the IgD- B cell compartment: identification of two major tonsillar B cell subsets. *Int. Immunol.* 5: 1259–1268.

Lane, P. (1996). Are polysaccharide antibody responses independent: the T cell enigma? *Clin. Exp. Immunol.* 105: 10–12.

Lane, P. (1997). Molecular mechanisms involved in T–B interactions. *Chem. Immunol.* 67: 1–13.

Lane, P., Traunecker, A., Hubele, S., Inui, S., Lanzavecchia, A. & Gray, D. (1992). Activated human T cells express a ligand for the human B cell associated antigen CD40 which participates in T cell-dependent activation of B lymphocytes. *Eur. J. Immunol.* 22: 2573–2578.

Lane, P., Burdet, C., McConnell, F., Lanzavecchia, A. & Padovan, E. (1995). CD40 ligand independent B cell activation revealed by CD40-ligand deficient T cell clones: evidence for distinct activation requirements for antibody formation and B cell proliferation. *Eur. J. Immunol.* 25: 1788–1793.

Larsen, C.P., Elwood, E.T., Alexander, D.Z. *et al.* (1996). Longterm acceptance of skin and cardiac allografts after blocking CD40 and CD28 pathways. *Nature* 381: 434–438.

Lassila, O., Vainio, O. & Matzinger, P. (1988). Can B cells turn on virgin T cells? *Nature* 334: 253–255.

Liu, Y.-J., Oldfield, S. & MacLennan, I. (1988). Memory B cells in T cell-dependent antibody responses colonize the splenic marginal zones. *Eur. J. Immunol.* 18: 355–362.

Liu, Y.-J., Joshua, D.E., Williams, G.T., Smith, C.A., Gordon, J. & MacLennan, I.C.M. (1989). Mechanism of antigen-driven-selection in germinal centres. *Nature* 342: 929–1931.

Liu, Y.J., Zhang, J., Lane, P.J., Chan, E.Y. & MacLennan, I.C. (1991). Sites of specific B cell activation in primary and secondary responses to T cell-dependent and T cell-independent antigens [published erratum appears in *Eur. J. Immunol.* (1992) 22, 615]. *Eur. J. Immunol.* 21: 2951–2962.

Luther, S., Gulbranson-Judge, A., AchaOrbea, H. & MacLennan, I. (1997). Viral superantigen drives extrafollicular and follicular B cell differentiation leading to virus-specific antibody production. *J. Exp. Med.* 185: 551–562.

Mackay, C.R., Marston, W.L. & Dudler, L. (1991). Naive and memory T cells show distinct pathways of lymphocyte recirculation. *J. Exp. Med.* 171: 801–817.

MacLennan, I.C.M., Liu, Y.J., Oldfield, S., Zhang, J. & Lane, P.J.L. (1990). The evolution of B cell clones. *Curr. Top. Microbiol. Immunol.* 159: 37–63.

Oxenius, A., Campbell, K.A., Maliszewski, C.R. *et al.* (1996). CD40–CD40 ligand interactions are critical in T–B cooperation but not for other antiviral CD4(+) T-cell functions. *J. Exp. Med.* 183: 2209–2218.

Pan, G., ORourke, K., Chinnaiyan, A.M. *et al.* (1997). The receptor for the cytotoxic ligand TRAIL. *Science* 276: 111–113.

Ranheim, E.A. & Kipps, T.J. (1993). Activated T cells induce expression of B7/BB1 on normal or leukemic B cells through a CD40-dependent signal. *J. Exp. Med.* 177: 925–935.

Sallusto, F. & Lanzavecchia, A. (1994). Efficient presentation of soluble antigen by cultured human dendritic cells is maintained by granulocyte/macrophage colony-stimulating factor plus interleukin 4 and downregulated by tumor necrosis factor alpha. *J. Exp. Med.* 179: 1109–1118.

Schittek, B. & Rajewsky, K. (1990). Maintenance of B-cell memory by long-lived cells generated from proliferating precursors. *Nature* 346: 749–751.

Smith, C.A., Farrah, T. & Goodwin, R.G. (1994). TNF receptor superfamily of cellular and viral proteins: activation, costimulation, and death. *Cell* 76: 959–962.

Soong, L., Xu, J.C., Grewal, I.S. *et al.* (1996). Disruption of CD40–CD40 ligand interactions results in an enhanced susceptibility to *Leishmania amazonensis* infection. *Immunity* 4: 263–273.

Trinchieri, G. (1995). Interleukin-12: a proinflammatory cytokine with immunoregulatory functions that bridge innate resistance and anitgen-specific adaptive immunity. *Annu. Rev. Immunol.* 13: 251–276.

van Essen, D., Kikutani, H. & Gray, D. (1995). CD40 ligand-transduced co-stimulation of T cells in the development of helper function. *Nature* 378: 620–623.

Xu, J., Foy, T.M., Laman, J.D. *et al.* (1994). Mice deficient for the CD40 ligand. *Immunity* 1: 423–431.

Yellin, M.J., Sipple, K.C., Inghirami, G. *et al.* (1994). CD40 molecules induce downmodulation and endocytosis of T-cell surface T-cell–B-cell activating molecule CD40–1: – potential role in regulating helper effector function. *J. Immunol.* 152: 598–608.

6

Manipulation of the T cell immune system via CD28 and CTLA-4

D. M. SANSOM and L. S. K. WALKER

Introduction

In order to provide protection from a vast array of infectious agents, the immune system has evolved a series of defences based on specialized immune cells. One component of this system, the T lymphocyte, is critical in organizing and effecting cellular responses by providing helper functions for B cells, as well as by generating direct cytotoxic actions. The major challenge faced in controlling T cell responses is how to generate a sufficiently large immune repertoire capable of recognizing any possible foreign antigen while at the same time maintaining T cells in an unresponsive state towards an equally large array of self-antigens. Clearly any breakdown in the barriers that prevent recognition and activation of T cells by self-antigens allows the possibility of developing autoimmune conditions, which include RA and SLE. In order to gain an understanding of potential disease mechanisms and to provide initiatives for novel therapeutic strategies, it is necessary to understand these mechanisms of T cell tolerance.

Since the late 1970s, substantial progress has been made in our understanding of the molecular basis of antigen recognition by T cells. Based on the observations of Zinkernagel and Doherty, who demonstrated that T cell recognition of foreign antigens requires appropriate (self) MHC antigens, it is now well established that the function of MHC class I and class II antigens is to bind and display both self and non-self peptide fragments on the cell surface (Zinkernagel & Doherty, 1974; 1975; Brown *et al.*, 1993). In the case of MHC class II molecules (HLA-DR, HLA-DQ and HLA-DP), expression is generally restricted to professional antigen-presenting cells, such as dendritic cells, monocytes, macrophages and activated B cells. MHC-displayed peptides thus form the central focus of T cell antigen recognition and it is, therefore, significant in the context of autoimmune conditions that diseases such as RA show strong selection for particular *HLA-DR* alleles such as *DR1* and *DR4* (Stastny, 1978;

Gregerson, Silver & Winchester, 1987) suggesting a possible T cell-driven aetiology.

Since antigens to both 'self' and 'non-self' are normally available for T cell recognition, T cell activation must be tightly controlled by self-tolerance, which involves both 'central' and 'peripheral' mechanisms. The central mechanism involves thymic selection, which has traditionally been seen as the major source of self-tolerance whereby the majority of T cells expressing clonally rearranged antigen receptors undergo apoptotic death (deletion) as a result of their expression of 'inappropriate' receptors (Kappler, Roehm & Marrack, 1987; Pullen, Kappler & Marrack, 1989; MacDonald & Lees, 1990). The details of this process are beyond the scope of this review; however, T cells that survive thymic selection emigrate from the thymus and then form the basis of the peripheral T cell pool. Despite the removal of large numbers of immature T cells during development in the thymus, there is increasing evidence that thymic selection is insufficient to completely account for self-tolerance and that other mechanisms must exist. Indeed evidence from mice that are defective in the control of peripheral tolerance mechanisms suggest these may be more important in preventing autoimmunity (Bluestone, 1997).

Our understanding of the mechanisms of peripheral self-tolerance was considerably advanced in the late 1980s when several lines of evidence began to show definitively that despite the expression of self-antigens and the presence of specific antigen-reactive T cells for these antigens immune activation did not necessarily ensue (Lo *et al.*, 1988; Markmann *et al.*, 1988; Ramensee, Kroschewski & Frangoulis, 1989; Schwartz, 1990). This underlined the existence of peripheral tolerance mechanisms and indicated that factors other than antigen recognition could determine the outcome of T cell receptor engagement. This review will focus on two molecules, CD28 and CTLA-4 (CD152), which are now known to play a key role in determining the fate of antigenically challenged T cells. Recent evidence suggests that while both CD28 and CTLA-4 interact with the same ligands (CD80 and CD86), CD28 and CTLA-4 function differentially to act as 'go' and 'stop' signals, respectively, for T cell activation and proliferation.

A general scheme for the interactions between these receptors and their ligands is shown in Fig. 6.1.

CD28 and CTLA-4

Structure of CD28 and CTLA-4

CD28 is a cell surface glycoprotein found on the majority of peripheral blood T cells, with preferential expression on CD4+ cells (95% positive) compared with

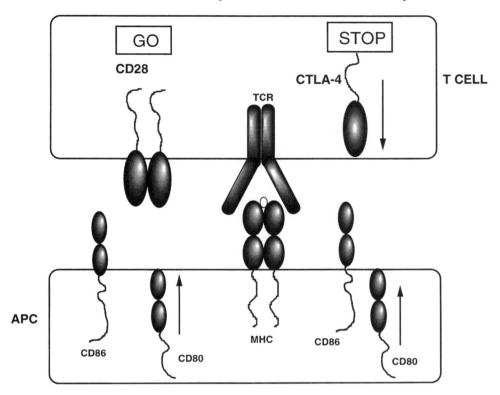

Fig. 6.1. Schematic representation of CD28 and CTLA-4 interactions. CD28 expressed on T cells initially interacts with the more abundantly expressed CD86 molecule on antigen-presenting cells. This provides positive 'go' signals for T cell proliferation and cytokine production in the context of antigenic stimulation via the MHC–TCR interaction. CD80 is induced upon activation of antigen-presenting cells and provides a second ligand capable of CD28 co-stimulation. In contrast, the higher-affinity CTLA-4 receptor is expressed intracellularly or in low abundance at the cell surface. Interaction of CTLA-4 with either CD80 or CD86 molecules initiates negative 'stop' signals' causing T cell cycle arrest and inhibition of T cell responses to antigen.

CD8[+] cells (50% positive) (Linsley & Ledbetter, 1993; June *et al.*, 1994). The gene for CD28 is a member of the immunoglobulin gene superfamily and expresses a protein containing a single extracellular 'V'-like domain. An initial polypeptide of M_r 23 000 is heavily glycosylated to give a mature glycoprotein of approximately 44 000, ultimately expressed at the cell surface as a 90 000 homodimer. The mature CD28 protein consists of 202 amino acid residues giving a single 134 residue extracellular domain, a transmembrane section and a 41 residue cytoplasmic tail responsible for signal transduction. This cytoplasmic domain contains a number of consensus amino acid motifs, including a YMNM motif, which are presumed to mediate interactions with signalling molecules inside the cell.

The CTLA-4 receptor, which is related to CD28, was initially isolated from a subtractive cDNA library screen for molecules expressed in activated T cells (Brunet *et al.*, 1987). The CTLA-4 gene is a member of the immunoglobulin superfamily encoding a single extracellular V-like domain polypeptide (approximately 20 kDa), which is reported to be expressed as a 40 kDa monomer at the cell surface (Lindsten *et al.*, 1993). Despite the fact that CD28 and CTLA-4 share only 30% amino acid identity, they are both located on chromosome 2 (2q33–34) in humans (Dariavach *et al.*, 1988) and share a similar intron/exon structure, suggesting that the two arose from a common ancestor (Harper *et al.*, 1991). Like CD28, CTLA-4 also contains a short cytoplasmic tail of some 36 amino acid residues, with a YVKM motif; this may be involved in its signalling functions and/or in control of cell surface CTLA-4 expression. Strikingly, the CTLA-4 cytoplasmic domain displays 100% evolutionary conservation in several species (June *et al.*, 1994; Harlan, Abe & June, 1995), indicating a highly conserved and essential function. Primary sequence comparisons and mutagenesis studies of the extracellular domains of CD28 and CTLA-4 have identified a conserved amino acid sequence (MYPPPY) present in the extracellular domains of both CTLA-4 and CD28 that appears to be required for their interactions with ligands (Peach *et al.*, 1994; Fargeas *et al.*, 1995; Morton *et al.*, 1996); however evidence suggests that CD80 and CD86 bind to discrete but overlapping sites.

Expression of CD28 and CTLA-4

The expression patterns of CD28 and CTLA-4 display marked differences. CD28 is constitutively expressed and is readily detected on the surface of the majority of resting T cells by flow cytometric analysis (FACS). In response to T cell activation, CD28 surface expression is subsequently modulated, during which both decreases and increases in expression can be observed. Currently, evidence suggests that initially CD28 is downregulated upon interaction with its ligand (Linsley *et al.*, 1993b). This downregulation occurs within a few hours of ligand engagement but is followed by re-expression during the following 24–48 hours. It has been suggested that the signalling capacity of CD28 may be compromised following re-expression, although this has not been confirmed. Our own observations indicate that while CD28 downregulation can be induced by ligand binding alone, re-expression of CD28 is contingent on TCR activation signals. Furthermore, in some circumstances, upon re-expression the levels of CD28 may be substantially higher, especially in cells that have encountered both antigen and

CD28 co-stimulation. This indicates that CD28 upregulation may be a consequence of correct activation and may possibly serve to adjust the balance between CD28 and CTLA-4 usage in activated T cells.

Expression data for CTLA-4 are more limited, since the protein is much less abundant than CD28 and, until recently, antibodies have not been widely available. Information from mRNA analysis surprisingly indicates similar levels of message for both CD28 and CTLA-4 in activated T cells yet CTLA-4 is found at much lower levels at the cell surface (Freeman *et al.*, 1992; Linsley *et al.*, 1993b). However, resting T cells do not express a detectable message for CTLA-4, in contrast to CD28 (Lindsten *et al.*, 1993). Activation signals via TCR and CD28 are also thought to enhance the surface expression of CTLA-4, which is reported to be maximal at 48–72 hours (Walunas *et al.*, 1994; Alegre *et al.*, 1996). However, it should be noted that even at maximal expression the surface levels of CTLA-4 are substantially lower than those of CD28. In line with these observations, current data indicate that CTLA-4 may be predominantly an intracellular protein that translocates to the surface following T cell activation (Alegre *et al.*, 1996; Wang *et al.*, 1996). This expression appears to be focally localized towards the contact site between the T cell and its target and is possibly regulated by a calcium-dependent mechanism (Linsley *et al.*, 1996). Recent studies have revealed that CTLA-4 is retained inside the cell via an association with the AP50 component of the clathrin-associated adaptor AP-2 (Chuang *et al.*, 1997; Shiratori *et al.*, 1997). This association is prevented by phosphorylation of the CTLA-4 YVKM motif, which thus allows surface CTLA-4 expression (Shiratori *et al.*, 1997). This observation is in agreement with mutagenesis studies on CTLA-4, which demonstrated that replacing tyrosine 164 in the YVKM motif with a phenylalanine residue also results in increased cell surface expression (Leung *et al.*, 1995).

Overall, the expression levels and mechanisms of expression of CD28 and CTLA-4 differ considerably, with much higher levels of CD28 being observed compared with CTLA-4. Both molecules are responsive to activation events and this may provide a way of altering the balance between these two receptors in order to maintain control of T cell activity. Given that both known ligands appear capable of binding either CTLA-4 or CD28, it seems likely that some mechanism must be required to allow interactions with either CTLA-4 or CD28 to predominate under appropriate circumstances. One possibility is that the mechanism which promotes CD28 downregulation enhances CTLA-4 expression. While there is little direct evidence for such a mechanism, the kinetics of CD28 downregulation and CTLA-4 expression as well as changes in mRNA levels (Lindsten *et al.*, 1993) are consistent with such a possibility.

CD80 and CD86

Currently, two ligands for CD28 and CTLA-4 have been cloned from humans and characterized (Freeman *et al.*, 1989; 1993; Azuma *et al.*, 1993a); both of which bind to CTLA-4 with higher affinity than to CD28. The first cloned ligand was originally termed B7 and renamed B7.1 when a second ligand B7.2/ B70 was identified. Subsequently, both B7.1 and B7.2/ B70 have been renamed CD80 and CD86, respectively. Like CD28 and CTLA-4, both CD80 and CD86 molecules are cell surface glycoprotein members of the immunoglobulin superfamily, which expresses two disulphide-linked extracellular domains. Similarly to CD28 and CTLA-4, the genes for both CD80 and CD86 are located to the same chromosomal region (3 Q13–Q23) in humans (Fernandez-Ruiz *et al.*, 1995), suggesting that they have also arisen via a gene duplication. The CD80 protein is a 262 amino acid residue, 30 kDa polypeptide that has a mature glycosylated mass of approximately 60 kDa. The CD86 molecule is slightly larger (34 kDa; 323 amino acid residues) because of an extended cytoplasmic tail, which is glycosylated to approximately 70 kDa, as determined by SDS–PAGE analysis (Azuma *et al.*, 1993a).

Despite only 23% sequence identity, both CD80 and CD86 were initially reported to have similar affinities for CD28 and CTLA-4 (Linsley *et al.*, 1994). However, more recent studies using surface plasmon resonance analysis have suggested that the affinity differences between CD80 and CD86 binding may be as large as 10-fold (Greene *et al.*, 1996). In addition, there are differences in the kinetics of binding to and dissociation from CTLA-4 (Linsley *et al.*, 1994; van der Merwe *et al.*, 1997). However, despite this, it has been difficult to demonstrate discrete functions for CD80 and CD86, as both are capable of effectively co-stimulating via CD28 (Lanier *et al.*, 1995). To date, the major differences between these two ligands appear to be mainly at the level and kinetics of surface expression. In this regard, CD86 is the most widely expressed and is found constitutively on professional antigen-presenting cells such as resting monocytes and dendritic cells (Azuma *et al.*, 1993a; Fleischer *et al.*, 1996). In addition, CD86 is upregulated by cytokines, such as IFN-γ upon activation, where increased levels are seen on monocytes and induction is found on activated T and B cells (Azuma *et al.*, 1993a; Stack *et al.*, 1994). Some reports have also suggested that CD86 may be expressed on resting T cells and that CD80 and CD86 may be reciprocally regulated following activation (Prabhu Das *et al.*, 1995). In contrast, CD80 has a much more limited expression profile, being virtually undetectable on peripheral blood mononuclear cells in the absence of activation (Koulova & Dupont, 1991; Azuma *et al.*, 1993a; Fleischer *et al.*, 1996). Following activation, CD80 is found on activated monocytes, albeit at lower levels than CD86, and is found on activated B cells and many B cell lines (Yokochi, Holly & Clark, 1982). Varying levels of CD80 are also found on T cells, depending on their state of activation (Sansom & Hall, 1993; Azuma *et al.*, 1993b). Therefore, in terms of providing initial CD28 ligation, CD86 appears to be the primary ligand, a view supported by the fact that anti-CD86 antibodies are more efficient inhibitors of T cell activation than anti-CD80. Furthermore, mice that are deficient for CD86 have a more severe immunodeficient phenotype than do mice which lack CD80 (Borriello *et al.*, 1997).

Given the interest in the CD28 pathway in controlling T cell activation, numerous studies have investigated the expression of these molecules in clinical conditions, including RA and SLE. Much of this work is still at the descriptive stage and there is not yet a consensus as to whether there are significant alterations in expression of these molecules in rheumatic diseases (Sfikakis *et al.*, 1995; Summers *et al.*, 1995; 1996; Balsa *et al.*, 1996; Garciacozar *et al.*, 1996; Schmidt, Goronzy & Weyand, 1996; Folzenlogen *et al.*, 1997; Sfikakis & Via, 1997). Accordingly, both increased expression and lack of expression has been reported for CD80/CD86 and CD28 molecules and the role of these proteins in causing or sustaining disease needs a more detailed functional analysis.

Functional aspects of CD28 and CTLA-4

CD28 co-stimulates T cell activation

During the late 1980s the two-signal model of T cell activation as proposed by Bretscher and Cohen received substantial experimental support from a number of sources, including a series of experiments by Jenkins *et al.* (Jenkins & Schwartz, 1987; Jenkins, Aswell & Schwartz, 1988; Mueller, Jenkins & Schwartz, 1989). These studies mainly involved the use of modified antigen-presenting cells and demonstrated that, by presenting antigen to T cells after fixation of the antigen-presenting cells, T cells could be made specifically unresponsive (anergic) to the presented peptide whereas normal antigen-presenting cells induced a proliferative response. The missing component from the fixed cells was identified as a cell surface molecule found on 'non-T' spleen cells, which could rescue from anergy if provided at the same time as TCR engagement. Similarly, studies using transgenic mice to study the autoimmune effects of ectopic expression of MHC class II molecules on pancreatic cells concluded that, instead of the predicted autoimmune attack on the class II-positive beta cells, T cells were instead made tolerant to the class II antigen (Lo *et al.*, 1988; 1989; Markmann *et al.*, 1988). Therefore, it emerged that both a TCR and a 'co-stimulatory' signal were required for T cell activation, and that in the absence of co-stimulatory signals T cells became unresponsive to antigen. The characteristics of this co-stimulatory signal were that it (i) was dependent on a cell surface molecule found on antigen-presenting cells; (ii) was required at the same time as TCR engagement; (iii) could be delivered by a cell distinct from the cell expressing the antigen target; and (iv) resulted in IL-2 production from the T cells.

Independently of these studies, cDNA cloning experiments had identified the genes for the B cell surface antigen B7 (Freeman *et al.*, 1989) and the gene for CD28 (Aruffo & Seed, 1987), culminating in the formal identification of B7 as a ligand for CD28 (Linsley *et al.*, 1991a) and the demonstration that this pathway fulfilled the above co-stimulatory criteria (Gimmi *et al.*, 1991; Jenkins *et al.*, 1991; Linsley *et al.*, 1991a; Razi-Wolf *et al.*, 1992; Sansom *et al.*, 1993). In particular, CD28 was found to be important in enhancement of cytokine production by T cells, an effect mediated by both increased transcription and stabilization of a number of cytokine mRNAs including those for IL-2, IL-4, IL-8, IL-13 and TNFγ (Lindsten *et al.*, 1989; Thompson *et al.*, 1993; June *et al.*, 1994). Furthermore, CD28 engagement was also shown to be capable of preventing T cell anergy, thus identifying it as a key second signal for T cell activation (Jenkins *et al.*, 1991; Harding *et al.*, 1992).

These experiments have resulted in a model of T cell activation where CD28 signals are thought to provide a check on T cell activation and only encounters with antigen in the context of CD80–CD86 interactions on professional antigen-presenting cells result in proliferation and cytokine production. Conversely, a lack of co-stimulatory signals is predicted to lead to an antigen-specific inactivation of the T cell (anergy), thereby providing a mechanism of peripheral self-tolerance. Whilst this view is most likely to be an oversimplification of the requirements of T cell activation, support for this model has been derived from a number of experimental systems.

In particular, considerable progress has been made using a recombinant chimaeric molecule (CTLA-4-Ig) generated by fusing the extracellular domain of CTLA-4 to an immunoglobulin heavy chain constant region (Linsley *et al.*, 1991b). The resulting protein is a soluble high-affinity antagonist of both CD80 and CD86. Results using this protein have demonstrated the tolerogenic potential of blocking CD28 interactions both *in vitro* (Tan *et al.*, 1993) and *in vivo* (Lenschow *et al.*, 1992). In particular, *in vivo* data have yielded impressive results in transplantation models, where CTLA-4-Ig treatment resulted not only in prevention of graft rejection but also in induced tolerance to subsequent grafts (Lenschow *et al.*, 1992; Blazar *et al.*, 1994; Pearson *et al.*, 1994; Ibrahim *et al.*, 1997). This suggests that blocking CD28 interactions is not only immunosuppressive but also that T cells manipulated in this way subsequently undergo a form of anergy. Clearly this mode of action has considerable therapeutic potential, and CTLA-4-Ig is currently under investigation as an immunotherapeutic agent.

CD28 promotes T cell survival

In addition to co-stimulating antigen-induced proliferation and stimulating cytokine production, CD28 signalling has also been increasingly associated with promoting T cell survival. Studies on CD28-deficient T cells have demonstrated that while proliferation can be initiated in the absence of CD28-derived signals the response cannot be sustained (Lucas *et al.*, 1995), which may be associated with decreased cell viability at late time points. Likewise *in vitro* studies indicate substantial T cell apoptosis following anti-CD3 engagement alone, which is prevented by co-stimulation with anti-CD28 (Boise *et al.*, 1995; Radvanyi *et al.*, 1996; Sperling *et al.*, 1996). Consistent with an anti-apoptotic role for CD28, studies in our own laboratory have analysed T cells that have received co-stimulatory signals and compared their survival with bystander-activated cells. This revealed a striking resistance to Fas-mediated apoptosis in those cells receiving co-stimulatory signals (McLeod *et al.*, 1998). The mechanisms that underlie CD28-mediated survival effects have not yet been clearly defined but two potential candidates are the production of anti-apoptotic lymphokines such as IL-2 and the induction of the anti-apoptotic protein Bcl-X_L. Whilst the role of CD28 enhancement of cytokine production by T cells is well established (Fraser *et al.*, 1991; Fraser & Weiss, 1992; Lindsten *et al.*, 1989; Thompson *et al.*, 1993), the role of IL-2 in survival is becoming less clear. The demonstration that IL-2-receptor knock-out mice exhibit lymphoproliferation and autoimmunity (Suzuki *et al.*, 1995) and a defect in Fas-mediated apoptosis indicates that IL-2 signalling may be involved in the maintenance of self-tolerance by facilitating programmed cell death.

The long splice variant of the *bcl-X* gene (*bcl-X_L*) (Boise *et al.*, 1993) has been found to prevent apoptosis induced by a diverse array of stimuli (Grillot, Merino & Nunez, 1995). Since CD28 stimulation upregulates *bcl-X_L*, this is potentially a major route for CD28 survival signals and has been observed in a number of studies (Boise *et al.*, 1995; Noel *et al.*, 1996; Radvanyi *et al.*, 1996; Sperling *et al.*, 1996). Therefore, there is considerable evidence that CD28 co-stimulation protects T cells from apoptosis and that this may involve Bcl-X_L; however it is likely that other routes also exist.

CTLA-4 acts as an inhibitor of T cell activation

While studies of CD28 interactions provide a clear picture of the co-stimulatory role of CD28, the role of CTLA-4 has been more difficult to elucidate. Our understanding is based on the use of anti-CTLA-4 monoclonal antibodies, and in spite of the fact that CTLA-4 is the higher affinity receptor for both ligands there are no functional data using ligands to stimulate CTLA-4. The interpretation of anti-CTLA-4 antibody data is somewhat complicated, since the various antibodies can be seen as (i) delivering a negative signal (decreasing T cell responses); (ii) blocking a negative signal (increasing responses); (iii) delivering a co-stimulatory signal (increasing responses); or (iv) blocking a co-stimulatory signal (decreasing responses). Interpretation of these experiments relies on the fact that intact antibodies generally deliver operative signals whereas using Fab fragments inhibits CTLA-4 interactions.

While initial studies utilizing CTLA-4 monoclonal antibodies appeared to indicate that CTLA-4 might play a role similar to CD28 in enhancing T cell activation (Linsley *et al.*, 1993a), more recent studies have indicated that CTLA-4 plays a role in inhibiting T cell activation. These experiments showed that blocking CTLA-4 enhances T cell proliferation whereas cross-linking agonistic antibodies to CTLA-4 revealed potent immunosuppression of T cell proliferation (Walunas *et al.*, 1994; Krummel & Allison, 1995; 1996; Walunas, Bakker & Bluestone, 1996). Most critically, CTLA-4 knock-out mice develop fatal lymphoproliferative disease (see below), indicating the importance of CTLA-4 in maintaining self-tolerance. The nature of this inhibitory pathway is, as yet, unidentified; however, data from two laboratories (Krummel & Allison, 1996; Walunas *et al.*, 1996) indicate that CTLA-4 can block T cell function at a relatively early stage (within 48 hours), preventing upregulation of activation markers, entry into the cell cycle and the generation of IL-2. Strikingly, these effects are seen when surface levels of CTLA-4 are undetectable. One further recent study has also suggested that CTLA-4 may be required for the induction of anergy (Perez *et al.*, 1997), again consistent with a negative role for CTLA-4 but suggesting that the induction of T cell unresponsiveness requires CTLA-4. This result is difficult to reconcile with the view that lack of CD80/CD86 during TCR engagement *in vitro* can also induce anergy, and it may reflect an additional mechanism for anergy induction.

The above data provide a convincing picture of CTLA-4 as an inhibitor of T cell activation; however, there are still studies that do not fit this general picture (Gribben *et al.*, 1995; Wu *et al.*, 1997). Furthermore, at present, there is little direct evidence of the ability of natural ligands to provide inhibitory signals in a similar manner to the anti-CTLA-4 antibodies and, most obviously, nearly all the inhibitory data are based on murine studies. While it is likely that natural ligands do stimulate CTLA-4 function, the circumstances under which CTLA-4 predominates have yet to be established. Likewise, the kinetics with which CTLA-4 is utilized by its natural ligands also remains unclear. To date, most

T cell experiments using transfected ligands indicate that engagement of CD80/CD86 in the presence of anti-CD3 appears effectively to deliver proliferative signals via CD28, with little evidence for CTLA-4 function under these circumstances (Linsley *et al.*, 1991a; Gjorloff Wingren *et al.*, 1993). Therefore, while the role of CTLA-4 as an inhibitory molecule appears to be of fundamental importance to the control of self-tolerance, a considerable amount remains to be learnt about how and when CTLA-4 is utilized *in vivo*.

Studies in knock-out mice

The use of transgenic and knock-out technologies has now been applied with considerable effect to the study of CD28/CTLA-4 interactions. Knock-out approaches have been successfully performed to generate CD28, CTLA-4, CD80, CD86 and CD80/CD86 double knock-out mice (Shahinian *et al.*, 1993; Green *et al.*, 1994; Tivol *et al.*, 1995; Waterhouse *et al.*, 1995; Borriello *et al.*, 1997). In general, results from these mice provide support for the conclusions reached from the above *in vitro* and *in vivo* studies.

CD28-deficient mice

Studies on mice deficient for CD28 reiterate the positive role played by CD28 in T cell activation. These mice have impaired responses to mitogens and super-antigens (Shahinian *et al.*, 1993); although proliferative T cell responses are seen in these mice, these responses appear to be of much lower magnitude and shorter duration (Lucas *et al.*, 1995). However, while CD28 clearly enhances and prolongs T cell responses, it does not appear to be strictly essential for all forms of T cell activation, providing support for the view that further important co-stimulatory ligands probably exist. For example, T cells from CD28-deficient mice display a number of surprisingly intact T cell responses, including the ability to reject skin allografts (Kawai *et al.*, 1996) and generate graft-versus-host reactions (Speiser *et al.*, 1997).

In addition to influencing whether or not a proliferative response is obtained, there is also evidence which suggests that CD28 may qualitatively affect the outcome of TCR engagement. In particular, CD28 co-stimulation may be involved in the ability to make T_H2 responses (Rulifson *et al.*, 1997). However, this may depend on the nature of the antigenic challenge (Gause *et al.*, 1997a,b).

CD28-deficient mice display profound deficiencies in antibody production in addition to their T cell defects. These mice lack germinal centres (Ferguson *et al.*, 1996) and have strongly impaired ability to generate class-switched antibody isotypes, showing similar defects as mice treated with CTLA-4-Ig (Linsley *et al.*, 1992). It would appear that one of the major functions of CD28 *in vivo* is to provide T cell help for antibody production, a function that most likely also involves the interaction between CD40 and its T cell ligand (CD40L), which has been shown to be dependent on CD28 for expression (Klaus *et al.*, 1994; Somoza & Lanier, 1995; Yang & Wilson, 1996). These data appear to confirm the roles of CD28 in initiating and sustaining T cell responses, protecting from T cell apoptosis and facilitating efficient B cell help.

CD80- and CD86-deficient mice

Perhaps unsurprisingly, mice deficient in CD80 or CD86 ligands have a phenotype that is highly reminiscent of the CD28 knock-out. For example, mice that lack CD80 or CD86 either singly or in combination demonstrate defects in immunoglobulin class switching and germinal centre formation. This is interpreted as highlighting the requirement for CD28-dependent T cell help in many of these responses. In addition, there is a spectrum of severity in these knock-out mice. Mice lacking CD80 have a relatively mild phenotype, consistent with the concept that CD86 is the major primary ligand, whereas mice deficient for CD86 have a more severe phenotype, again affecting antibody class switching. This is especially noticeable when immunizations occur in the absence of adjuvant, suggesting that CD80 can compensate when induced by inflammation. However, mice lacking both CD80 and CD86 have the most severe phenotype, which is very similar to that found in mice defective for CD28 in that they lack germinal centres and have highly defective T cell-dependent antibody responses as well as defects in T cell activation (Sharpe, 1995; Borriello *et al.*, 1997; Schweitzer *et al.*, 1997). Interestingly, these mice are not specifically defective in either T_H1 or T_H2 responses, suggesting no obligatory role for either CD80 or CD86 in these responses.

CTLA-4-deficient mice

The most revealing in this series of knock-out mice have been mice deficient for CTLA-4. These animals provide powerful evidence that CTLA-4 is a negative regulator of T cell function since they develop a spectacular lymphoproliferative disease that proves fatal a few weeks after birth (Tivol *et al.*, 1995; Waterhouse *et al.*, 1995). Analysis of the T cell compartment reveals a dramatic expansion of mature CD25+ activated T cells, consistent with an unchecked expansion of activated T cells. One possibility is that these mice fail to downregulate TCR and/or CD28 activation signals following antigenic stimulation. This hypothesis is supported by the fact that these mice can be effectively treated with CTLA-

4-Ig, suggesting that the lymphoproliferation is CD80/CD86 co-stimulation dependent (Tivol *et al.*, 1997). This implies that CTLA-4 can negatively regulate either or both the TCR and CD28 pathways. Biochemical analysis of these mice is still in its early stages but hyperactivation of *src* kinases has been suggested as one possible mechanism (Marengere *et al.*, 1996). However, given that this study investigated T cells that were clearly activated, this may be an effect of uncontrolled T cell expansion rather than the cause. This study also indicated that CTLA-4 may interact with the Syp phosphatase, and that this may be involved in inhibition of activation (Marengere *et al.*, 1996); however, this work has yet to be confirmed. Therefore, despite significant gaps in our understanding of the mechanism of CTLA-4 function, the importance of this receptor in negatively regulating T cells is beyond doubt. Clearly, given the essential role of CTLA-4, a complete understanding of its functions will provide significant opportunities for immune intervention and therapies for autoimmune disease.

CD28/CTLA-4 signalling mechanisms

A detailed understanding of the signalling mechanisms utilized by CD28 and CTLA-4 is still being elucidated and has been the subject of several extensive reviews (June *et al.*, 1994; Ward, June & Olive, 1996; Sansom *et al.*, 1997). To date, there is little information on the mechanisms used by CTLA-4 and, therefore, only the salient features of CD28 signalling will be reviewed here.

The cytoplasmic domains of CD28 and CTLA-4 are 41 and 36 amino acids residues long, respectively, and, in common with many receptors of the immune system, do not contain any intrinsic enzymatic activity. The most obvious and intensively studied region of interest is the YMNM motif based around tyrosine (Y) 173 in CD28. This motif has been identified as a binding site for protein SH-2 domains, which interact with phosphorylated tyrosine residues. In particular, this motif effectively recruits the p85 subunit of the enzyme phosphatidylinositol 3-kinase (PI_3K) and it has been established that CD28 recruits and activates this lipid kinase (Ward *et al.*, 1993; 1995; Pages *et al.*, 1994; Prasad *et al.*, 1994; Cai *et al.*, 1995) upon ligand binding. The role of PI_3K in the downstream events of CD28 signalling is still controversial, in particular with respect to its requirement in IL-2 responses (Crooks *et al.*, 1995). Nonetheless, given the increasing evidence that CD28 is required for cell survival and proliferation, it is likely that these may provide important targets for PI_3K. This possibility is strengthened by the fact that recently elucidated downstream targets include protein kinase B and p70 S6kinase, which are essential for cell proliferation (Burgering & Coffer, 1995; Downward, 1995; Franke *et al.*, 1995). Given that the YMNM motif requires tyrosine phosphorylation before it can interact with

PI$_3$K, there have been a number of efforts to identify the kinase responsible. These have largely concentrated on *src*-coded kinases, such as Lck and Fyn as well as Tec family kinases such as Itk. At present, the best evidence suggests that Lck is capable of phosphorylating CD28; however, it is not yet clear whether this occurs *in vivo* (Raab *et al.*, 1995). Interestingly, while Itk has been shown to be phosphorylated following CD28 activation (August *et al.*, 1994), recent data suggest that Itk performs a negative regulatory role in T cell proliferation and is, therefore, not a likely candidate for CD28 co-stimulatory signals (Liao *et al.*, 1997).

Further downstream targets for CD28 signals include the activation of Jun amino terminal kinase, and it has been suggested that activation of this kinase may be a point of integration between signals from the TCR and CD28 (Su *et al.*, 1994). Other studies of CD28 have suggested a role for the enzyme acidic sphingomyelinase, which results in the subsequent production of ceramide (Boucher *et al.*, 1995). This pathway is a candidate for transmitting signal to Jun kinase as it is clear that other potent activators of Jun kinase such as TNFα also trigger sphingomyelinase activation (Wiegmann *et al.*, 1994).

Since a major effect of CD28 signalling is on cytokine production, transcription factor targets that bind to cytokine promoters have been sought which are responsive to CD28 signals. In this respect, a number of transcription factors have been observed to be regulated by CD28, including a putative CD28-response element (CD28RE) as well as other targets such as AP-1 and NFκB (Fraser *et al.*, 1991; Verweij, Geerts & Aarden, 1991; Fraser & Weiss, 1992; Edmead *et al.*, 1996). Interestingly, one of the major features of CD28 signalling is its resistance to the drug cyclosporin A, which is a potent inhibitor of the transcription factor NFAT. The fact that CD28 can still induce proliferation in the presence of cyclosporin suggests that CD28 signals may provide an alternative pathway to NFAT activation (Ghosh *et al.*, 1996).

Relevance of CD28 and CTLA-4 to rheumatic diseases

The role of T cells in RA

Given that a major hypothesis of the aetiology of many autoimmune conditions invokes a breakdown in T cell self-tolerance provoked by an environmental antigenic stimulus, then manipulation of the CD28/CTLA-4 system is an attractive target for therapeutic intervention. While there is a solid basis suggesting an autoimmune component in the development of RA, the aetiology of this disorder is largely unknown, and the relative contribution of T lymphocytes to disease has been controversial (Firestein & Zvaifler, 1990). In particular, the evidence that inflammatory cytokines such as TNFα and IL-1 are clearly involved in joint inflammation, and the relative lack of T cell cytokines such as IL-2, has prompted questions about the role of T cells (Feldman, Brennan & Maini, 1996). To some extent, this may result from problems of timing, since analysis of patients with classical RA may occur well after incitement of disease and observations will predominantly reflect inflammatory sequelae. Alternatively, it may be that expectations of T cell infiltration by a limited number of causative T cell clones in affected joints is over optimistic. Nonetheless, it is evident that in virtually all models where joint disease initiation can be studied, T lymphocytes play a central, causative role (Kadowaki *et al.*, 1994; Mima *et al.*, 1995; Sakata *et al.*, 1996; Tada *et al.*, 1996; Stasiuk *et al.*, 1997).

This evidence is strengthened by the classical observation that the major genetic predisposition to RA development maps to the HLA region (Stastny, 1978; Sansom *et al.*, 1987; 1989; Lanchbury *et al.*, 1991). Detailed studies of the protein sequences of the HLA susceptibility alleles gave rise to the 'shared epitope theory' proposed by Gregersen and colleagues (Gregerson *et al.*, 1987) in which the protein sequence of the polymorphic third hypervariable region (HVR) of the HLA-DR1 and HLA-DR4 appears to predispose to disease. Since the only known function of HLA-DR molecules is the presentation of peptide fragments to T cells, this has been used to support a central role for antigen-specific T cell activation in RA aetiology.

The recent identification by Mathis and co-workers of a novel animal model of spontaneous arthritis has provided a new perspective on the initiation and progression of autoimmune conditions (Kouskoff *et al.*, 1996). In this model, a novel mouse strain was generated by breeding a TCR transgenic line (KRN) onto the NOD background. This strain spontaneously develops a symmetrical erosive arthritis that is characterized by features highly reminiscent of RA. Analysis of this strain indicated a mechanism involving the recognition of a specific mouse class II molecule and yet, significantly, despite having a definitive T cell-MHC allele-dependent disease, T cells from diseased animals displayed poor proliferative responses and were difficult to detect in affected joints. Therefore, the lack of obvious T cell activity in the RA synovial compartment does not preclude a causative role for T cells in RA. Accordingly, there is still considerable scope for therapeutic approaches based on manipulating the CD28/CTLA-4 system.

Manipulation of CD28 interactions in autoimmune disease

A significant number of studies have now been carried out to investigate the effects of CD28/CTLA-4 manipulations in disease situations, including several autoimmune models as well as transplantation and tumour therapy settings. Initial successes using CTLA-4-Ig in transplant models, suggested that blocking both CD80 and CD86 could be used as an effective means to prevent graft rejection as well as to generate subsequent tolerance (Lenschow *et al.*, 1992; Linsley *et al.*, 1992). Subsequently, CTLA-4-Ig has been utilized in a number of auto-immune conditions. Particularly striking has been the treatment of lupus-prone NZB/NZW (F1) mice with soluble murine CTLA-Ig. This effectively inhibited T-dependent primary immune responses, leading to suppression of autoantibody production, decreased renal disease and enhanced survival rates (Finck, Linsley & Wofsy, 1994). Encouragingly, initiation of CTLA4-Ig therapy late on in disease progression (when lupus-associated mortality had reached 40%) still inhibited further production of autoantibodies and markedly prolonged life (Finck *et al.*, 1994), indicating significant efficacy even in the context of a well-established immune response. CTLA-4-Ig has also been utilized successfully in the amelioration of collagen-induced arthritis (Webb, Walmsley & Feldmann, 1996). Here again, administration at the time of antigen challenge was effective at preventing arthritis and effects were apparent even when CTLA-4-Ig was administered later in disease progression.

While studies in models of rheumatic diseases are still limited, more detailed work has been carried out in the context of other autoimmune conditions. In general, studies in experimental allergic encephalomyelitis (EAE) have shown similar results in that early administration of CTLA-4-Ig prevented disease onset (Miller *et al.*, 1995; Perrin *et al.*, 1995; 1996; Racke *et al.*, 1995). Therefore, blocking CD80 and CD86 interactions necessary for the activation of T cells, and consequently B cells, can establish effective immunosuppressive regimens. Similarly, initial experiments in the NOD mouse have established that administration of CTLA-4-Ig blocked the establishment of full blown diabetes (Lenschow *et al.*, 1995). Therefore, CTLA-4-Ig has been generally found to be efficient at suppressing and treating a variety of T cell-driven autoimmune diseases.

However, the NOD model has also revealed unexpected complexity in manipulating the CD28/CTLA-4 system. In particular, breeding of the NOD mouse onto a CD28 knock-out mouse resulted in increased incidence and severity of disease instead of the predicted amelioration (Lenschow *et al.*, 1996). Strikingly, the CD28-negative background allowed 80% of the male mice, which are normally largely unaffected, to become diseased. Furthermore, the use of anti-CD80/CD86 antibodies has also had mixed results, including both suppression and exacerbation of disease (Lenschow *et al.*, 1995; 1996). One hypothesis is that this relates to the requirements for CD80 and CD86 to influence differentially T_H1 and T_H2 cell development. In some diseases T_H2 responses may be protective, and, therefore, blocking CD28-related T_H2 effects may exacerbate disease. While a differential signalling role of CD80 versus CD86 is unlikely in view of the data from CD80 and CD86 knock-out mice (Borriello *et al.*, 1997; Schweitzer *et al.*, 1997), an alternative view is that T_H2 development is dependent on the 'strength of signal' (Sperling & Bluestone, 1996). Accordingly, T cells that receive CD28 co-stimulation either via CD80 or CD86 have a greater propensity to develop T_H2 responses, as indicated by increased IL-4 production. This hypothesis has received some experimental support, which indicates that co-stimulation may indeed be influential in development of T_H2 responses (Seder *et al.*, 1994; Freeman *et al.*, 1995; Thompson, 1995; Gause *et al.*, 1997b; Rulifson *et al.*, 1997). However, this finding is not universal and may depend on the nature of the antigenic challenge (Brown *et al.*, 1996; Gause *et al.*, 1997a; Schweitzer *et al.*, 1997).

At first sight, it is difficult to reconcile the preventative effects of CTLA-4-Ig treatment with the exacerbation in NOD × CD28 knock-out mice. However, re-evaluation of the treatment of NOD mice with CTLA-4-Ig has revealed that the timing of CTLA-4-Ig administration has a critical influence on disease outcome and that CD28 functions may differ at different times of treatment (Sperling & Bluestone, 1996).

In principle, the molecule with the most obvious therapeutic potential in autoimmune disease is CTLA-4. Since this molecule is a potent 'off switch' for T cells, CTLA-4 agonists may prove very useful for downregulating auto-immune responses. As yet, however, there are few data studying the effects of CTLA-4 agonists in autoimmune disease models. Encouragingly, however, where antagonists of CTLA-4 have been used, they have had spectacular and predicted results. Most striking is the enhancement of anti-tumour immunity following the blockade of CTLA-4. Here, mice rejected unmanipulated tumour cells when treated with anti-CTLA-4, whereas control mice universally succumbed to tumours (Leach, Krummel & Allison, 1996). More recently, other studies have shown that blocking CTLA-4 exacerbates autoimmune EAE models, again suggesting CTLA-4 is involved in downregulating autoimmune responses (Perrin *et al.*, 1996; Hurwitz *et al.*, 1997). Finally perhaps the most vivid demonstration that CTLA-4 may normally be involved in preventing autoimmunity is the fatal disease seen in CTLA-4 knock-out mice in which destructive myocarditis, pancreatitis and infiltration of lungs and liver have been described.

The notable successes of manipulating the CD28/CTLA-4 system in many disease models indicate that this pathway has excellent potential as a route for controlling autoimmune disease. However, the fact that some manipulations lead to disease exacerbation and the fact that CD80/CD86 ligands operate both inhibitory and stimulatory controls over T cells suggests the need for a cautious approach driven by a more detailed understanding of the system. Nonetheless, the benefits offered in terms of potential long-term tolerance, as well as the ability to manipulate only activated T cells, make this system an extremely promising area for developing future therapy.

References

Alegre, M.-L., Noel, P.J., Eisfelder, B.J. *et al.* (1996). Regulation of surface and intracellular expression of CTLA-4 on mouse T cells. *J. Immunol.* 157: 4762–4770.

Aruffo, A. & Seed, B. (1987). Molecular cloning of a CD28 cDNA by a high efficiency COS cell expression system. *Proc. Natl. Acad. Sci., USA* 84: 8573–8577.

August, A., Gibson, S., Kawakami, Y. *et al.* (1994). CD28 is associated with and induces the immediate tyrosine phosphorylation and activation of the Tec family kinase ITK/EMT in the human leukaemic T cell line. *Proc. Natl. Acad. Sci., USA* 91: 9347–9351.

Azuma, M., Ito, D., Yagita, H. *et al.* (1993a). B70 antigen is a second ligand for CTLA-4 and CD28. *Nature* 366: 76–79.

Azuma, M., Yssel, H., Phillips, J., Spits, H. & Lanier, L. (1993b). Functional expression of B7/BB1 on activated T lymphocytes. *J. Exp. Med.* 177: 845–850.

Balsa, A., Dixey, J., Sansom, D.M., Maddison, P.J. & Hall, N.D. (1996). Differential expression of the costimulatory molecules B7.1 (CD80) and B7.2 (CD86) in rheumatoid synovial tissue. *Br. J. Rheumatol.* 35: 33–37.

Blazar, B.R., Taylor, P.A., Linsley, P.S. & Vallera, D.A. (1994). In-vivo blockade of CD28/CTLA-4-B7/BB1 interaction with CTLA-4-Ig reduces lethal murine graft-versus-host disease across the major histocompatibility complex barrier in mice. *Blood* 83: 3815–3825.

Bluestone, J.A. (1997). Is CTLA-4 a master switch for peripheral tolerance. *J. Immunol.* 158: 1989–1993.

Boise, L.H., Gonzalez-Garcia, M., Postema, C. *et al.* (1993). bcl-X, a bcl-2-related gene that functions as a dominant regulator of apoptotic cell death. *Cell* 74: 597–608.

Boise, L.H., Minn, A.J., Noel, P.J. *et al.* (1995). CD28 costimulation can promote T cell survival by enhancing expression of Bcl-X$_L$. *Immunity* 3: 87–98.

Borriello, F., Sethna, M.P., Boyd, S.D. *et al.* (1997). B7-1 and B7-2 have overlapping, critical roles in immunoglobulin class switching and germinal center formation. *Immunity* 6: 303–313.

Boucher, L.-M., Wiegmann, K., Futterer, A. *et al.* (1995). CD28 signals through acidic sphingomyelinase. *J. Exp. Med.* 181: 2059–2068.

Brown, D.R., Green, J.M., Moskowitz, N.H., Davis, M., Thompson, C.B. & Reiner, S.L. (1996). Limited role of CD28-mediated signals in T-helper subset differentiation. *J. Exp. Med.* 184: 803–810.

Brown, J., Jardetzky, T., Gorga, J. *et al.* (1993). Three dimensional structure of the human class II histocompatibility antigen HLA-DR1. *Nature* 364: 33–39.

Brunet, J.F., Denziot, F., Luciani, M.F. *et al.* (1987). A new member of the immunoglobulin superfamily – CTLA-4. *Nature* 328: 267–270.

Burgering, B.M.T. & Coffer, P.J. (1995). Protein kinase B (c-Akt) in phosphatidylinositol-3-OH kinase signal transduction. *Nature* 376: 599–602.

Cai, Y., Cefai, D., Schneider, H. Raab, M., Nabavi, N. & Rudd, C.E. (1995). Selective CD28pYMNM mutations implicate phosphatidyl inositol 3-kinase in CD86-CD28 mediated costimulations. *Immunity* 3: 417–426.

Chuang, E., Alegre, M.L., Duckett, C.S. *et al.* (1997). Interaction of CTLA-4 with the clathrin-associated protein AP50 results in ligand-independent endocytosis that limits cell surface expression. *J. Immunol.* 159: 144–151.

Crooks, M.E.C., Littman, D.R., Carter, R.H., Fearon, D.T., Weiss, A. & Stein, P.H. (1995). CD28-mediated costimulation in the absence of phosphatidylinositol 3-kinase association and activation. *Mol. Cell. Biol.* 15: 6820–6828.

Dariavach, P., Matthei, M.-G., Golstein, P. & Lefranc, M.-P. (1988). Human Ig superfamily CTLA4 gene: chromosomal localisation and identification of protein sequence between murine and human CTLA4 cytoplasmic domains. *Eur. J. Immunol.* 18: 1901–1900.

Downward, J. (1995). A target for PI$_3$ kinase. *Nature* 376: 553–554.

Edmead, C.E., Patel, Y.I., Wilson, A.J. *et al.* (1996). Induction of NFκB and AP-1 by CD28 signalling involves both PI-3 kinase and acidic sphingomyelinase signals. *J. Immunol.* 57: 3290–3297.

Fargeas, C.A., Truneh, A., Reddy, M., Hurle, M., Sweet, R. & Sekaly, R.P. (1995). Identification of residues in the V-domain of CD80 (B7-1) implicated in functional interactions with CD28 and CTLA-4. *J. Exp. Med.* 182: 667–675.

Feldmann, M., Brennan, F.M. & Maini, R.N. (1996). Rheumatoid arthritis. *Cell* 85: 307–310.

Ferguson, S.E., Han, S.H., Kelsoe, G. & Thompson, C.B. (1996). CD28 is required for germinal center formation. *J. Immunol.* 156: 4576–4581.

Fernandez-Ruiz, E., Somoza, C., Sanchez-Madrid, F. & Lanier, L. (1995). CD28/CTLA-4 ligands – the genes encoding CD86 (B70/B7.2) maps to the same region as CD80 (B7/B7.1) gene in human chromosome 3Q13–Q23. *Eur. J. Immunol.* 25: 1453–1456.

Finck, B.K., Linsley, P.S. & Wofsy, D. (1994). Treatment of murine lupus with CTLA4-Ig. *Science* 265: 1225–1227.

Firestein, G.S. & Zvaifler, N.J. (1990). How important are T cells in chronic rheumatoid arthritis? *Arthritis Rheum.* 33: 768–773.

Fleischer, J., Soeth, E., Reiling, N. *et al.* (1996). Differential expression and function of CD80 (B7-1) and CD86(B7-2) on human peripheral blood monocytes. *Immunology* 89: 592–598.

Folzenlogen, D., Hofer, M.F., Leung, D.Y.M. *et al.* (1997). Analysis of CD80 and CD86 expression on peripheral blood B lymphocytes reveals increased expression of CD86 in lupus patients. *Clin. Immunol. Immunopathol.* 83: 199–204.

Franke, T.F., Yang, S., Chan, T.O. *et al.* (1995). The protein kinase encoded by the Akt proto-oncogene is a target of the PDGF-activated phosphoinositol 3-kinase. *Cell* 81: 727–736.

Fraser, J.D. & Weiss, A. (1992). Regulation of T cell lymphokine gene transcription by the accessory molecule CD28. *Mol. Cell. Biol.* 12: 4357–4363.

Fraser, J., Irving, B., Crabtree, G. & Weiss, A. (1991). Regulation of interleukin-2 gene enhancer activity by the T cell accessory molecule CD28. *Science* 251: 313–316.

Freeman, G.J., Freedman, A.S., Segil, J.M., Lee, G., Whitman, J.F. & Nadler, L.M. (1989). B7 a new member of the Ig superfamily with unique expression on activated and neoplastic B cells. *J. Immunol.* 143: 2710–2714.

Freeman, G.J., Lombard, D.B., Gimmi, C.D. *et al.* (1992). CTLA-4 and CD28 mRNA are coexpressed in most T cells after activation. *J. Immunol.* 149: 3795–3801.

Freeman, G.J., Gribben, J.G., Boussiotis, V.A. *et al.* (1993). Cloning of B7–2: a CTLA-4 counter-receptor that costimulates human T cell proliferation. *Science* 262: 909–912.

Freeman, G.J., Boussiotis, V.A., Anumanthan, A. *et al.* (1995). B7-1 and B7–2 do not deliver identical costimulatory signals, since B7–2 but not B7–1 preferentially costimulates the initial production of IL-4. *Immunity* 2: 523–532.

Garciacozar, F.J., Molina, I.J., Cuadrado, M.J. *et al.* (1996). Defective B7 expression on antigen-presenting cells underlying T-cell activation abnormalities in systemic lupus-erythematosus (SLE) patients. *Clin. Exp. Immunol.* 104: 72–79.

Gause, W.C., Chen, S.J., Greenwald, R.J. *et al.* (1997a). CD28 dependence of T cell differentiation to IL-4 production varies with the particular type 2 immune response. *J. Immunol.* 158: 4082–4087.

Gause, W.C., Halvorson, M.J., Lu, P. *et al.* (1997b). The function of costimulatory molecules and the development of IL-4-producing T cells. *Immunol. Today* 18: 115–120.

Ghosh, P., Sica, A., Cippitelli, M. *et al.* (1996). Activation of nuclear factor of activated T-cells in a cyclosporin A-resistant pathway. *J. Biol. Chem.* 271: 7700–7704.

Gimmi, C.D., Freeman, G.J., Gribben, J.G. *et al.* (1991). B-cell surface antigen B7 provides a costimulatory signal that induces T cells to proliferate and secrete interleukin 2. *Proc. Natl. Acad. Sci., USA* 88: 6575–6579.

Gjorloff Wingren, A., Dahlenborg, K., Bjorklund, M. *et al.* (1993). Monocyte regulated IFNγ production in human T cells involves CD2 signalling. *J. Immunol.* 151: 1328–1336.

Green, J.M., Noel, P.J., Sperling, A.I. *et al.* (1994). Absence of B7-dependent responses in CD28-deficient mice. *Immunity* 1: 501–508.

Greene, J.L., Leytze, G.M., Emswiler, J. *et al.* (1996). Covalent dimerisation of CD28/CTLA-4 and oligomerisation of CD80/CD86 regulate costimulatory interactions. *J. Biol. Chem.* 271: 26 762–26 771.

Gregerson, P.K., Silver, J. & Winchester, R.J. (1987). The shared epitope hypothesis: an approach to understanding the molecular genetics of susceptibility to rheumatoid arthritis. *Arthritis Rheum.* 30: 1205–1213.

Gribben, J.G., Freeman, G.J., Boussiotis, V.A. *et al.*, (1995). CTLA-4 mediates antigen-specific apotosis of human T cells. *Proc. Natl. Acad. Sci., USA* 92: 811–815.

Grillot, D.A.M., Merino, R. & Nunez, G. (1995). Bcl-xL displays restricted distribution during T cell development and inhibits multiple forms of apoptosis but not clonal deletion in transgenic mice. *J. Exp. Med.* 182: 1973–1983.

Harding, F., McArthur, J.G., Gross, J.A., Roulet, D.H. & Allison, J.P. (1992). CD28-mediated signalling co-stimulates murine T cells and prevents the induction of anergy in T cell clones. *Nature* 356: 607–609.

Harlan, D.M., Abe, R., Lee, K. *et al.* (1995). Potential roles of the B7 and CD28 receptor families in autoimmunity and immune evasion. *Clin. Immunol. Immunopathol.* 75: 99–111.

Harper, K., Balzano, C., Rouvier, E., Mattei, M., Luciani, M. & Golstein, P. (1991). CTLA-4 and CD28 activated lymphocyte molecules are closely related in both mouse and human as to sequence, message expression, gene structure and chromosomal location. *J. Immunol.* 147: 1037–1044.

Hurwitz, A.A., Sullivan, T.J., Krummel, M.F., Sobel, R.A. & Allison, J.P. (1997). Specific blockade of CTLA-4/B7 interactions results in exacerbated clinical and histologic disease in an actively-induced model of experimental allergic encephalomyelitis. *J. Neuroimmunol.* 73: 57–62.

Ibrahim, S., Jakobs, F., Linsley, P.S., Sanfilippo, F. & Baldwin, W.H. (1997). CTLA-

4-Ig inhibits alloantibody responses to transfusions and transplants. *Transplant. Proc.* 29: 1025.

Jenkins, M.K. & Schwartz, R.H. (1987). Antigen presentation by chemically modified splenocytes induces antigen-specific T cell unresponsiveness in vitro and in vivo. *J. Exp. Med.* 165: 302–319.

Jenkins, M.K., Aswell, J.D. & Schwartz, R.H. (1988). Allogeneic non-T spleen cells restore the responsiveness of normal T cell clones stimulated with antigen and chemically modified antigen presenting cells. *J. Immunol.* 140: 3324–3330.

Jenkins, M.K., Taylor, P.S., Norton, S.D. & Urdahl, K.B. (1991). CD28 delivers a costimulatory signal involved in antigen specific IL-2 production by human T cells. *J. Immunol.* 147: 2461–2466.

June, C.H., Bluestone, J.A., Nadler, L.M. & Thompson, C.B. (1994). The B7 and CD28 receptor families. *Immunol. Today* 15: 321–331.

Kadowaki, K.M., Matsuno, H., Tsuji, H. & Tunru, I. (1994). CD4+ T-cells from collagen-induced arthritic mice are essential to transfer arthritis into severe combined immunodeficient mice. *Clin. Exp. Immunol.* 97: 212–218.

Kappler, J.W., Roehm, N. & Marrack, P. (1987). T-cell tolerance by clonal elimination in the thymus. *Cell* 49: 273–280.

Kawai, K., Shahinian, A., Mak, T.W. & Ohashi, P.S. (1996). Skin allograft-rejection in CD28-deficient mice. *Transplantation* 61: 352–355.

Klaus, S.J., Pinchuk, L.M., Ochs, H.D. et al. (1994). Costimulation through CD28 enhances T-cell-dependent B-cell activation via CD40–CD401 interaction. *J. Immunol.* 152: 5643–5652.

Koulova, L. & Dupont, B. (1991). The CD28 ligand B7/BB1 provides costimulatory signal for alloactivation of CD4+ T cells. *J. Exp. Med.* 173: 759–762.

Kouskoff, V., Korganow, A., Duchatelle, V., Benoist, C. & Mathis, D. (1996). Organ-specific disease provoked by systemic autoimmunity. *Cell* 87: 811–822.

Krummel, M.F. & Allison, J.P. (1995). CD28 and CTLA-4 have opposing effects on the response of T cells to stimulation. *J. Exp. Med.* 182: 459–465.

Krummel, M.F. & Allison, J.P. (1996). CTLA-4 engagement inhibits IL-2 accumulation and cell cycle progression upon activation of resting T cells. *J. Exp. Med.* 183: 2533–2540.

Lanchbury, J.S.S., Jaeger, E.E.M., Sansom, D.M. et al. (1991). Strong primary selection for the Dw4 subtype of DR4 accounts for the HLA-DQw7 association with Felty's syndrome. *Hum. Immunol.* 32: 56–64.

Lanier, L., O'Fallon, S., Somoza, C. et al. (1995) CD80(B7) and CD86(B70) provide similar costimulatory signals for T cell proliferation, cytokine production and generation of CTL. *J. Immunol.* 154: 97–105.

Leach, D.R., Krummel, M.F. & Allison, J.P. (1996). Enhancement of antitumour immunity by CTLA-4 blockade. *Science* 271: 1734–1736.

Lenschow, D., Zeng, Y., Thistlethwaite, J. et al. (1992). Longterm survival of xenogeneic pancreatic islet grafts induced by CTLA4Ig. *Science* 257: 789–780.

Lenschow, D.J., Ho, S.C., Sattar, H. et al. (1995). Differential effects of anti-B7-1 and B7-2 monoclonal antibody treatment on the development of diabetes in the nonobese diabetic mouse. *J. Exp. Med.* 181: 1145–1155.

Lenschow, D.J., Herold, K.C., Rhee, L. et al. (1996). CD28/B7 regulation of Th-1 and Th-2 subsets in the development of autoimmune diabetes. *Immunity* 5: 285–293.

Leung, H.T., Bradshaw, J., Cleaveland, J.S. & Linsley, P.S. (1995). Cytotoxic T-lymphocyte-associated molecule-4, a high avidity receptor for CD80 and CD86, contains an intracellular-localization motif in its cytoplasmic tail. *J. Biol. Chem.* 270: 25 107–25 114.

Liao, X.C., Fournier, S., Killeen, N., Weiss, A., Allison, J.P. & Littman, D.R. (1997). Itk negatively regulates induction of T cell proliferation by CD28 costimulation. *J. Exp. Med.* 186: 221–228.

Lindsten, T., June, J., Ledbetter, J., Stella, G. & Thompson, C. (1989). Regulation of lymphokine mRNA stability by a surface-mediated T cell activation pathway. *Science* 244: 339–345.

Lindsten, T., Lee, K.P., Harris, E.S. *et al.* (1993). Characterisation of CTLA-4 structure and expression on human T cells. *J. Immunol.* 151: 3489–3499.

Linsley, P.S. & Ledbetter, J.A. (1993). The role of the CD28 receptor during T cell responses to antigen. *Annu. Rev. Immunol.* 11: 191–212.

Linsley, P.S., Brady, W., Grosmaire, L., Aruffo, A., Damle, N.K. & Ledbetter, J.A. (1991a). Binding of the B cell activation antigen B7 to CD28 costimulates T cell proliferation and interleukin 2 mRNA accumulation. *J. Exp. Med.* 173: 721–730.

Linsley, P.S., Brady, W., Urnes, M., Grosmaire, L., Damle, N.K. & Ledbetter, J.A. (1991b). CTLA-4 is a second receptor for the B cell activation antigen B7. *J. Exp. Med.* 174: 561–569.

Linsley, P.S., Wallace, P.M., Johnson, J. *et al.* (1992). Immunosuppression *in vivo* by a soluble form of the CTLA-4 T cell activation molecule. *Science* 257: 792–795.

Linsley, P.S., Greene, J., Tan, P. *et al.* (1993a). Co-expression and functional cooperativity of CTLA-4 and CD28 on activated T lymphocytes. *J. Exp. Med.* 176: 1595–1604.

Linsley, P., Bradshaw, J., Urnes, M., Grosmaire, L. & Ledbetter, J. (1993b). CD28 engagement by B7/BB1 induces transient down-regulation of CD28 synthesis and prolonged unresponponiveness to CCD28 signalling. *J. Immunol.* 150: 3161–3169.

Linsley, P.S., Greene, J.L., Bradey, W., Bajorth, J., Ledbetter, J.A. & Peach, R. (1994). Human B7-1 (CD80) and B7-2 (CD86) bind with similar avidities but distinct kinetics to CD28 and CTLA-4 receptors. *Immunity* 1: 793–801.

Linsley, P.S., Bradshaw, J., Greene, J. *et al.* (1996). Intracellular trafficking of CTLA-4 and focal localisation towards sites of TCR engagement. *Immunity* 4: 535–543.

Lo, D., Burkly, L.C., Cowing, C., Flavell, R.A., Palmiter, R.D. & Brinster, R.L. (1988). Diabetes and tolerance in transgenic mice expressing class II MHC molecules in pancreatic beta cells. *Cell* 53: 159–168.

Lo, D., Burkly, L.C., Flavell, R.A., Palmiter, R.D. & Brinster, R.L. (1989). Tolerance in transgenic mice expressing class II major histocompatibility complex on pancreatic acinar cells. *J. Exp. Med.* 170: 87–104.

Lucas, P.J., Negishi, I., Nakayama, K., Fields, L.E. & Loh, D.Y. (1995). Naive CD28 deficient T cells can initiate but not sustain an *in vitro* antigen specific immune response. *J. Immunol.* 154: 5757–5768.

MacDonald, H.R. & Lees, R. (1990). Programmed death of autoreactive thymocytes. *Nature* 343: 642–644.

Marengere, L.E.M., Waterhouse, P., Duncan, G., Mittrucker, H., Feng, G. & Mak, T.W. (1996). Regulation of T cell receptor signalling by tyrosine phosphatase SYP association with CTLA-4. *Science* 272: 1170–1173.

Markmann, J., Lo, D., Naji, A., Palmiter, R.D., Brinster, R.L. & Heber-Katz, E. (1988). Antigen presenting function of class II MHC expressing pancreatic beta cells. *Nature* 336: 476–479.

McLeod, J.D., Walker, L.S.K., Ellwood, C. *et al.* (1998). Activation of human T cells with superantigen and CD28 confers resistance to apoptosis by CD95. *J. Immunol.* 160: 2072–2079.

Miller, S.D., Vnaderlugt, C.L., Lenschow, D.J. *et al.* (1995). Blockade of CD28/B7-1 interaction prevents epitope spreading and clinical relapses in murine EAE.

Immunity 3: 739–745.

Mima, T., Saeki, Y., Ohshima, S. *et al.* (1995). Transfer of rheumatoid-arthritis into severe combined immunodeficient mice – the pathogenetic implications of T-cell populations oligoclonally expanding in the rheumatoid joints. *J. Clin. Invest.* 96: 1746–1758.

Morton, P.A., Fu, X.T., Stewart, J.A. *et al.* (1996). Differential-effects of CTLA-4 substitutions on the binding of human CD80 (B7–1) and CD86 (B7–2). *J. Immunol.* 156: 1047–1054.

Mueller, D.L., Jenkins, M.K. & Schwartz, R.H. (1989). Clonal expansion versus functional clonal inactivation: a costimulatory signalling pathway determines the outcome of T cell antigen receptor occupancy. *Annu. Rev. Immunol.* 7: 445–480.

Noel, P.J., Boise, L.H., Green, J.M. & Thompson, C.B. (1996). CD28 costimulation prevents cell death during primary T cell activation. *J. Immunol.* 157: 636–642.

Pages, F., Ragueneau, M., Rottapel, R. *et al.* (1994). Binding of phosphatidylinositol-3-OH kinase to CD28 is required for T cell signalling. *Nature* 369: 327–329.

Peach, R.J., Bajorath, J., Brady, W. *et al.* (1994). Complementarity-determining region-1 (CDR1)-analogous and CDR3-analogous regions in CTLA-4 and CD28 determine the binding to B7-1. *J. Exp. Med.* 180: 2049–2058.

Pearson, T.C., Alexander, D.Z., Winn, K.J., Linsley, P.S., Lowry, R.P. & Larsen, C.P. (1994). Transplantation tolerance induced by CTLA-4-Ig. *Transplantation* 57: 1701–1706.

Perez, V.L., van Parijs, L., Biuckians, A., Zheng, X.X., Strom, T.B. & Abbas, A.K. (1997). Induction of peripheral T cell tolerance in vivo requires CTLA-4 engagement. *Immunity* 6: 411–417.

Perrin, P.J., Scott, D., Quigley, L. *et al.* (1995). Role of B7/ CD28 CTLA-4 in the induction of chronic relapsing experimental allergic encephalomyelitis. *J. Immunol.* 154: 1481–1490.

Perrin, P.J., Maldonado, J.H., Davis, T.A., June, C.H. & Racke, M.K. (1996). CTLA-4 blockade enhances clinical disease and cytokine production during experimental allergic encephalomyelitis. *J. Immunol.* 157: 1333–1336.

Prabhu Das, M.R., Zamvil, S.S., Weiner, H.L., Sharpe, A.H. & Kuchroo, V.K. (1995). Reciprocal expression of costimulatory molecules B7–1 and B7–2 on murine T cells following activation. *Eur. J. Immunol.* 25: 207–211.

Prasad, K.V.S., Cai, Y., Raab, M. *et al.* (1994). T cell antigen CD28 interacts with the lipid kinase phosphatidylinositol 3-kinase by a cytoplasmic Tyr(p)-met-Xaa-Met motif. *Proc. Natl. Acad. Sci., USA* 91: 2834–2838.

Pullen, A.M., Kappler, J.W. & Marrack, P. (1989). Tolerance to self antigens shapes the T-cell repertoire. *Immunol. Rev.* 107: 125–139.

Raab, M., Cai, Y.C., Bunnell, S.C., Heyeck, S., Berg, L.J. & Rudd, C.E. (1995). p56lck and p59fyn regulate CD28 binding to PI3 kinase, growth factor receptor bound GRB-2 and T cell specific PTK, ITK: implications for T cell costimulation. *Proc. Natl. Acad. Sci., USA* 92: 8891–8895.

Racke, M.K., Scott, D.E., Quigley, L. *et al.* (1995). Distinct roles for B7–1 (CD-80) and B7–2 (CD-86) in the initiation of experimental allergic encephalomyelitis. *J. Clin. Invest.* 96: 2195–2203.

Radvanyi, L.G., Shi, Y., Vaziri, H. *et al.* (1996). CD28 costimulation inhibits TCR induced apoptosis during a primary T cell response. *J. Immunol.* 156: 1788–1798.

Ramensee, H.G., Kroschewski, R. & Frangoulis, B. (1989). Clonal anergy induced in mature Vb6[+] T lymphocytes on immunising Mls-1[b] mice with Mls-1[a] expressing cells. *Nature* 339: 541–545.

Razi-Wolf, Z., Freeman, G.J., Galvin, F., Benacerraf, B., Nadler, L. & Reiser, H.

(1992). Expression and function of the murine B7 antigen, the major costimulatory molecule expressed on peritoneal exudate cells. *Proc. Natl. Acad. Sci., USA* 89: 4210–4214.

Rulifson, I.C., Sperling, A.I., Fields, P.E., Fitch, F.W. & Bluestone, J.A. (1997). CD28 costimulation promotes the production of T_h2 cytokines. *J. Immunol.* 158: 658–665.

Sakata, A., Sakata, K., Ping, H., Omura, T., Tsukano, M. & Kakimoto, K. (1996). Successful induction of severe destructive arthritis by the transfer of in-vitro activated synovial fluid T cells from patients with rheumatoid arthritis in severe combined immunodeficient (SCID) mice. *Clin. Exp. Immunol.* 104: 247–254.

Sansom, D.M. & Hall, N.D. (1993). B7/BB1, the ligand for CD28 is expressed on repeatedly activated human T cells *in vitro*. *Eur. J. Immunol.* 23: 295–298.

Sansom, D.M., Bidwell, J.L, Maddison, P.J., Campion, G., Klouda, P.T. & Bradley, B.A. (1987). HLA-DQ alpha and DQ beta restriction fragment length polymorphisms associated with Felty's syndrome and DR4-positive rheumatoid arthritis. *Hum. Immunol.* 19: 269–278.

Sansom, D.M., Amin, S.N., Bidwell, J.L. *et al.* (1989). HLA-DQ-related restriction fragment length polymorphisms in rheumatoid arthritis: evidence for a link with disease expression. *Br. J. Rheumatol.* 28: 374–378.

Sansom, D.M., Wilson, A., Boshell, M., Lewis, J. & Hall, N.D. (1993). B7/CD28 but not LFA-3 CD2 interactions can provide third party costimulation for human T cell activation. *Immunology* 80: 242–247.

Sansom, D.M., Edmead, C., Parry, R. & Ward, S.G. (1997). The T cell costimulatory molecule CD28 couples to multiple signalling pathways. In *Lymphocyte Signalling*, ed. M.M. Harnett & K.P. Rigley, pp. 91–106. Chichester, UK: Wiley.

Schmidt, D., Goronzy, J. & Weyand, C. (1996). CD4(+)CD7(–)CD28(–) T cells are expanded rheumatoid arthritis and are characterised by autoreactivity. *J. Clin. Invest.* 97: 2027–2037.

Schwartz, R.H. (1990). A cell culture model for T lymphocyte clonal anergy. *Science* 248: 1349–1356.

Schweitzer, A.N., Borriello, F., Wong, R.C.K., Abbas, A.K. & Sharpe, A.H. (1997). Role of costimulators in T cell differentiation – studies using antigen-presenting cells lacking expression of CD80 or CD86. *J. Immunol.* 158: 2713–2722.

Seder, R.A., Germain, R.N., Linsley, P.S. & Paul, W.E. (1994). CD28-mediated costimulation of interleukin-2 (IL-2) production plays a critical role in T-cell priming for IL-4 and interferon-gamma production. *J. Exp. Med.* 179: 299–304.

Sfikakis, P.P. & Via, C.S. (1997). Expression of CD28, CTLA-4, CD80, and CD86 molecules in patients with autoimmune rheumatic diseases: implications for immunotherapy. *Clin. Immunol. Immunopathol.* 83: 195–198.

Sfikakis, P.P., Zografou, A., Viglis, V. *et al.* (1995). CD28 expression on T-cell subsets in-vivo and CD28-mediated T-cell response in-vitro in patients with rheumatoid-arthritis. *Arthritis Rheum.* 38: 649–654.

Shahinian, A., Pfeffer, K., Lee, K.P. *et al.* (1993). Differential T cell costimulatory requirements in CD28 deficient mice. *Science* 261: 609–612.

Sharpe, A.H. (1995). Analysis of lymphocyte costimulation in-vivo using transgenic and knockout mice. *Curr. Opin. Immunol.* 7: 389–395.

Shiratori, T., Miyatake, S., Ohno, H. *et al.* (1997). Tyrosine phosphorylation controls internalization of CTLA-4 by regulating its interaction with clathrin-associated adaptor complex AP-2. *Immunity* 6: 583–589.

Somoza, C. & Lanier, L.L. (1995). T-cell costimulation via CD28–CD80/CD86 and CD40–CD40 ligand interactions. *Res. Immunol* 146: 171–176.

Speiser, D.E., Bachmann, M.F., Shahinian, A., Mak, Tiwi & Ohashi, P.S. (1997). Acute graft-versus-host disease without costimulation via CD28. *Transplantation* 63: 1042–1044.

Sperling, A.I. & Bluestone, J.A. (1996). The complexities of T-cell co-stimulation: CD28 and beyond. *Immunol. Rev.* 153: 155–182.

Sperling, A.I., Auger, J.A., Ehst, B.D. *et al.* (1996). CD28/B7 interactions deliver a unique signal to naive T cells that regulates cell survival but not early proliferation. *J. Immunol.* 157: 3909–3917.

Stack, R.M., Lenschow, D.J., Gray, G.S., Bluestone, J.A. & Fitch, F.W. (1994). IL-4 treatment of small splenic B-cells induces costimulatory molecules B7–1 and B7–2. *J. Immunol.* 152: 5723–5733.

Stasiuk, L.M., Ghoraishian, M., Elson, C.J. & Thompson, S.J. (1997). Pristane-induced arthritis is CD4(+) T-cell independent. *Immunology* 90: 81–86.

Stastny, P. (1978). Association of B cell alloantigen DRw4 with rheumatoid arthritis. *N. Eng. J. Med.* 298: 869–871.

Su, B., Jacinto, E., Hibi, M., Kallunki, T., Karin, M. & Ben-Neriah, Y. (1994). JNK is involved in signal integration during costimulation of T lymphocytes. *Cell* 77: 727–736.

Summers, K.L., Daniel, P.B., Odonnell, J.L. & Hart, D.N.J. (1995). Dendritic cells in synovial-fluid of chronic inflammatory arthritis lack CD80 surface expression. *Clin. Exp. Immunol.* 100: 81–89.

Summers, K.L., Odonnell, J.L., Williams, L.A. & Hart, D.N.J. (1996). Expression and function of CD80 and CD86 costimulator molecules on synovial dendritic cells in chronic arthritis. *Arthritis Rheum.* 39: 1287–1291.

Suzuki, H., Kundig, T.M., Furlonger, C. *et al.* (1995). Deregulated T-cell activation and autoimmunity in mice lacking interleukin-2 receptor-beta. *Science* 268: 1472–1476.

Tada, Y., Ho, A., Koh, D.R. & Mak, T.W. (1996). Collagen-induced arthritis in CD4-deficient or CD8-deficient mice – CD8(+) T-cells play a role in initiation and regulate recovery phase of collagen-induced arthritis. *J. Immunol.* 156: 4520–4526.

Tan, P., Anasetti, C., Hansen, J. *et al.* (1993). Induction of alloantigen specific hyporesponsiveness in human T lymphocytes by blocking interaction of CD28 with its natural ligand B7/BB1. *J. Exp. Med.* 177: 165–173.

Thompson, C.B. (1995). Distinct roles for the costimulatory ligands B7-1 and B7-2 in T helper cell differentiation. *Cell* 81: 979–970.

Thompson, C., Lindsten, T., Ledbetter, J. *et al.* (1993). CD28 activation pathway regulates the production of multiple T cell-derived lymphokines/cytokines. *Proc. Natl. Acad. Sci., USA* 86: 1333–1337.

Tivol, E.A., Borriello, F., Schweitzer, A.N., Lynch, W.P., Bluestone, J.A. & Sharpe, A.H. (1995). Loss of CTLA-4 leads to massive lymphoproliferation and fatal multiorgan tissue destruction, revealing a critical negative regulatory role of CTLA-4. *Immunity* 3: 541–547.

Tivol, E.A., Boyd, S.D., McKeon, S. *et al.* (1997). CTLA-4-Ig prevents lymphoproliferation and fatal multiorgan tissue destruction in CTLA-4-deficient mice. *J. Immunol.* 158: 5091–5094.

van der Merwe, P.A., Bodian, D.L., Daenke, S., Daenke, S., Linsley, P. & Davis, S.J. (1997) CD80 (B7–1) binds both J CD28 and CTLA-4 with a low affinity and very fast kinetics. *J. Exp. Med.* 185: 393–403.

Verweij, C.L, Geerts, M. & Aarden, L.A (1991). Activation of interleukin-2 gene transactivation via the T cell surface molecule CD28 is mediated through an NFκB-like response element. *J. Biol. Chem.* 266: 14 179–14 182.

Walunas, T.L., Lenschow, D.J., Bakker, C.Y. *et al.* (1994). CTLA-4 can function as a negative regulator of T cell activation. *Immunity* 1: 405–413.

Walunas, T.L., Bakker, C.Y. & Bluestone, J.A. (1996). CTLA-4 ligation blocks CD28-dependent T cell activation. *J. Exp. Med.* 183: 2541–2550.

Wang, H., Balderas, R., Rosenberg, J. Huang, E.C.M. & Chen, Z. (1996). Expression and function of CTLA-4 on human T-cells. *Tissue Antigens* 48: TC203.

Ward, S., Westwick, J., Hall, N. & Sansom, D. (1993). CD28 ligation elevates PtdIns(3,4)P_2 and PtdIns(3,4,5)P_3 in T cells. *Eur. J. Immunol.* 23: 2572–2577.

Ward, S.G., Wilson, A., Turner, L., Westwick, J. & Sansom, D.M. (1995). Inhibition of CD28-mediated T cell costimulation by the phosphoinositide 3-kinase inhibitor wortmannin. *Eur. J. Immunol.* 25: 526–532.

Ward, S.G., June, C.H. & Olive, D. (1996). PI_3 kinase: a pivotal pathway in T cell activation? *Immunol. Today* 17: 187–197.

Waterhouse, P., Penninger, J.M., Timms, E. *et al.* (1995). Lymphoproliferative disorders with early lethality in mice deficient in CTLA-4. *Science* 270: 985–988.

Webb, L.M.C., Walmsley, M.J. & Feldmann, M. (1996). Prevention and amelioration of collagen induced arthritis by blockade of the CD28 co-stimulatory pathway: requirement for both B7-1 and B7-2. *Eur. J. Immunol.* 26: 2320–2328.

Wiegmann, K., Schutze, S., Machleidt, T., Witte, D. & Kronke, M. (1994). Functional dichotomy of neutral and acidic sphingomyelinases in tumour necrosis factor signalling. *Cell* 78: 1005–1015.

Wu, Y., Guo, Y., Huang, A., Zheng, P. & Liu, Y. (1997). CTLA-4-B7 interaction is sufficient to costimulate T cell clonal expansion. *J. Exp. Med.* 185: 1327–1335.

Yang, Y.P. & Wilson, J.M. (1996). CD40 ligand-dependent T-cell activation – requirement of B7-CD28 signaling through CD40. *Science* 273: 1862–1864.

Yokochi, T., Holly, R.D. & Clark, E.A. (1982). B-lymphoblast antigen (BB1) expressed on Epstein-Barr virus-activated cell blasts, B lymphoblastoid cell lines, and Burkitt's lymphomas. *J. Immunol.* 128: 823–827.

Zinkernagel, R.M. & Doherty, P.C. (1974). Restriction of in vitro T cell-mediated cytotoxicity in lymphocytic choriomeningitis within a syngeneic or semiallogenic system. *Nature* 248: 702–710.

Zinkernagel, R.M. & Doherty, P.C. (1975). H-2 compatibility requirement for T cell mediated lysis of target cells infected with lymphocytic choriomeningitis virus: different cytotoxic specificities associated with structures coded for in H-2K or H-2D. *J. Exp. Med.* 141: 1427–1436.

7

Lymphocyte antigen receptor signal transduction

D. R. ALEXANDER

Introduction

Lymphocytes can be separated into thymus-derived cells (T cells) that are specialized for protecting the body against intracellular pathogens (cell-mediated immunity) and the bone-marrow derived cells (B cells, originally described in the bursa of Fabricius in the chicken) that protect against extracellular pathogens (humoral immunity). The specificity of these responses is achieved by the expression of clonotypic B and T cell antigen-specific receptors on the lymphocyte surface, known as the BCR and TCR, respectively. The BCR is specialized for the recognition, capture and internalization of antigens for processing and presentation on the cell surface in association with MHC class II molecule. The TCR is specialized for the recognition of small peptides presented on antigen-presenting cells in association with MHC class I or class II molecules. The peptides are typically 8–10 amino acid residues long when in association with class I molecules and rather more variable in length (typically 10–20 residues) when in association with class II molecules.

The outcome of BCR or TCR engagement by ligands depends on the avidity of the interaction, the length of time for which ligands bind, the lymphocyte differentiation state and the nature of other co-stimulatory signals being received by the cell. A fascinating aspect of antigen receptor signalling is that the same receptor can mediate signals resulting in apoptosis, activation or cellular non-responsiveness ('anergy') depending on the interplay between these four variables. During T cell development in the thymus, for example, selection events occur at the CD4+CD8+ stage of differentiation that define which T cells will mature and eventually exit to the periphery as CD4+ and CD8+ cells. High-avidity interactions between MHC–peptides and the TCR expressed on CD4+CD8+ thymocytes cause their deletion by apoptosis. When ligand–receptor interactions of equivalent avidity occur on mature peripheral T cells, however, the result is the activation and clonal expansion of the T cell population. In the absence of the correct cohort of co-stimulatory signals, the same ligand–TCR engagement could result in a state of peripheral T cell non-responsiveness. A similar diversity of outcomes characterizes BCR engagement. For example, when cell-bound polyvalent antigens bind to the BCR on immature B cells, then the cells die by apoptosis, whereas the same stimulus leads to a proliferative response in mature B cells.

The differences in the signalling pathways that mediate these radically different outcomes still remain poorly understood. Elucidation of these differences is critical for our understanding of tolerance, autoimmunity and immunosuppression, not least in the context of lymphocyte pathology in the inflamed synovium. From the practical point of view, it is also important to remember when assessing the rapidly growing literature on lymphocyte signalling pathways that the BCR and TCR do not necessarily mediate identical signals in any particular B or T cell. These will depend on the variables already listed above. Relevant questions to ask about any study of lymphocyte signalling, therefore, include the following: 'Are the lymphocytes being used primary cells or transformed cell lines?'; 'What is the differentiation state of the cells?'; 'Are the lymphocytes being triggered with antibodies or with physiological ligands?'; and 'Are co-receptors being stimulated at the same time as engagement of antigen receptors?'.

This chapter will focus mainly on the signals mediated by antigen receptors expressed on mature lymphocytes and on the regulation of receptor thresholds by CD45. The role of co-receptors such as CD4/CD8 on T cells, and CD22 and CD19/CD21 on B cells, which are intimately involved in antigen receptor signal transduction, will also be briefly summarized. Extensive reviews are available describing signalling pathways in T cells (Chan, Desai & Weiss, 1994a; Cantrell, 1996; Wange & Samelson, 1996; Alexander, 1997; Berridge, 1997; Frearson & Alexander, 1997) and in B cells (Cambier, Pleiman & Clark, 1994a; Pleiman, Dambrosio & Cambier, 1994; DeFranco, 1997; Kurosaki, 1997; O'Rourke, Tooze & Fearon, 1997).

It should be noted that at the level of lymphocyte cell biology the immediate consequences of ligand binding to the BCR and TCR are distinct. Thus, engagement of the BCR expressed on mature quiescent B cells by multimeric antigens results directly in cell proliferation in a T cell-independent manner. Engagement of the TCR on mature quiescent T cells, however, does not provide a proliferative signal, *per se*, but rather promotes the entry of the cells into the cell cycle, known as the G_0 to G_1 transition (Fig. 7.1). During this transition TCR-mediated signals cause the induction of IL-2 and IL-2 receptor-α (CD25) genes with the consequent secretion of IL-2 and expression of high-affinity IL-2 receptors on the cell surface. The subsequent autocrine or paracrine binding of IL-2 to IL-

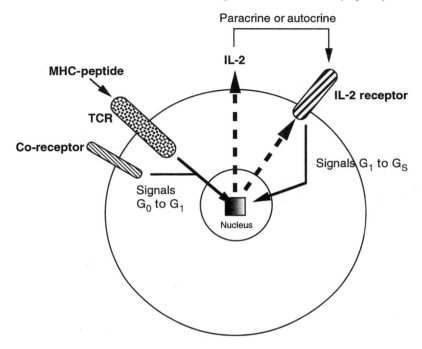

Fig. 7.1. The two major phases of T cell activation.

2 receptors then induces a panoply of signals that cause DNA synthesis and T cell proliferation. Many of these signals are quite distinct from those mediated by the TCR. Thus B cell activation is a one-phase process whereby engagement of the BCR by appropriate antigens triggers the full gamut of proliferative signals, whereas T cell activation is a two-phase process comprising antigen-driven entry into the cell cycle followed by cytokine-induced proliferation.

The structure of antigen receptors

Characterization of the molecular structures of the BCR and TCR have provided critical insights into the way these receptors couple to intracellular signalling pathways. The TCR comprises the polymorphic α and β subunits, which recognize MHC-associated peptides, in non-covalent association with the invariant transmembrane CD3 γ, δ and ε chains and the TCR-ς chain homodimer (Fig. 7.2a) (Weiss, 1993). These invariant polypeptides are responsible for stabilizing the assembly of the receptor to enable its expression at the cell surface, and for coupling the TCR to intracellular signalling pathways. The equivalent antigen-recognizing component of the BCR is surface immunoglobulin (sIg), a tetrameric complex of immunoglobulin heavy and light chains (Fig. 7.2b) that are extensively

122   *D. R. Alexander*

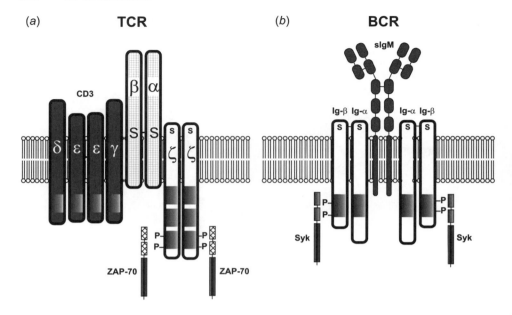

Fig. 7.2. The structures of the TCR and BCR.

homologous to the immunoglobulins which are secreted by differentiated daughter cells (Cambier *et al.*, 1993). These polymorphic chains are non-covalently associated with an invariant disulphide-linked transmembrane heterodimer of Ig-α (CD79a) and Ig-β (CD79b) polypeptides, which are encoded by the immunoglobulin superfamily genes *mb-1* and *B29*, respectively. The same Ig-α/Ig-β heterodimer is associated with all of the five different heavy (H) chain classes of sIg molecules (Venkitaraman *et al.*, 1991), and plays an analogous role to that of the CD3/TCR-ζ chains in both receptor assembly and signal transduction. In addition, the cytoplasmic tails of Ig-α and Ig-β are involved in the internalization of proteins bound to the BCR and their subsequent targeting to endosomal compartments for processing (Bonnerot *et al.*, 1995). Interestingly, however, the short cytoplasmic tails of sIg H chains, which vary in length from 3 to 28 amino acid residues, are also involved in targeting receptor-bound antigens to endosomes (Weiser *et al.*, 1997), and, in some cases, antigen internalization and presentation in memory B cells is largely independent of Ig-α and Ig-β expression (Tarlinton, 1997). It is, therefore, possible that sIg exists in two pools, either with or without association with Ig-α/Ig-β. Upon sIg ligation by antigen, both receptor pools would mediate antigen internalization and processing, whereas only the pool containing Ig-α/Ig-β would induce intracellular signals.

The invariant chains of the TCR and BCR contain 'immunoreceptor tyrosine-based activation motifs' (ITAMs) comprising the sequence

E/DX$_2$YX$_2$L/IX$_7$YX$_2$L/I (single-letter code for amino acids where X represents any amino acid). The TCR-ς chain contains three ITAMs, whereas the CD3, Ig-α and Ig-β chains each contain one ITAM. Upon binding of ligands to the TCR or BCR, the tyrosine residues of the ITAMs are phosphorylated by tyrosine kinases, so forming high-affinity binding sites for signalling proteins, which engage the phosphorylated sequences by means of their Src homology type 2 (SH2) domains. In this way, protein complexes are recruited to the receptors, which, in turn, activate intracellular signalling pathways involved in transcription factor regulation. It is not yet clear whether each phosphorylated ITAM *in vivo* has a selective binding capacity for different proteins or whether the ITAMs of a receptor bind the same proteins, thereby providing a signal amplification system. Evidence is available for both scenarios.

Engagement of the TCR or BCR by ligands does not necessarily induce optimal ITAM phosphorylation. For example, the binding of altered peptide ligands (APLs) to the TCR expressed on T cell clones can cause the generation of abnormal phosphoisomers of TCR-ς, which are probably incompletely phosphorylated (Sloan-Lancaster *et al.*, 1994; Madrenas *et al.*, 1995). Such signals correlate with the induction of states of cellular non-responsiveness in which cells do not proliferate or secrete IL-2 upon subsequent challenge with an MHC-peptide (Sloan-Lancaster & Allen, 1996). Abnormal ITAM phosphorylation states may, therefore, be involved in the induction of cellular non-responsiveness.

Tyrosine kinases and antigen receptors

In contrast to growth factor receptors, such as the epidermal growth factor receptor, in which tyrosine kinase activity is expressed within the receptor cytoplasmic tail, antigen receptor polypeptides do not possess any kinase activity. Instead they utilize cytosolic tyrosine kinases for phosphorylating their ITAM motifs and for triggering a cascade of phosphorylation events that involve the regulation of serine/threonine protein kinases.

Tyrosine kinases and TCR signalling

The role of tyrosine kinases in TCR signalling is more clearly defined than for BCR signalling. There are four families of tyrosine kinases now known to be involved in TCR signal transduction (Chan *et al.*, 1994a; Qian & Weiss, 1997). The first comprises the p59[fyn] and p56[lck] members of the Src family of tyrosine kinases. As Fig. 7.3 illustrates, these kinases share the same domain structure, with myristoylated and palmitylated amino terminal domains which tether the kinases to the plasma membrane, and which also bear receptor-binding sequences.

The SH3 domain interacts with proteins carrying proline-rich motifs and the SH2 domain interacts by an intramolecular association with a regulatory phosphorylated tyrosine residue in the carboxy-terminus of the kinase. Upon dephosphorylation of this tyrosine residue, the SH2 domain is then available to engage with other tyrosine phosphorylated proteins. The p59^{fyn} kinase associates directly with rather weak affinity and low stoichiometry with the TCR (Samelson *et al.*, 1990). The p56^{lck} kinase associates with the CD4 and CD8 co-receptors with a considerably higher affinity and stoichiometry (Rudd *et al.*, 1988). The expression of CD4 is characteristic of helper T cells whereas CD8 expression is a marker of cytotoxic T cells. It is thought that when an MHC–peptide engages the TCR, the class I or class II molecule simultaneously binds to CD8 or CD4, respectively, thereby bringing the associated p56^{lck} kinase into association with the CD3/TCR-ç ITAMs, so causing their phosphorylation. The marked reduction in TCR-ç and CD3-ε phosphorylation observed in mice lacking p56^{lck} expression is consistent with such a model (van Oers, Killeen & Weiss, 1996a). Furthermore, there is a correlation between the ability of TCR antibodies to stimulate T cell activation and their efficiency at promoting CD4–TCR association and TCR-ç phosphorylation (Janeway, 1992). In contrast, in mice lacking p59^{fyn}, TCR-ç phosphorylation is normal (van Oers *et al.*, 1996b), suggesting that the role of p56^{lck} is more critical than that of p59^{fyn} in regulating ITAM phosphorylation. This conclusion is supported by the severe defects in thymic development observed in Lck$^{-/-}$ mice, which contrast with the normal thymic development that occurs in Fyn$^{-/-}$ mice (Molina *et al.*, 1992). Interestingly, however, in mice lacking both p56^{lck} and p59^{fyn} the block in T cell development is more severe than in Lck$^{-/-}$ mice (van Oers *et al.*, 1996b), suggesting that there could be some overlapping functions between these two kinases. Furthermore, the proliferation of mature T cells is not completely ablated in Lck$^{-/-}$ mice, suggesting that p56^{lck} is not the only kinase involved in coupling the TCR to activation pathways. Therefore, a role for p59^{fyn} in phosphorylating ITAMs in certain contexts cannot yet be excluded.

The second family of kinases involved in TCR signal transduction is represented by Csk (C-Src kinase). As shown in Fig. 7.3, this kinase phosphorylates the regulatory carboxy terminal tyrosine residues in Src kinase family members, thereby inhibiting their ability to phosphorylate relevant substrates.

The third family of kinases is represented by ZAP-70 (ç-associated protein-70) and its homologue Syk (Fig. 7.4.). ZAP-70 is more important than Syk in TCR signalling, whereas ZAP-70 is not expressed in B cells. The critical role of ZAP-70 in TCR signalling is illustrated by patients with severe combined immunodeficiency (SCID) carrying mutations of ZAP-70 resulting in deficient ZAP-70 protein levels or loss of its kinase activity (Arpaia *et al.*, 1994). Whereas

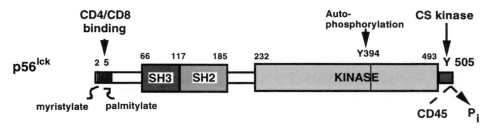

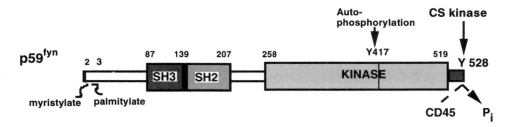

Fig. 7.3. The structure and regulation of the p56lck and p59fyn tyrosine kinases. CS kinase, C-Src kinase. The numbers refer to amino acids that demarcate domains or which are phosphorylated.

CD4+CD8+ thymocytes are present in these patients, only CD4+ and not CD8+ T cells emerge to the periphery. The peripheral CD4+ cells do not proliferate in response to TCR stimulation, fail to secrete IL-2 and have markedly reduced TCR-induced protein tyrosine phosphorylation, suggesting that ZAP-70 plays a central role in mediating T cell activation. Mice deficient in ZAP-70 expression have an even more severe phenotype in which there is a failure of both positive and negative selection events so that neither CD4+ nor CD8+ T cells exit to the periphery (Negishi *et al.*, 1995). The residual ZAP-70 function that may remain in SCID patients could explain why their phenotype is less severe than that of ZAP-70$^{-/-}$ mice, and the bias to maturation of CD4+ T cells in these patients most likely results from the greater affinity of p56lck binding to CD4 than to CD8. The secondary importance of Syk for T cell signal transduction is illustrated by the normal T cell development which occurs in Syk$^{-/-}$ mice (Turner *et al.*, 1995).

ZAP-70 and Syk both possess two SH2 domains but lack the carboxy terminal regulatory tyrosine residues that are characteristic of the Src kinases. Upon TCR stimulation, ZAP-70 and Syk engage via both their SH2 domains with doubly phosphorylated TCR-ç ITAMs (Iwashima *et al.*, 1994; Isakov *et al.*, 1995), thereby facilitating their phosphorylation by kinases such as p56lck and

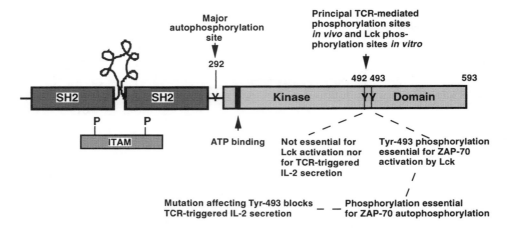

Fig. 7.4. The structure and regulation of the ZAP-70 tyrosine kinase. The major sites of tyrosine phosphorylation are indicated.

p59[fyn]. The crystal structure of two ZAP-70 SH2 domains bound to a phosphorylated ITAM motif has revealed the importance of this interaction for the conformation of the kinase (Hatada *et al.*, 1995). Thus, the binding pocket for the amino terminal phosphorylated tyrosine in the ITAM is formed by the carboxy terminal SH2 domain alone of ZAP-70. In contrast, the formation of the binding pocket for the carboxy terminal phosphorylated tyrosine in the ITAM requires residues provided by both SH2 domains, in the process facilitating a coiled-coil structure in the interdomain region between the two SH2 domains. The dual interaction between the two SH2 domains and the two phosphorylated ITAM tyrosine residues helps to explain the high affinity of interaction between ZAP-70 and TCR-ς.

The binding of ZAP-70 to phosphorylated ITAM motifs *per se* is insufficient to cause kinase activation. This has been confirmed both by *in vitro* peptide-binding studies and by the observation that in murine thymocytes ZAP-70 is constitutively associated with the ς-chain without activation (van Oers *et al.*, 1994). In fact activation of ZAP-70 requires phosphorylation by p56[lck] at Tyr-493 on the putative regulatory loop of its kinase domain (Chan *et al.*, 1995), which is followed by further phosphorylation of the kinase (Fig. 7.4.), involving both positive and negative regulatory sites, some of which results from transphosphorylation ('autophosphorylation') between the activated ZAP-70 molecules (Wange *et al.*, 1995). An actual increase in ZAP-70 kinase activity is critical for coupling the TCR to intracellular signals (Wiest *et al.*, 1997). There is some evidence that several ZAP-70 molecules need to be juxtaposed on adjacent phosphorylated ITAM motifs (Fig. 7.5), in order for effective ZAP-70 trans-

(a) **ζ-chain**

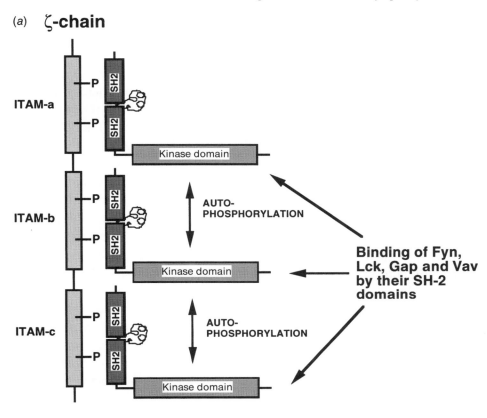

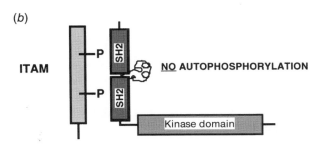

Fig. 7.5. The aggregation model of ZAP-70 regulation. (*a*) Some evidence suggests that when several ZAP-70 molecules are bound in tandem to the three phosphorylated ITAMs present in TCR-ζ then ZAP-70 autophosphorylation (more strictly transphosphorylation) proceeds more efficiently, so generating binding sites for SH2-domain-containing proteins (Neumeister *et al*., 1995). (*b*) In contrast, when only a single ZAP-70 molecule is bound to one phosphorylated ITAM, ZAP-70 autophosphorylation is inefficient.

phosphorylation to occur (Neumeister *et al.*, 1995). Phosphorylation of ZAP-70 results in the generation of binding sites for SH2 domain-containing proteins, leading to the further recruitment of signalling proteins (Neumeister *et al.*, 1995). It has also been suggested that ZAP-70 phosphorylation results in the recruit-ment of p56[lck] via its SH2 domain, so providing a mechanism whereby the asso-ciation of CD4/CD8-p56[lck] with the TCR could be stabilized (Duplay *et al.*, 1994). Overall, therefore, ZAP-70 is critical for coupling the TCR to intracel-lular signalling pathways. When ZAP-70 is absent, Syk is able to substitute for its functions to a certain extent, suggesting some redundancy between these two kinases (Gelfand *et al.*, 1995). In normal T cells, however, it is not yet clear whether Syk has any actions in TCR signalling distinct from those of ZAP-70. Interestingly, Syk expression is relatively high in thymocytes, whereas it is expressed at low levels in mature peripheral T cells, pointing to a possible selec-tive function in thymocytes (Chan *et al.*, 1994b).

The fourth family of tyrosine kinases implicated in T cell signalling is the Tec family, and the member of this kinase preferentially expressed in T cells is Itk (Siliciano, Morrow & Desiderio, 1992). The Tec family of kinases share some homology with the Src kinase family but lack the amino-terminal myristoylation consensus sequence and carboxy terminal tyrosine residues that characterize the Src kinases. The Tec family of kinases are cytosolic but their pleckstrin homol-ogy (PH) domains may be involved in targeting them to membranes and/or in mediating their regulation by phospholipids. Mice lacking Itk have a reduced number of mature thymocytes, implicating Itk in T cell development, and their mature T cells proliferated poorly in response to antigenic stimulation, suggest-ing that Itk is involved in TCR signal transduction (Liao & Littman, 1995). The molecular mechanism of action of Itk in this context remains to be elucidated.

Tyrosine kinases and BCR signalling

The same four families of tyrosine kinases involved in TCR signalling have also been implicated in BCR signalling (Bolen, 1995; Kurosaki, 1997). The Src fam-ily members Blk, Lyn, Fgr and Fyn have been reported to associate with the BCR and to be activated following sIg cross-linking (Yamanashi *et al.*, 1991; Cambier *et al.*, 1993). Binding studies *in vitro* suggest that these kinases bind to resting receptors through an association of their amino terminal residues with the Ig-α chain (Clark *et al.*, 1992), an association that does not appear to require ITAM phosphorylation (Clark, Johnson & Cambier, 1994). Upon BCR ligation, the ITAMs within the Ig-α and Ig-β chains become phosphorylated and this is thought to result in further recruitment of Src family kinases via their SH2 domains, so promoting kinase activation (Clark *et al.*, 1994). An attractive model, therefore, involves the relatively weak association of Src family kinases with the BCR in resting B cells, which then become activated upon engagement of their SH2 domains with phosphorylated ITAMs (Pleiman *et al.*, 1994). Whether the Ig-α and Ig-β ITAMs are initially phosphorylated by a member of the Src family or by Syk is an issue that awaits a clear resolution. Of the various Src kinase family members implicated in BCR signalling, p59^{lyn} has received the most attention since peripheral B cells appear to be hyperresponsive in Lyn$^{-/-}$ mice, which develop circulating autoantibodies despite apparently normal B cell development (Hibbs *et al.*, 1995). One possible explanation for this finding is that the dominant role of p59^{lyn} is to phosphorylate a tyrosine residue in the cytoplasmic tail of CD22, which normally exerts a negative action on BCR signalling (see below). In the absence of this phosphorylation event, BCR signalling might then be amplified (Kurosaki, 1997). Such an interpretation does not exclude a role for p59^{lyn} in phosphorylating Ig-α or Ig-β ITAMs, or indeed other substrates.

The role of Csk in suppressing the activity of Src kinases is the same in B cells as in T cells. As far as the third family of tyrosine kinases is concerned, Syk is clearly the key player in BCR signalling. In mice deficient for Syk, there is a developmental block in the pro-B to pre-B cell transition and, despite the production of small numbers of immature B cells, mature B cells fail to accumulate, suggesting a role for Syk in the production or maintenance of mature B cells (Turner *et al.*, 1995). Overall BCR signal transduction appears to be as dependent upon the actions of Syk as, for example, TCR signalling is dependent upon the actions of ZAP-70.

The way in which Syk is activated also appears to be different from the mechanism of ZAP-70 activation. Engagement of the two SH2 domains of Syk by phosphorylated ITAM peptides causes a change in conformation of Syk and kinase activation, but under these conditions ZAP-70 activation does not occur (Shiue, Zoller & Brugge, 1995; Kimura *et al.*, 1996). Upon BCR stimulation *in situ*, Syk is, therefore, recruited to phosphorylated Ig-α/Ig-β ITAMs, which causes its activation and transphosphorylation together with further phosphorylation by a Src family tyrosine kinase (Kurosaki *et al.*, 1994; Rowley *et al.*, 1995). Tyrosine-phosphorylated Syk then dissociates from the BCR by a process that is itself regulated by a tyrosine phosphorylation event within the Syk molecule (Keshvara *et al.*, 1997). As with ZAP-70, the phosphorylation of Syk leads to the formation of signal transduction complexes with other SH2 domain-containing proteins.

The fourth tyrosine kinase family is well illustrated in B cells by the important role played by Btk (Bruton's tyrosine kinase). Defects in the *btk* gene are associated with X-linked agammaglobulinaemia (XLA), the first primary immunodeficiency to be identified (by Bruton). Affected males have decreased levels of circulating immunoglobulins and a severe deficit in the number of B cells; however, the patients have normal myeloid and T cell function as well as intact cellular immunity, consistent with the lack of Btk expression in T cells. Ligation of the BCR in Btk-deficient splenic B cells results in severely defective proliferation when compared with wild-type cells (Khan *et al.*, 1995). The Src family kinases appear to be necessary for the BCR-mediated regulation of Btk activation (Afar *et al.*, 1996; Rawlings *et al.*, 1996) and Btk interacts via a proline-rich motif within its Tec homology domain with the SH3 domains of Src family kinases (Yang *et al.*, 1995). Analysis of signal transduction pathways in a B cell line lacking Btk has implicated the kinase in the coupling of the BCR to increased phosphatidylinositol hydrolysis and calcium signalling (see below) (Takata & Kurosaki, 1996). The downstream signals regulated by Btk in primary cells remain the focus of active research (Kurosaki, 1997).

The regulation of tyrosine kinases by the CD45 phosphotyrosine phosphatase

CD45 is a transmembrane phosphotyrosine phosphatase that regulates the threshold of TCR and BCR signal transduction (Fig. 7.6) (Frearson & Alexander, 1996; Alexander, 1997). CD45 has a large ectodomain with a receptor-like structure, although physiologically relevant ligand(s) remain to be identified. Studies utilizing mutant cell lines and transgenic mice have established that CD45 exerts a positive regulatory role on both TCR- and BCR-mediated signals (Pingel & Thomas, 1989; Koretzky *et al.*, 1990; Justement *et al.*, 1991; Kishihara *et al.*, 1993). In CD45 mice there are severe defects in T cell development, particularly in the positive selection of CD4$^+$CD8$^+$ thymocytes (Byth *et al.*, 1996). The few mature T cells that exit to the periphery in these mice do not proliferate upon TCR stimulation (Stone *et al.*, 1997). Studies using mutant cell lines and CD45$^{-/-}$ mice have established that in T cells p56^{lck} and p59^{fyn} are substrates for CD45 (Ostergaard *et al.*, 1989; Shiroo *et al.*, 1992; Stone *et al.*, 1997). In the absence of CD45, these kinases are hyperphosphorylated at their regulatory carboxy terminal tyrosine residues and are in their closed 'inactive' conformations (Sieh, Bolen & Weiss, 1993; Stone *et al.*, 1997). As a consequence, there are extensive defects in TCR signal transduction coupling. For example, TCR ς chain phosphorylation is much reduced in the absence of CD45, consistent with an important role for CD45-activated p56^{lck} in phosphorylating the TCR ς chain. Furthermore, upon TCR ligation an abnormally phosphorylated form of the ς chain is generated (Stone *et al.*, 1997), which is reminiscent of the partial signals induced upon engagement of the TCR with altered peptide ligands (Sloan-Lancaster *et al.*, 1994; Madrenas *et al.*, 1995). As a result, ZAP-70 fails to be

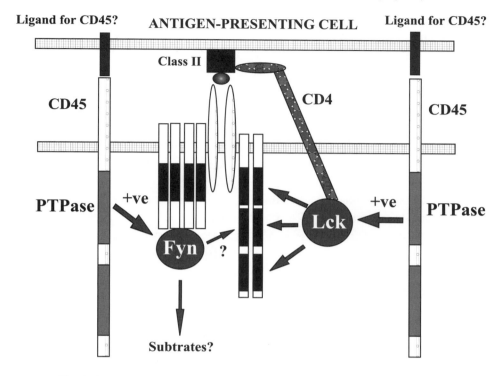

Fig. 7.6. Regulation of p56^{lck} by the CD45 phosphotyrosine phosphatase is critical for phosphorylation of TCR-ζ and CD3-ε ITAMs and subsequent recruitment of signal transduction complexes.

recruited efficiently to TCR-ς. Interestingly, however, TCR-mediated Syk phosphorylation is normal or even increased in the absence of CD45, underlining the relative independence of Syk regulation from regulation by the Src family kinases (Chu *et al.*, 1996). Not surprisingly in light of the early point in the signal transduction cascade at which CD45 acts, there are multiple downstream signalling defects in cells lacking CD45 (Shiroo *et al.*, 1992). However, it should be noted that in primary CD45$^{-/-}$ thymocytes, some TCR-mediated signals still occur, and at high ligand concentrations calcium signals, for example, are only partially defective (Stone *et al.*, 1997). Therefore, in T cells, CD45 appears to act like a 'gatekeeper' to modulate the intensity of signals mediated by the TCR by regulating the actions of Src family kinases (Frearson & Alexander, 1997).

The role of CD45 in B cells appears less stringent than in T cells, perhaps reflecting the importance of CD45-regulated p56^{lck} in T cell development and activation, in contrast to any comparable role for a single CD45-dependent kinase in B cells. However, B cell maturation is defective in CD45$^{-/-}$ mice, leading to a relative deficit of IgM-low, IgD-high B cells and an accumulation of the more immature IgM-high, IgD-low B cells. Furthermore, splenic B cells fail to prolif-erate in response to sIg cross-linking in the absence of CD45 (Byth *et al.*, 1996). The defects in BCR signalling observed in primary CD45$^{-/-}$ B cells are quite subtle. Whereas major changes in BCR-triggered protein tyrosine phosphoryla-tion have not been observed in CD45$^{-/-}$ spleen cells, the BCR is selectively uncoupled from activation of the MAP kinase pathway (see below for more details of this pathway) (Cyster *et al.*, 1996) and from calcium influx (Benatar *et al.*, 1996). Such defects are likely to explain the increased threshold for BCR signal transduction that has been noted in CD45$^{-/-}$ B cells (Cyster *et al.*, 1996; Cyster, 1997).

Other tyrosine phosphatases are also involved in lymphocyte signal transduc-tion. Some of these, like the SH2-domain-containing SHP-2 phosphatase, appear to exert a positive regulatory action on antigen receptor-mediated signals, whereas others, such as SHP-1, exert negative effects (Frearson & Alexander, 1997). The early events of antigen receptor signalling are, therefore, regulated by a fine bal-ance between the actions of tyrosine kinases and phosphatases.

Antigen receptors and signal transduction complexes

As already noted, ligation of the TCR and BCR causes the recruitment of recep-tor-associated 'signal transduction complexes' that couple the receptors to sig-nalling pathways. As the kinase activation cascade continues, cytosolic 'docking proteins' also become tyrosine phosphorylated, recruiting proteins in the process via SH2 domains and other types of protein–protein interaction to form signal transduction complexes that are not necessarily associated with receptors (Wange & Samelson 1996; DeFranco, 1997). One function of such docking proteins is to activate or inhibit associated enzymes or exchange factors, and to target them to their relevant substrates.

An interesting example of such a 'signal transduction complex' is provided by the interaction that occurs in T cells between molecules known as Grb-2, Vav, SLP-76 (SH2 domain-containing leukocyte protein of 76 kDa) and SLAP-130 (also called Fyb), as illustrated in Fig. 7.7. Grb-2 is an adaptor protein contain-ing two SH3 domains and one SH2 domain. The role of Grb-2 is to bind to pro-teins bearing proline-rich motifs via its two SH3 domains and to bring these proteins into association with tyrosine-phosphorylated proteins via its SH2 domain. Vav is a docking protein that contains a single SH2 and two SH3 domains, as well as a PH domain, which together mediate its interactions with other proteins (Bustelo, Ledbetter & Barbacid, 1992). Furthermore, Vav contains an enzymatic domain which catalyses guanine nucleotide exchange on the Rho/Rac/CDC42 family of low-molecular-weight Ras-like GTP-binding pro-

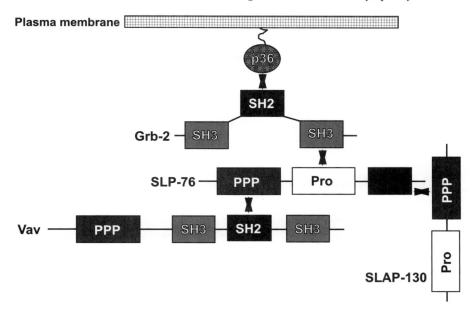

Fig. 7.7. The Vav–SLP-76–Grb-2 signal transduction complex. Note that only certain domains of the molecules are shown to illustrate the way in which mul-timolecular complexes are assembled upon TCR engagement. The p36 mole-cule is membrane associated and upon tyrosine phosphorylation engages with the adaptor protein Grb-2, which in turn is associated with SLP-76 by an inter-action that does not require tyrosine phosphorylation. Tyrosine phosphorylation of SLP-76 leads to its interaction with Vav; another tyrosine phosphorylated protein, SLAP-130 (Fyb), also binds to SLP-76. Such complexes provide a way in which several molecules may be brought to the plasma membrane in a func-tionally active form.

teins. Mature T and B cells lacking Vav proliferate poorly and, in the case of T cells, produce little IL-2 in response to TCR stimulation (Tarakhovsky *et al.*, 1995). Vav is rapidly phosphorylated by tyrosine kinases upon TCR engagement and then acts to promote Rac-1 to the active GTP-bound state (Crespo *et al.*, 1997). Another protein called SLP-76 is also tyrosine phosphorylated, probably by ZAP-70 (Wardenburg *et al.*, 1996) and binds to Vav via its SH2 domain, an interaction that appears to be critical for signals leading to IL-2 gene induction (Wu *et al.*, 1996; Raab *et al.*, 1997). SLP-76 also contains an SH2 domain and in turn binds via this domain to a further tyrosine-phosphorylated protein called SLAP-130 (also called Fyb), which may be a negative regulator of signal trans-duction (Musci *et al.*, 1997). There is evidence that this Grb-2/Vav/SLP-76/SLAP-130 complex is involved in coupling ZAP-70 activation to the Ras and calcium-signalling pathways (described further below). The rate of dissoci-ation of such complexes is probably as important as the rate at which they associate, since such rates presumably determine how long specific signalling pathways continue to be activated. It is, therefore, of interest that therapeutic reagents which suppress T cell activation may act by preventing the formation of such signal transduction complexes (Jabado *et al.*, 1997).

Signal transduction pathways induced by antigen receptors

Lymphocyte activation involves three major signalling pathways that lead from antigen receptors to the regulation of nuclear events and which are now beginning to be understood in some detail. These pathways involve the elevation of intracellular calcium, the activation of protein kinase C (PKC) and the activation of the Ras/MAP kinase pathway and are illustrated for T cells in Fig. 7.8. The same pathways are also activated in B cells, but results from T cells will be used to describe these pathways and the way in which they integrate to regulate the IL-2 gene by means of transcription factors such as AP-1, NFκB and nuclear factor of activated T cells (NFAT).

The calcium-signalling pathway

TCR stimulation causes the tyrosine phosphorylation and activation of phospholipase-Cγl (PLCγl) (Secrist, Karnitz & Abraham, 1991) followed by its recruitment to the plasma membrane, possibly by means of an associated tyrosine-phosphorylated 36 kDa molecule (Motto *et al.*, 1996). Activated PLCγl then hydrolyses its substrate phosphatidylinositol 4,5-bisphosphate, which is located in the membrane, to generate diacylglycerol (DAG) and inositol 1,4,5-trisphosphate (IP_3). DAG activates PKC whereas IP_3 binds to IP_3 receptors, calcium-release channels on the endoplasmic reticulum that open to cause the release of calcium from intracellular stores (Berridge, 1993). TCR stimulation causes the tyrosine phosphorylation of IP_3 receptors by a process involving the p59[fyn] tyrosine kinase (Jayaraman *et al.*, 1996). The depletion of these stores in turn triggers the opening of calcium channels in the plasma membrane, known as store operated channels (SOCs), causing an influx of calcium ions from outside the cell (Zweifach & Lewis, 1993; Berridge, 1995). The opening of the SOCs depends upon the membrane potential, which is kept hyperpolarized by both voltage-gated and calcium-sensitive potassium channels (Lewis & Cahalan, 1995). If the potassium channels are blocked using inhibitors, then the membrane is depolarized, calcium influx no longer occurs and T cell proliferation is inhibited. For full activation and proliferation to occur, the prolonged elevation of intracellular calcium ions that results is essential (Goldsmith & Weiss, 1988; Wacholtz & Lipsky, 1993). For example, a T cell line lacking type 1 IP_3 receptors was unable to increase the

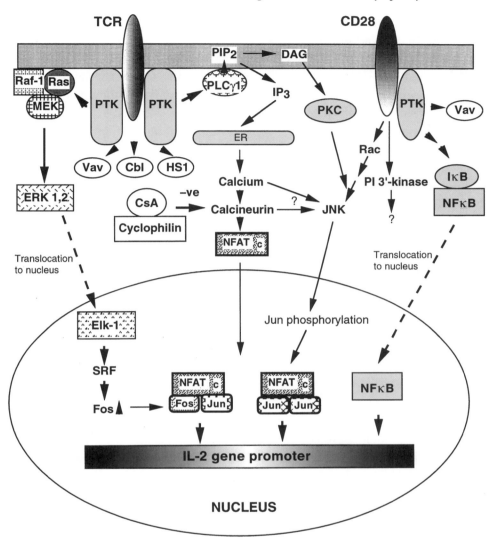

Fig. 7.8. The integration of TCR and CD28-mediated signal transduction pathways in T cells. CsA, cyclosporin A; IκB, inhibitor-κB; NFAT, nuclear factor of activated T cells; SRF, serum response factor; JNK, Jun kinase.

intracellular calcium concentration or produce IL-2 following TCR stimulation, demonstrating the critical role of this pathway in T cell activation (Jayaraman *et al.*, 1995). A patient with a severe immunodeficiency has been described with defective T cell SOCs (Ledeist *et al.*, 1995) and in T cell-lines expressing various SOC mutations a close correlation was found between the level of calcium influx and calcium-dependent gene transcription (Fanger *et al.*, 1995).

An important consequence of the increased intracellular calcium ion concentration is the activation of a calcium-dependent phosphoserine/threonine phosphatase called calcineurin. Calcineurin activation results in the rapid translocation (within minutes) to the nucleus of NFAT proteins, which are located in the cytosol in primary resting T cells (Luo *et al.*, 1996). There they combine with AP-1 to form a functional transcriptional factor complex (Rao, Luo & Hogan, 1997). Translocation requires two nuclear localization motifs found in the NFAT molecule, one of which is in an intramolecular association with phosphoserines located at its amino terminus. Dephosphorylation by calcineurin exposes these motifs so that NFAT moves into the nucleus (Beals *et al.*, 1997a). In the nucleus, NFAT is then rephosphorylated by the serine/threonine kinase glycogen synthase kinase-3, so promoting its return to the cytsolic compartment after several hours, providing that the calcium ion level has declined to resting levels (Loh *et al.*, 1996; Beals *et al.*, 1997b). Therefore, just as the earliest events of antigen receptor–signal transduction coupling are regulated by the balance between the actions of *tyrosine* kinases and phosphatases, so downstream signalling pathways are controlled by the balance between *serine* kinases and phosphatases. The antigen receptor–calcium–calcineurin–NFAT pathway also provides a good example of the way in which tyrosine kinases 'translate' the effects of receptor occupation into protein serine phosphorylation/dephosphorylation, so in turn regulating nuclear events.

The immunosuppressive drugs cyclosporin A (CsA) and FK506 (tacrolimus) exert their inhibitory effects by binding to immunophilins known as cyclophilin and the FK506-binding protein (FKBP), respectively (Liu *et al.*, 1991; Fruman *et al.*, 1992). The CsA–cyclophilin and FK506–FKBP complexes then bind in a calcium-dependent manner to calcineurin, so inhibiting its phosphatase activity. Thus, the addition of these drugs to lymphocytes blocks NFAT dephosphorylation and translocation to the nucleus, thereby preventing IL-2 gene induction by inhibiting the formation of functional transcription factor complexes (Rao *et al.*, 1997).

Other consequences of increased intracellular calcium ions are mediated by the binding of calcium to a binding protein called calmodulin, which leads to the activation of calcium-sensitive serine/threonine kinases such as calmodulin-activated kinase IV (CaM kinase IV) (Park & Soderling, 1995). CaM kinase IV has been implicated in regulation of the AP-1 gene (Ho, Gullberg & Chatila, 1996) and in cell-cycle regulation (Larsson *et al.*, 1995).

Protein kinase C activation

It has long been known that a full T cell activation programme can be induced by the addition of phorbol esters, which activate PKC, and calcium ionophores, which greatly increase the concentration of intracellular calcium, so bypassing the early events of TCR signal transduction coupling (Truneh *et al.*, 1985). It is now realised, however, that the pharmacological activation of PKC has multiple effects, including the activation of the Ras/MAP kinase pathway (see below), whereas the TCR *in situ* does not couple to the Ras pathway using PKC (Cantrell, 1996). The fact that phorbol esters have effects on certain pathways does not mean that the same TCR-stimulated pathways are mediated by PKC *in vivo*. Furthermore, multiple PKC isoforms are present in lymphocytes, some of which are activated by the combination of calcium ions plus DAG, whereas the regulation of others is calcium independent. One characteristic of PKC enzymes is that they are translocated to membranes upon activation, so bringing them into contact with their membrane-localized substrates. Interestingly, although six different PKC isoforms were detected in antigen-specific T cell clones, only one of these, PKCθ, was found to translocate to the site of cell contact between antigen-presenting cells and T cells; the increased activity of PKCθ correlated well with T cell activation (Monks *et al.*, 1997). Thus specific PKC isoforms may have highly selective effects during lymphocyte activation; in fact, active forms of PKC isoforms transfected into T cell lines demonstrate different effects on gene regulation (Genot, Parker & Cantrell, 1995). The selectivity of PKC isoform actions is also illustrated by the phenotype of mice lacking PKCβ, in which T cell development and TCR-triggered proliferation was normal whereas B cell development was perturbed and the proliferation of B cells in response to BCR ligation was much reduced (Leitges *et al.*, 1996). Furthermore, another PKC isoform, PKCμ, has been found to associate with the BCR and is activated upon BCR engagement (Sidorenko *et al.*, 1996).

The function of PKC in T cell signal transduction pathways has been investigated by the use of inhibitors. A selective PKC inhibitor inhibits IL-2 secretion and T cell proliferation (Birchall *et al.*, 1994), but only the TCR stimulation of NFκB induction is inhibited, not that of NFAT or AP-1 (Williams *et al.*, 1995). Since the binding of NFκB to a site on the IL-2 gene promoter is necessary for IL-2 gene induction (Fig. 7.8), these results point to a role for PKC in regulating IL-2 secretion via NFκB. Like NFAT, NFκB is present in the cytosol in an inactive complex. NFκB consists of a heterodimer of p50 (NFκB-1) and p65 (RelA) polypeptides in complex with an inhibitory subunit (IκB), which, when proteolytically degraded, unmasks a nuclear localization motif on RelA, so promoting the translocation of NFκB to the nucleus (Baldwin, 1996). The important role of NFκB for T cell activation is well illustrated by the actions of immunosuppressive glucocorticoids, which act by inhibiting NFκB induction, possibly by inducing the synthesis of IκB (Auphan *et al.*, 1995). Signals from the CD28 receptor also appear to be involved in NFκB activation (Lai & Tan,

1994). The precise role of TCR/CD28 stimulation and PKC activation in the regulation of NFκB awaits further elucidation.

The Ras/MAP kinase pathway

Ras is a low-molecular-weight (21 000) guanine nucleotide-binding protein localized in the plasma membrane that can exist in an active GTP-bound form or an inactive GDP-bound form. In resting T cells, Ras exists in its inactive GDP-bound form but is rapidly converted to its active form upon TCR stimulation (Downward *et al.*, 1990). The equilibrium between these two forms involves the action of exchange factors such as Sos and C3G, which catalyse the conversion of Ras–GDP to Ras–GTP, and the activation of the GTPase activity of Ras by the Ras–GTPase activating protein (Ras–GAP), which hydrolyses Ras-bound GTP so converting Ras back to its inactive form. The exact way in which TCR stimulation causes Ras activation is not yet understood but appears to involve both inhibition of Ras–GAP (Downward *et al.*, 1990) and the recruitment of Grb2–Sos and Crk–C3G complexes to the membrane, possibly by means of a membrane-associated p36 tyrosine-phosphorylated protein (Buday *et al.*, 1994; Pastor, Reif & Cantrell, 1995; Sawasdikosol *et al.*, 1995) (the same p36 protein as illustrated in Fig. 7.7). Like Grb-2, Crk is an adaptor protein and contains three SH3 domains and a single SH2 domain. Similar mechanisms couple the BCR to Ras activation, although in this context the Shc adaptor protein is thought to be involved in bringing Sos into association with its Ras–GDP substrate (DeFranco, 1997).

An important function of Ras is to couple the TCR to the mitogen-activated protein kinase (MAP kinase) pathway (also known as the extracellular signal regulated kinase pathway, ERK), which comprises a cascade of kinases leading from the plasma membrane to the nucleus (Fig. 7.8). The MAP kinase kinase kinase (MAPKKK) Raf-1 binds directly to Ras–GTP, which thereby recruits Raf-1 to the membrane where it is activated by a complex series of events (Morrison & Cutler, 1997). Activated Raf-1 in turn activates a MAP kinase kinase (MAPKK or MEK), which then phosphorylates and stimulates the MAP kinases Erk1 and Erk2, which translocate to the nucleus where they phosphorylate transcription factors (Robinson & Cobb, 1997). An important substrate for Erk2 is the transcription factor Elk1, which forms a ternary complex with the transcriptional activator serum response factor, so playing an important role in expression of *fos* (Hunter & Karin, 1992). Fos and Jun together form complexes (AP-1) that bind to sites in the IL-2 gene promoter. The multimolecular AP-1/NFAT$_c$ complex ('NFAT') also binds to a further site in this promoter. Studies using both active and inactive mutants of Ras have shown that Ras does indeed synergize with calcium to induce active NFAT complexes (Cantrell, 1996), although the MAP kinase cascade is probably not the only pathway whereby Ras regulates NFAT (Genot *et al.*, 1996). Furthermore, the CD28 signalling pathway synergizes with TCR-mediated signals in the activation of the Jun kinase (JNK) member of the MAP kinase family, which is activated by a cascade analogous to that which regulates Erk1/2 (Su *et al.*, 1994). JNK is thought to phosphorylate Jun and thereby promote the formation of active Fos–Jun (AP-1) complexes, illustrating the way in which the signals from the TCR and CD28 can integrate at the transcription factor level. In contrast to the TCR, physiological ligands for CD28 do not appear to activate Ras (Nunes *et al.*, 1994).

An important issue that is not yet fully resolved is the extent to which Erk1/2 activation is important in mature peripheral T cells. It should be noted that many of the data available on Ras function in T cells have been generated using cell lines as well as transgenic mice. The expression of dominant-negative mutant forms of Ras and of MEK-1 in transgenic mice has unambiguously demonstrated that the Ras/MAP kinase pathway is essential for the positive selection but not the negative selection of CD4+CD8+ thymocytes (Alberolaila *et al.*, 1995; 1996; Swan *et al.*, 1995). However, whereas the dominant-negative Ras completely inhibits proliferative responses to TCR stimulation (Swan *et al.*, 1995), the overexpression of dominant-negative MEK-1 does not perturb TCR-stimulated proliferation of, or IL-2 secretion from, mature splenic T cells, despite the inability of the TCR to trigger Erk1/2 activation under such conditions (Alberolaila *et al.*, 1995). Therefore, the possibility remains that Ras activation is essential for T cell proliferation but the critical Ras-mediated pathway that mediates T cell proliferation does not involve Erk1/2 activation in mature T cells.

The role of co-receptors in antigen receptor signalling

The term 'co-receptor' is sometimes restricted in use to molecules such as CD4/CD8, which are intimately involved in TCR functions, but in other contexts the word is used more widely to refer to any receptor that either upmodulates or downmodulates antigen receptor signal transduction. The term here is used in this second more general sense. The important role of CD4 and CD8 in TCR signalling has already been summarized, and the signalling functions of CD28 and CTLA-4 expressed on T cells are described in Chapter 6. On B cells, there are two important co-receptors that either upregulate (CD19) or downregulate (CD22) BCR-mediated signals, thereby playing important roles in establishing signalling thresholds (Fig. 7.9) (O'Rourke *et al.*, 1997).

CD19 is a member of the immunoglobulin superfamily that is expressed on B cells in association with CD21 and CD81 (Tedder, Inaoki & Sato, 1997a). CD21

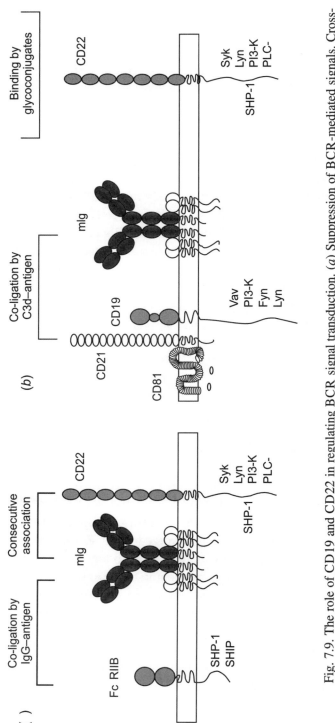

Fig. 7.9. The role of CD19 and CD22 in regulating BCR signal transduction. (*a*) Suppression of BCR-mediated signals. Cross-linking of mIg induces tyrosine phosphorylation of CD22, recruitment of SHP-1 and downregulation of signal transduction. (*b*) Enhancement of BCR-mediated signals. Co-ligation of CD19/CD21/CD81 complex to mIg by C3d–antigen recruits positive signal transduction effectors that augment B cell activation. Ligation of CD22 by glycoconjugates in lymphoid organs releases mIg and prevents the negative effects of CD22. (From O'Rourke *et al.*, 1997.)

is the complement receptor type 2 and binds the cleavage products of the third complement component (C3). If an antigen has covalently bound C3 molecules, it will bind to the BCR and simultaneously engage the CD19/CD21 complex, so promoting an association between CD19 and the BCR. For example, hen egg lysozyme becomes 10 000-fold more immunogenic when it is attached to the C3d complement protein (Dempsey *et al.*, 1996). This amplification system is mediated by synergistic interactions occurring between CD19 and the BCR. CD19 is a signalling molecule with a long cytoplasmic tail, containing nine conserved tyrosine residues that become phosphorylated upon engagement of CD19 with activating mAbs or ligation of the BCR. If CD19 is cross-linked with the BCR, then the signals induced are greater than those triggered by either receptor alone (Carter & Fearon, 1992), and BCR-associated tyrosine kinases such as Syk may be responsible for CD19 phosphorylation (Carter *et al.*, 1997). Upon phosphorylation, a number of SH2 domain-containing proteins are recruited to the CD19 cytoplasmic tail, including p59^{fyn}, p56^{lck}, p59^{lyn}, Vav and the p85 regulatory subunit of phosphoinositide (PI) 3'-kinase, which generates the important second messenger phosphoinositide trisphosphate (Tedder *et al.*, 1997a). p59^{fyn} binds CD19 at a different site from PI 3'-kinase and so both molecules are probably bound simultaneously. This may allow the involvement of the p59^{fyn} SH3 domain in activating PI 3'-kinase. A CD19-recruited complex involving Vav and PI 3'-kinase is, therefore, likely to be important in triggering intracellular pathways, although the downstream consequences are not yet well understood.

The nature of CD19 as an amplification system for BCR signal transduction has been confirmed by the study of CD19-deficient mice in which there is a severe deficit in mature B cells (B-1), the cells which normally have the highest levels of cell-surface CD19 expression (Rickert, Rajewsky & Roes, 1995). In these mice, B cells no longer proliferate upon BCR engagement, whereas in mice overexpressing CD19, B cells demonstrate increased proliferative responses, underlining the key role that CD19 plays in altering BCR signalling thresholds.

In contrast to CD19, CD22 is thought to exert a negative action on BCR signal transduction (O'Rourke *et al.*, 1997; Tedder *et al.*, 1997b). CD22 becomes associated with the BCR upon BCR cross-linking and is phosphorylated on tyrosine residues within its cytoplasmic tail (Schulte *et al.*, 1992). Three of the six tyrosine residues located in the tail are found within immunoreceptor tyrosine-based inhibitory motifs (ITIMs), which have the sequence V/I-X-Y-X-X-L. These motifs have also been found in the FcγRllb receptor, which likewise has a negative regulatory role in BCR signalling (Muta *et al.*, 1994). Upon phosphorylation, an SH2 domain-containing tyrosine phosphatase called SHP-1 is recruited to an ITIM within the CD22 tail, where it is activated (Doody *et al.*, 1995). The negative effects of SHP-1 in lymphocyte signalling are well established (Frearson & Alexander, 1997). The phosphatase may exert its effects by dephosphorylating one or more tyrosine-phosphorylated proteins required for coupling the BCR to the calcium-signalling pathway, although the uncoupling effects of other molecules recruited to CD22 cannot yet be excluded. This model is supported by results obtained from CD22-deficient mice in which B cell development is normal but splenic B cells were found to be hyperresponsive to BCR signalling, with increased and prolonged calcium signals and proliferative responses (O'Keefe *et al.*, 1996; Nitschke *et al.*, 1997). Interestingly, B cells from 'motheaten mice', which have defects in SHP-1, display a similar phenotype to CD22–/– mice and likewise have elevated calcium responses to B cell antigens (Cyster & Goodnow, 1995). In neither CD22–/– nor in motheaten mice, however, are there global defects in the coupling of the BCR to intracellular protein tyrosine-phosphorylation events (Nitschke *et al.*, 1997). It seems likely, therefore, that the negative actions of the CD22 co-receptor result from the highly selective effects of SHP-1 and perhaps other CD22-recruited molecules on the BCR signalling apparatus.

The balance between the positive and negative effects of CD28 and CTLA-4 on T cell function, and the parallel types of effect of CD19 and CD22 on B cell function, illustrate the complex way in which the responses of antigen receptor-mediated signals are 'fine tuned' to respond appropriately to a very broad spectrum of antigens encountered within a wide range of cellular contexts.

Pharmaceutical intervention in lymphocyte signalling pathways

The present available range of immunosuppressive drugs are of great value in the clinic but suffer from various harmful side effects. Cyclosporin A and FK506, for example, have the disadvantage that their target (calcineurin) is widely expressed in non-haematopoietic tissues, thereby facilitating deleterious effects of these drugs in organs such as the kidney and heart. An enormous amount of research is, therefore, being carried out by pharmaceutical companies to target molecules in lymphocyte activation pathways that would provide a more selective means of immunosuppression. Several of the key enzymes already identified, such as ZAP-70, p56[lck], p56[lck] and CD45, are largely restricted in their expression to haematopoietic cells, making such molecules attractive targets for pharmaceutical intervention. Monoclonal antibodies against cell-surface antigens such as CD4 have also been used with some success to suppress the inappropriate activation of T cells in autoimmune diseases such as RA. By humanizing such antibodies, that is by engineering the antibody to mimic human immunoglobulin as much as possible, the risk of the recipient undergoing an immune response to the therapeutic reagent is lessened.

The ability of receptors such as CD28 and CTLA-4 to induce signals that modulate the proliferative and survival responses of T cells has also aroused great interest in the pharmaceutical industry, since hopes have been raised that in the future it will prove possible using appropriate drugs to raise and lower T cell activation levels at will. The temporary upregulation of T cell responses could be invaluable in promoting, for example, the cytotoxic actions of tumour-infiltrating lymphocytes, or in boosting the immune system to attack residual malignant cells following surgical removal of cancerous tissue. The temporary suppression of T cell responses is clearly important in the context of organ transplantation, autoimmunity and inflammation.

Such pharmaceutical hopes lie largely in the future. Nevertheless, it is very likely that the basic research carried out on lymphocyte signal transduction pathways in the late twentieth century will pave the way for a rational approach to drug-induced manipulation of the immune system that will reach its fruition during the course of the twenty-first century.

Acknowledgements

I am grateful to Dr Julie Frearson and to Dr Martin Turner for their helpful suggestions on an earlier draft of this chapter.

References

Afar, D.E.H., Park, H., Howell, B.W., Rawlings, D.J., Cooper, J. & Witte, O.N. (1996). Regulation of Btk by Src family tyrosine kinases. *Mol. Cell. Biol.* 16: 3465–3471.

Alberolaila, J., Forbush, K.A., Seger, R., Krebs, E.G. & Perlmutter, R.M. (1995). Selective requirement for MAP kinase activation in thymocyte differentiation. *Nature* 373: 620–623.

Alberolaila, J., Hogquist, K.A., Swan, K.A., Bevan, M.J. & Perlmutter, R.M. (1996). Positive and negative selection invoke distinct signaling pathways. *J. Exp. Med.* 184: 9–18.

Alexander, D.R. (1997). The role of the CD45 phosphatase in lymphocyte signalling. In *Lymphocyte Signalling: Mechanisms, Subversion and Manipulation*, eds. M.M. Harnett and K.P. Rigley, pp. 107–140. Chichester, UK: Wiley.

Arpaia, E., Shahar, M., Dadi, H., Cohen, A. & Roifman, C.M. (1994). Defective T cell receptor signaling and CD8+ thymic selection in humans lacking ZAP-70 kinase. *Cell* 76: 947–958.

Auphan, N., Didonato, J.A., Rosette, C., Helmberg, A. & Karin, M. (1995). Immunosuppression by glucocorticoids – inhibition of NF-Kappa-B activity through induction of I-Kappa-B synthesis. *Science* 270: 286–290.

Baldwin, A.S. (1996). The NF-κB and IκB proteins: new discoveries and insights. *Annu. Rev. Immunol.* 14: 649–681.

Beals, C.R., Clipstone, N.A., Ho, S.N. & Crabtree, G.R. (1997a). Nuclear localization of NF-ATc by a calcineurin-dependent, cyclosporin-sensitive intramolecular interaction. *Genes Devel.* 11: 824–834.

Beals, C.R., Sheridan, C.M., Turck, C.W., Gardner, P. & Crabtree, G.R. (1997b). Nuclear export of NF-ATc enhanced by glycogen synthase kinase-3. *Science* 275: 1930–1933.

Benatar, T., Carsetti, R., Furlonger, C., Kamalia, N., Mak, T. & Paige, C.J. (1996). Immunoglobulin-mediated signal transduction in B-cells from CD45-deficient mice. *J. Exp. Med.* 183: 329–334.

Berridge, M.J. (1993). Inositol trisphosphate and calcium signaling. *Nature* 361: 315–325.

Berridge, M.J. (1995). Capacitative calcium-entry. *Biochem. J.* 312: 1–11.

Berridge, M.J. (1997). Lymphocyte activation in health and disease. *Crit. Rev. Immunol.* 17: 155–178.

Birchall, A.M., Bishop, J., Bradshaw, D., Cline, A., Coffey, J., Elliott, L.H., Gibson, V.M., Greenham, A., Hallam, T.J., Harris, W., Hill, C.H., Hutchings, A., Lamont, A.G., Lawton, G., Lewis, E.J., Maw, A., Nixon, J.S., Pole, D., Wadsworth, J. & Wilkinson, S.E. (1994). Ro-32-0432, a selective and orally-active inhibitor of protein kinase-C prevents T-cell activation. *J. Pharmacol. Exp. Therapeut.* 268: 922–929.

Bolen, J.B. (1995). Protein-tyrosine kinases in the initiation of antigen receptor signaling. *Curr. Opin. Immunol.* 7: 306–311.

Bonnerot, C., Lankar, D., Hanau, D., Spehner, D., Davoust, J., Salamero, J. & Fridman, W.H. (1995). Role of B-cell receptor Ig-alpha and Ig-beta subunits in MHC class II-restricted antigen presentation. *Immunity* 3: 335–347.

Buday, L., Egan, S.E., Viciana, P.R., Cantrell, D.A. & Downward, J. (1994). A complex of Grb2 adapter protein, Sos exchange factor, and a 36-kDA membrane-bound tyrosine phosphoprotein is implicated in Ras activation in T-cells. *J. Biol. Chem.* 269: 9019–9023.

Bustelo, X.R., Ledbetter, J.A. & Barbacid, M. (1992). Product of *vav* protooncogene defines a new class of tyrosine protein-kinase substrates. *Nature* 356: 68–71.

Byth, K.F., Conroy, L.A., Howlett, S., Smith, A.J.H., May, J., Alexander, D.R. & Holmes, N. (1996). CD45-null transgenic mice reveal a positive regulatory role for CD45 in early thymocyte development, in the selection of CD4(+)CD8(+) thymocytes, and in B-cell maturation. *J. Exp. Med.* 183: 1707–1718.

Cambier, J.C., Bedzyk, W., Campbell, K., Chien, N., Friedrich, J., Harwood, A., Jensen, W., Pleiman, C. & Clark, M.R. (1993). The B-cell antigen receptor – structure and function of primary, secondary, tertiary and quaternary components. *Immunol. Rev.* 132: 85–106.

Cambier, J.C., Pleiman, C.M. & Clark, M.R. (1994). Signal-transduction by the B-cell antigen receptor and its coreceptors. *Annu. Rev. Immunol.* 12: 457–486.

Cantrell, D. (1996). T cell antigen receptor signal transduction pathways. *Annu. Rev. Immunol.* 14: 259–274.

Carter, R.H. & Fearon, D.T. (1992). CD19: lowering the threshold for antigen receptor stimulation of B lymphocytes. *Science* 256: 105–107.

Carter, R.H., Doody, G.M., Bolen, J.B. & Fearon, D.T. (1997). Membrane IgM-induced tyrosine phosphorylation of CD19 requires a CD19 domain that mediates association with components of the B cell antigen receptor complex. *J. Immunol.* 158: 3062–3069.

Chan, A.C., Desai, D.M. & Weiss, A. (1994a). The role of protein-tyrosine kinases and protein-tyrosine phosphatases in T-cell antigen receptor signal-transduction. *Annu. Rev. Immunol.* 12: 555–592.

Chan, A.C., Van Oers, N.S.C., Tran, A., Turka, L., Law, C.L., Ryan, J.C., Clark, E.A. & Weiss, A. (1994b). Differential expression of ZAP-70 and Syk protein-tyrosine kinases, and the role of this family of protein-tyrosine kinases in TCR signaling. *J. Immunol.* 152: 4758–4766.

Chan, A.C., Dalton, M., Johnson, R., Kong, G.H., Wang, T., Thoma, R. & Kurosaki, T. (1995). Activation of ZAP-70 kinase-activity by phosphorylation of tyrosine-493 is required for lymphocyte antigen receptor function. *EMBO J.* 14: 2499–2508.

Chu, D.H., Spits, H., Peyron, J.-F., Rowley, R.B., Bolen, J.B. & Weiss, A. (1996). The Syk protein tyrosine kinase can function independently of CD45 or Lck in T cell antigen receptor signaling. *EMBO J.* 15: 6251–6261.

Clark, M.R., Campbell, K.S., Kazlauskas, A., Johnson, S.A., Hertz, M., Potter, T.A., Pleiman, C. & Cambier, J.C. (1992). The B-cell antigen receptor complex – association of Ig-alpha and Ig-beta with distinct cytoplasmic effectors. *Science* 258: 123–126.

Clark, M.R., Johnson, S.A. & Cambier, J.C. (1994). Analysis of Ig-alpha–tyrosine kinase interaction reveals 2 levels of binding-specificity and tyrosine-phosphorylated Ig-alpha stimulation of Fyn activity. *EMBO J.* 13: 1911–1919.

Crespo, P., Schuebel, K.E., Ostrom, A.A., Gutkind, J.S. & Bustelo, X.R (1997). Phosphotyrosine-dependent activation of Rac-1 GDP/GTP exchange by the *vav* proto-oncogene product. *Nature* 385: 169–172.

Cyster, J.G. (1997). Signaling thresholds and interclonal competition in preimmune B-cell selection. *Immunol. Rev.* 156: 87–101.

Cyster, J.G. & Goodnow, C.C. (1995). Protein-tyrosine-phosphatase 1C negatively regulates antigen receptor signaling in B-lymphocytes and determines thresholds for negative selection. *Immunity* 2: 13–24.

Cyster, J.G., Healy, J.I., Kishihara, K., Mak, T.W., Thomas, M.L. & Goodnow, C.C. (1996). Regulation of B-lymphocyte negative and positive selection by tyrosine phosphatase CD45. *Nature* 381: 325–328.

DeFranco, A.L. (1997). The complexity of signaling pathways activated by the BCR. *Curr. Opin. Immunol.* 9: 296–308.

Dempsey, P.W., Allison, M.E.D., Akkaraju, S., Goodnow, C.C. & Fearon, D.T. (1996). C3d of complement as a molecular adjuvant – bridging innate and acquired immunity. *Science* 271: 348–350.

Doody, G.M., Justement, L.B., Delibrias, C.C., Matthews, R.J., Lin, J.J., Thomas, M.L. & Fearon, D.T. (1995). A role in B-cell activation for CD22 and the protein-tyrosine-phosphatase Shp. *Science* 269: 242–244.

Downward, J., Graves, J.D., Warne, P.H., Rayter, S. & Cantrell, D.A. (1990). Stimulation of P21*ras* upon T-cell activation. *Nature* 346: 719–723.

Duplay, P., Thome, M., Herve, F. & Acuto, O. (1994). P56(Lck) interacts via its Src homology-2 domain with the ZAP-70 kinase. *J. Exp. Med.* 179: 1163–1172.

Fanger, C.M., Hoth, M., Crabtree, G.R. & Lewis, R.S. (1995). Characterization of T-cell mutants with defects in capacitative calcium-entry – genetic evidence for the physiological roles of Crac channels. *J. Cell Biol.* 131: 655–667.

Frearson, J.A. & Alexander, D.R. (1996). The role of phosphotyrosine phosphatases in T-lymphocyte development, apoptosis and signalling. *Immunol. Today* 17: 385–391.

Frearson, J.A. & Alexander, D.R. (1997). The role of phosphotyrosine phosphatases in haematopoietic cell signal transduction. *Bioessays* 19: 417–427.

Fruman, D.A., Klee, C.B., Bierer, B.E. & Burakoff, S.J. (1992). Calcineurin phosphatase activity in lymphocytes-T is inhibited by FK-506 and cyclosporine-A. *Proc. Natl. Acad. Sci., USA* 89: 3686–3690.

Gelfand, E.W., Weinberg, K., Mazer, B.D., Kadlecek, T.A. & Weiss, A. (1995). Absence of ZAP-70 prevents signaling through the antigen receptor on peripheral-blood T-cells but not on thymocytes. *J. Exp. Med.* 182: 1057–1065.

Genot, E.M., Parker, P.J. & Cantrell, D.A. (1995). Analysis of the role of protein-kinase-C-alpha, protein-kinase-epsilon, and protein-kinase-zeta in T-cell activation. *J. Biol. Chem.* 270: 9833–9839.

Genot, E., Cleverley, S., Henning, S. & Cantrell, D. (1996). Multiple p21*ras* effector pathways regulate nuclear factor of activated T cells. *EMBO J.* 15: 3923–3933.

Goldsmith, M.A. & Weiss, A. (1988) Early signal transduction by the antigen receptor without commitment to T-cell activation. *Science* 240: 1029–1031.

Hatada, M.H., Lu, X.D., Laird, E.R., Green, J., Morgenstern, J.P., Lou, M.Z., Marr, C.S., Phillips, T.B., Ram, M.K., Theriault, K., Zoller, M.J. & Karas, J.L. (1995). Molecular-basis for interaction of the protein-tyrosine kinase ZAP-70 with the T-cell receptor. *Nature* 377: 32–38.

Hibbs, M.L., Tarlinton, D.M., Armes, J., Grail, D., Hodgson, G., Maglitto, R., Stacker, S.A. & Dunn, A.R. (1995). Multiple defects in the immune system of Lyn-deficient mice, culminating in autoimmune disease. *Cell* 83: 301–311.

Ho, N., Gullberg, M. & Chatila, T. (1996). Activation protein 1-dependent transcriptional activation of interleukin-2 gene by Ca^{2+}/calmodulin kinase type IV/GR. *J. Exp. Med.* 184: 101–112.

Hunter, T. & Karin, M. (1992). The regulation of transcription by phosphorylation. *Cell* 70: 375–387.

Isakov, N., Wange, R.L., Burgess, W.H., Watts, J.D., Aebersold, R. & Samelson, L.E. (1995). ZAP-70 binding-specificity to T-cell receptor tyrosine-based activation motifs – the tandem SH2 domains of ZAP-70 bind distinct tyrosine-based activation motifs with varying affinity. *J. Exp. Med.* 181: 375–380.

Iwashima, M., Irving, B.A., Vanoers, N.S.C., Chan, A.C. & Weiss, A. (1994). Sequential interactions of the TCR with 2 distinct cytoplasmic tyrosine kinases. *Science* 263: 1136–1139.

Jabado, N., Pallier, A., Le Deist, F., Bernard, F., Fischer, A. & Hivroz, C. (1997). CD4 ligands inhibit the formation of multifunctional transduction complexes involved in T cell activation. *J. Immunol.* 158: 94–103.

Janeway, C.A. (1992). The T-cell receptor as a multicomponent signaling machine – CD4/CD8 coreceptors and CD45 in T-cell activation. *Annu. Rev. Immunol.* 10: 645–674.

Jayaraman, T., Ondriasova, E., Ondrias, K., Harnick, D.J. & Marks, A.R. (1995). The inositol 1,4,5-trisphosphate receptor is essential for T-cell receptor signaling. *Proc. Natl. Acad. Sci., USA* 92: 6007–6011.

Jayaraman, T., Ondrias, K., Ondriasova, E. & Marks, A.R. (1996). Regulation of the inositol 1,4,5-trisphosphate receptor by tyrosine phosphorylation. *Science* 272: 1492–1494.

Justement, L.B., Campbell, K.S., Chien, N.C. & Cambier, J.C. (1991). Regulation of B-cell antigen receptor signal transduction and phosphorylation by CD45. *Science* 252: 1839–1842.

Keshvara, L.M., Isaacson, C., Harrison, M.L. & Geahlen, R.L. (1997). Syk activation and dissociation from the B-cell antigen receptor is mediated by phosphorylation of tyrosine 130. *J. Biol. Chem.* 272: 10 377–10 381.

Khan, W.N., Alt, F.W., Gerstein, R.M., Malynn, B.A., Larsson, I., Rathbun, G., Davidson, L., Muller, S., Kantor, A.B., Herzenberg, L.A., Rosen, F.S. & Sideras,

P. (1995). Defective B-cell development and function in Btk-deficient mice. *Immunity* 3: 283–299.

Kimura, T., Sakamoto, H., Appella, E. & Siraganian, R.P. (1996). Conformational-changes induced in the protein-tyrosine kinase P72(Syk) by tyrosine phosphorylation or by binding of phosphorylated immunoreceptor tyrosine-based activation motif peptides. *Mol. Cell. Biol.* 16: 1471–1478.

Kishihara, K., Penninger, J., Wallace, V.A., Kundig, T.M., Kawai, K., Wakeham, A., Timms, E., Pfeffer, K., Ohashi, P.S., Thomas, M.L., Furlonger, C., Paige, C.J. & Mak, T.W. (1993). Normal B-lymphocyte development but impaired T-cell maturation in CD45-exon 6 protein-tyrosine-phosphatase deficient mice. *Cell* 74: 143–156.

Koretzky, G.A., Picus, J., Thomas, M.L. & Weiss, A. (1990). Tyrosine phosphatase CD45 is essential for coupling T-cell antigen receptor to the phosphatidyl inositol pathway. *Nature* 346: 66–68.

Kurosaki, T. (1997). Molecular mechanisms in B cell antigen receptor signaling. *Curr. Opin. Immunol.* 9: 309–318.

Kurosaki, T., Takata, M., Yamanashi, Y., Inazu, T., Taniguchi, T., Yamamoto, T. & Yamamura, H. (1994). Syk activation by the Src-family tyrosine kinase in the B-cell receptor signaling. *J. Exp. Med.* 179: 1725–1729.

Lai, J.H. & Tan, T.H. (1994). CD28 signaling causes a sustained down-regulation of 1-kappa-B-alpha which can be prevented by the immunosuppressant rapamycin. *J. Biol. Chem.* 269: 30 007–30 080.

Larsson, N., Melander, H., Marklund, U., Osterman, O. & Gullberg, M. (1995). G2/M transition requires multisite phosphorylation of oncoprotein-18 by distinct protein-kinase systems. *J. Biol. Chem.* 270: 14 175–14 183.

Ledeist, F., Hivroz, C., Partiseti, M., Thomas, C., Buc, H.A., Oleastro, M., Belohradsky, B., Choquet, D. & Fischer, A. (1995). A primary T-cell immunodeficiency associated with defective transmembrane calcium influx. *Blood* 85: 1053–1062.

Leitges, M., Schmedt, C., Guinamard, R., Davoust, J., Schaal, S., Stabel, S. & Tarakhovsky, A. (1996). Immunodeficiency in protein kinase Cβ-deficient mice. *Science* 273: 788–791.

Lewis, R.S. & Cahalan, M.D. (1995). Potassium and calcium channels in lymphocytes. *Annu. Rev. Immunol.* 13: 623–653.

Liao, X.C. & Littman, D.R. (1995). Altered T-cell receptor signaling and disrupted T-cell development in mice lacking Itk. *Immunity.* 3: 757–769.

Liu, J., Farmer, J.D., Lane, W.S., Friedman, J., Weissman, I. & Schreiber, S.L. (1991). Calcineurin is a common target of cyclophilin–cyclosporin A and FKBP–FK506 complexes. *Cell* 66: 807–815.

Loh, C., Carew, J.A., Kim, J., Hogan, P.G. & Rao, A. (1996). T-cell receptor stimulation elicits an early phase of activation and a later phase of deactivation of the transcription factor NFatl. *Mol. Cell. Biol.* 16: 3945–3954.

Luo, C., Burgeon, E., Carew, J.A., McCaffrey, P.G., Badalian, T.M., Lane, W.S., Hogan, P.G. & Rao, A. (1996). Recombinant NFatl (Nfatp) is regulated by calcineurin in T-cells and mediates transcription of several cytokine genes. *Mol. Cell. Biol.* 16: 3955–3966.

Madrenas, J., Wange, R.L., Wang, J.L., Isakov, N., Samelson, L.E. & Germain, R.N. (1995). Zeta-phosphorylation without ZAP-70 activation-induced by TCR antagonists or partial agonists. *Science* 267: 515–518.

Molina, T.J., Kishihara, K., Siderovski, D.P., Vanewijk, W., Narendran, A., Timms, E., Wakeham, A., Paige, C.J., Hartmann, K.U., Veillette, A., Davidson, D. & Mak,

T.W. (1992). Profound block in thymocyte development in mice lacking p56[lck]. *Nature* 357: 161–164.

Monks, C.R.F., Kupfer, H., Tamir, I., Barlow, A. & Kupfer, A. (1997). Selective modulation of protein kinase C-theta during T-cell activation. *Nature* 385: 83–86.

Morrison, D.K. & Cutler, R.E. (1997). The complexity of Raf-1 regulation. *Curr. Biol.* 9: 174–179.

Motto, D.G., Musci, M.A., Ross, S.E. & Koretzky, G.A. (1996). Tyrosine phosphorylation of Grb2-associated proteins correlates with phospholipase C-gamma-1 activation in T-cells. *Mol. Cell. Biol.* 16: 2823–2829.

Musci, M.A., Hendricks Taylor, L.R., Motto, D.G., Paskind, M., Kamens, J., Turck, C.W. & Koretzky, G.A. (1997). Molecular cloning of SLAP-130, an SLP-76-associated substrate of the T cell antigen receptor-stimulated protein tyrosine kinases. *J. Biol. Chem.* 272: 11 674–11 677.

Muta, T., Kurosaki, T., Misulovin, Z., Sanchez, M., Nussenzweig, M.C. & Ravetch, J.V. (1994). A 13-amino-acid motif in the cytoplasmic domain of Fc-gamma-Riib modulates B-cell receptor signaling. *Nature* 368: 70–73.

Negishi, I., Motoyama, N., Nakayama, K., Nakayama, K., Senju, S., Hatakeyama, S., Zhang, Q., Chan, A.C. & Loh, D.Y. (1995). Essential role for ZAP-70 in both positive and negative selection of thymocytes. *Nature* 376: 435–438.

Neumeister, E.N., Zhu, Y.X., Richard, S., Terhorst, C., Chan, A.C. & Shaw, A.S. (1995). Binding of ZAP-70 to phosphorylated T-cell receptor-zeta and receptor-eta enhances its autophosphorylation and generates specific binding-sites for SH2 domain-containing proteins. *Mol. Cell. Biol.* 15: 3171–3178.

Nitschke, L., Carsetti, R., Ocker, B., Kohler, G. & Lamers, M.C. (1997). CD22 is a negative regulator of B-cell receptor signalling. *Curr. Biol.* 7: 133–143.

Nunes, J.A., Collette, Y., Truneh, A., Olive, D. & Cantrell, D.A. (1994). The role of p21(Ras) in CD28 signal-transduction – triggering of CD28 with antibodies, but not the ligand B7-1, activates P21(Ras). *J. Exp. Med.* 180: 1067–1076.

O'Rourke, L., Tooze, R. & Fearon, D.T. (1997). Co-receptors of B lymphocytes. *Curr. Opin. Immunol.* 9: 324–329.

O'Keefe, T.L., Williams, G.T., Davies, S.L. & Neuberger, M.S. (1996). Hyperresponsive B-cells in CD22–deficient mice. *Science* 274: 798–801.

Ostergaard, H.L., Shackelford, D.A., Hurley, T.R., Johnson, P., Hyman, R., Sefton, B.M. & Trowbridge, I.S. (1989). Expression of CD45 alters phosphorylation of the Lck-encoded tyrosine protein-kinase in murine lymphoma T-cell lines. *Proc. Natl. Acad. Sci., USA* 86: 8959–8963.

Park, I.K. & Soderling, T.R. (1995). Activation of Ca^{2+}/calmodulin-dependent protein-kinase (cam-kinase) – IV by Cam-kinase kinase in Jurkat T-lymphocytes. *J. Biol. Chem.* 270: 30 464–30 469.

Pastor, M.I., Reif, K. & Cantrell, D. (1995). The regulation and function of p21(Ras) during T-cell activation and growth. *Immunol. Today* 16: 159–164.

Pingel, J.T. & Thomas, M.L. (1989). Evidence that the leukocyte–common antigen is required for antigen-induced lymphocyte-T proliferation. *Cell* 58: 1055–1065.

Pleiman, C.M., Dambrosio, D. & Cambier, J.C. (1994). The B-cell antigen receptor complex – structure and signal transduction. *Immunol. Today* 15: 393–399.

Qian, D.P. & Weiss, A. (1997). T cell antigen receptor signal transduction. *Curr. Opin. Cell Biol.* 9: 205–212.

Raab, M., daSilva, A.J., Findell, P.R. & Rudd, C.E. (1997). Regulation of Vav-SLP-76 binding by ZAP-70 and its relevance to TCR zeta/CD3 induction of interleukin-2. *Immunity* 6: 155–164.

Rao, A., Luo, C. & Hogan, P.G. (1997). Transcription factors of the NFAT family: regulation and function. *Annu. Rev. Immunol.* 15: 707–747.

Rawlings, D.J., Scharenberg, A.M., Park, H., Wahl, M.I., Lin, S.Q. Kato, R.M., Fluckiger, A.C., Witte, O.N. & Kinet, J.P. (1996). Activation of Btk by a phosphorylation mechanism initiated by Src family kinases. *Science* 271: 822–825.

Rickert, R.C., Rajewsky, K. & Roes, J. (1995). Impairment of T-cell-dependent B-cell responses and B-1 cell development in CD19-deficient mice. *Nature* 376: 352–355.

Robinson, M.J. & Cobb, M.H. (1997). Mitogen-activated protein kinase pathways. *Curr. Biol.* 9: 180–186.

Rowley, R.B., Burkhardt, A.L., Chao, H.G., Matsueda, G.R. & Bolen, J.B. (1995). Syk protein-tyrosine kinase is regulated by tyrosine-phosphorylated Ig-alpha Ig-beta immunoreceptor tyrosine activation motif binding and autophosphorylation. *J. Biol. Chem.* 270: 11 590–11 594.

Rudd, C.E., Trevillyan, J.M., Dasgupta, J.D., Wong, L.L. & Schlossman, S.F. (1988). The CD4 receptor is complexed in detergent lysates to a protein-tyrosine kinase (Pp58) from human lymphocytes-T. *Proc. Natl. Acad. Sci., USA* 85: 5190–5194.

Samelson, L.E., Phillips, A.F., Luong, E.T. & Klausner, R.D. (1990). Association of the Fyn protein-tyrosine kinase with the T-cell antigen receptor. *Proc. Natl. Acad. Sci., USA* 87: 4358–4362

Sawasdikosol, S., Ravichandran, K.S., Lee, K.K., Chang, J.-H. & Burakoff, S.J. (1995). Crk interacts with tyrosine-phosphorylated p116 upon T cell activation. *J. Biol. Chem.* 270: 2893–2896.

Schulte, R.J., Campbell, M.A., Fischer, W.H. & Sefton, B.M. (1992). Tyrosine phosphorylation of CD22 during B-cell activation. *Science* 258: 1001–1004.

Secrist, J.P., Karnitz, L. & Abraham, R.T. (1991). T-cell antigen receptor ligation induces tyrosine phosphorylation of phospholipase C-gamma-1. *J. Biol. Chem.* 266: 12 135–12 139.

Shiroo, M., Goff, L., Biffen, M., Shivnan, E. & Alexander, D. (1992). CD45-tyrosine phosphatase-activated p59Fyn couples the T-cell antigen receptor to pathways of diacylglycerol production, protein-kinase-C activation and calcium influx. *EMBO J.* 11: 4887–4897.

Shiue, L., Zoller, M.J. & Brugge, J.S. (1995). Syk is activated by phosphotyrosine containing peptides representing the tyrosine-based activation motifs of the high affinity receptor for IgE. *J. Biol. Chem.* 270: 10 498–10 502.

Sidorenko, S.P., Law, C.L., Klaus, S.J., Chandran, K.A., Takata, M., Kurosaki, T. & Clark, E.A. (1996). Protein-kinase-C-mu (PKC-mu) associates with the B-cell antigen receptor complex and regulates lymphocyte signaling. *Immunity* 5: 353–363.

Sieh, M., Bolen, J.B. & Weiss, A. (1993). CD45 specifically modulates binding of Lck to a phosphopeptide encompassing the negative regulatory tyrosine of Lck. *EMBO J.* 12: 315–321.

Siliciano, J.D., Morrow, T.A. & Desiderio, S.V. (1992). Itk, a T-cell-specific tyrosine kinase gene inducible by interleukin- 2. *Proc. Natl. Acad. Sci., USA* 89: 11 194–11 198.

Sloan-Lancaster, J. & Allen, P.M. (1996). Altered peptide ligand-induced partial T cell activation: molecular mechanisms and role in T cell biology. *Annu. Rev. Immunol.* 14: 1–27.

Sloan-Lancaster, J., Shaw, A.S., Rothbard, J.B. & Allen, P.M. (1994). Partial T cell signaling – altered phospho-Zeta and lack of ZAP 70 recruitment in APl-induced T-cell anergy. *Cell* 79: 913–922.

Stone, J.D., Conroy, L.A., Byth, K.F., Hederer, R.A., Howlett, S, Takemoto, Y., Holmes, N. & Alexander, D.R. (1997). Aberrant TCR-mediated signalling in CD45-null thymocytes involves dysfunctional regulation of Lck, Fyn, TCR-ς and ZAP-70. *J. Immunol.* 158: 5773–5782.

Su, B., Jacinto, E., Hibi, M., Kallunki, T., Karin, M. & Benneriah, Y. (1994). Jnk is involved in signal integration during costimulation of T-lymphocytes. *Cell* 77: 727–736.

Swan, K.A., Alberolaila, J., Gross, J.A., Appleby, M.W., Forbush, K.A., Thomas, J.F. & Perlmutter, R.M. (1995). Involvement of p21 ras distinguishes positive and negative selection in thymocytes. *EMBO J.* 14: 276–285.

Takata, M. & Kurosaki, T. (1996). A role for Brutons tyrosine kinase in B-cell antigen receptor-mediated activation of phospholipase C-gamma-2. *J. Exp. Med.* 184: 31–40.

Tarakhovsky, A., Turner, M., Schaal, S., Mee, P.J., Duddy, L.P., Rajewsky, K. & Tybulewicz, V.L.J. (1995). Defective antigen receptor-mediated proliferation of B-cells and T-cells in the absence of Vav. *Nature* 374: 467–470.

Tarlinton, B. (1997). Antigen presentation by memory B cells: the sting is in the tail. *Science* 276: 374–375.

Tedder, T.F., Inaoki, M. & Sato, S. (1997a). The CD19–CD21 complex regulates signal transduction thresholds governing humoral immunity and autoimmunity. *Immunity* 6: 107–118.

Tedder, T.F., Tuscano, J., Sato, S. & Kehrl, J.H. (1997b). CD22, a B lymphocyte-specific adhesion molecule that regulates antigen receptor signaling. *Annu. Rev. Immunol.* 15: 481–504.

Truneh, A., Albert, F., Golstein, P. & Schmitt-Verhulst, A.-M. (1985). Early steps of lymphocyte activation bypassed by synergy between calcium ionophores and phorbol ester. *Nature* 313: 318–320.

Turner, M., Mee, P.J., Costello, P.S., Williams, O., Price, A.A., Duddy, L.P., Furlong, M.T., Geahlen, R.L. & Tybulewicz, V.L.J. (1995). Perinatal lethality and blocked B-cell development in mice lacking the tyrosine kinase Syk. *Nature* 378: 298–302.

van Oers, N.S.C., Killeen, N. & Weiss, A. (1994). ZAP-70 is constitutively associated with zeta in murine thymocytes and lymph-node T-cells. *Immunity* 1: 675–685.

van Oers, N.S.C., Killeen, N. & Weiss, A. (1996a). Lck regulates the tyrosine phosphorylation of the T-cell subunits and ZAP-70 in murine thymocytes. *J. Exp. Med.* 183: 1053–1062.

van Oers, N.S.C., Lowinkropf, B., Finlay, D., Connolly, K. & Weiss, A. (1996b). Alpha-beta-T-cell development is abolished in mice lacking both Lck and Fyn protein-tyrosine kinases. *Immunity* 5: 429–436.

Venkitaraman, A.R., Williams, G.T., Dariavach, P. & Neuberger, M.S. (1991). The B-cell antigen receptor of the 5 immunoglobulin classes. *Nature* 352: 777–781.

Wacholtz, M.C. & Lipsky, P.E. (1993). Anti-CD3-stimulated Ca^{2+} signal in individual human peripheral T-cells – activation correlates with a sustained increase in intracellular Ca^{2+}. *J. Immunol.* 150: 5338–5349.

Wange, R.L. & Samelson, L.E. (1996). Complex complexes: signaling at the TCR. *Immunity* 5: 197–205.

Wange, R.L., Guitian, R., Isakov, N., Watts, J.D., Aebersold, R. & Samelson, L.E. (1995). Activating and inhibitory mutations in adjacent tyrosines in the kinase domain of ZAP-70. *J. Biol. Chem.* 270: 18 730–18 733.

Wardenburg, J.B., Fu, C., Jackman, J.K., Flotow, H., Wilkinson, S.E., Williams, D.H., Johnson, R., Kong, G.H., Chan, A.C. & Findell, P.R. (1996). Phosphorylation of

Slp-76 by the ZAP-70 protein-tyrosine kinase is required for T-cell receptor function. *J. Biol. Chem.* 271: 19 641–19 644.

Weiser, P., Muller, R., Braun, U. & Reth, M. (1997). Endosomal targeting by the cytoplasmic tail of membrane immunoglobulin. *Science* 276: 407–409.

Weiss, A. (1993). T-cell antigen receptor signal transduction – a tale of tails and cytoplasmic protein-tyrosine kinases. *Cell* 73: 209–212.

Wiest, D.L., Ashe, J.M., Howcroft, T.K., Lee, H.-M., Kemper, D.M., Negishi, I., Singer, D.S., Singer, A. & Abe, R. (1997). A spontaneously arising mutation in the DLAARN motif of murine ZAP-70 abrogates kinase activity and arrests thymocyte development. *Immunity* 6: 663–671.

Williams, D.H., Woodrow, M., Cantrell, D.A. & Murray, E.J. (1995). Protein–Kinase-C is not a downstream effector of p21(Ras) in activated T-cells. *Eur. J. Immunol.* 25: 42–47.

Wu, J., Motto, D.G., Koretzky, G.A. & Weiss, A. (1996). Vav and Slp-76 interact and functionally cooperate in Il-2 gene activation. *Immunity* 4: 593–602.

Yamanashi, Y., Kakiuchi, T., Mizuguchi, J., Yamamoto, T. & Toyoshima, K. (1991). Association of b-cell antigen receptor with protein tyrosine kinase Lyn. *Science* 251: 192–194.

Yang, W.Y., Malek, S.N. & Desiderio, S. (1995). An SH3-binding site conserved in Brutons tyrosine kinase and related tyrosine kinases mediates specific protein interactions in-vitro and in-vivo. *J. Biol. Chem.* 270: 20 832–20 840.

Zweifach, A. & Lewis, R.S. (1993). Mitogen-regulated Ca^{2+} current of T-lymphocytes is activated by depletion of intracellular Ca^{2+} stores. *Proc. Natl. Acad. Sci., USA* 90: 6295–6299.

8

The role of adhesion mechanisms in inflammation

C. PITZALIS

Introduction

Adhesion mechanisms play extraordinarily diverse roles in many biological phenomena. These range from physiological events in early life, when they are crucial for the development of the embryo, to pathological processes, including tumour growth and metastasis. In some cases, adhesion molecules act as receptors for infective agents such as viruses and parasites. From the immunological point of view, they are involved in virtually every process involving cell contact from thymic selection to antigen processing, from antigen priming to cell activation, from cytotoxicity to lymphocyte recirculation. The last process is part of a sophisticated system that allows efficient surveillance of the various tissues in the body for the presence of infectious pathogens and 'dangerous' exogenous or endogenous antigens. However, when the immune response goes astray, these same mechanisms are often responsible for the perpetuation of inflammation. A classical example is provided by RA and the other chronic inflammatory arthropathies, where the persistent synovial inflammation is maintained, among other factors, by the continuous migration of inflammatory cells from the bloodstream into the joint. Adhesion mechanisms further contribute to the perpetuation of the inflammatory response by the retention of these cells within the tissues, through interactions with extracellular matrix components, and by facilitating contact-dependent immunological events.

In this review, I will concentrate firstly on the general mechanisms that regulate the process of leukocyte extravasation from the blood into the tissues. Secondly, I will discuss the additional mechanisms that finely tune this process to allow the selective migration of distinct leukocyte populations in specific conditions and into different organs. Thirdly, I will consider some of the mechanisms involved in cell migration, spatial orientation and retention within the tissues. Finally, I will focus on the current therapeutic developments that target adhesion mechanisms.

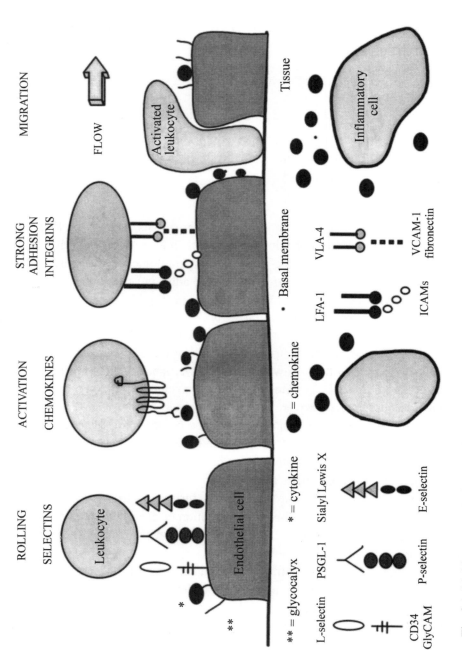

Fig. 8.1. Multistep model of migration.

Regulation of leukocyte migration: general mechanisms

The initial stage in the process of cell extravasation into the tissues is the inter-action of circulating leukocytes with vascular endothelium. As initially shown by Gowans and co-workers (Gowans & Knight, 1964; Marchesi & Gowans, 1964), and subsequently confirmed by others (Anderson & Anderson, 1976; Smith & Ford, 1983), cell migration into lymphoid tissues occurs at specialized postcap-illary vascular sites called high endothelial venules (HEV) because of the par-ticular cuboidal morphology of the endothelial cells. In non-lymphoid tissues, migration takes place also in postcapillary venules, where blood flow velocity is reduced, but, unlike lymphoid HEV, the vessels are lined by flat endothelium. Interestingly, in cronically inflamed tissues such as the rheumatoid synovium, HEV-like vessels are also formed (Freemont *et al.*, 1983; Freemont, 1988; Yanni *et al.*, 1993). Here, HEV are localized in areas where the infiltrating lympho-cytes are organized in lymphoid follicle-like structures, in contrast to areas with a diffuse lymphocytic infiltrate, where the endothelium remains flat (Yanni *et al.*, 1993; van Dinther-Janssen *et al.*, 1990). This suggests that HEV formation can be induced outside the lymphoid tissues in response to local factors such as inflammatory cytokines and in association with an increase in lymphocyte traf-fic. Similar factors also appear to be important for the maintenance of HEV in lymphoid tissues, as lymph node HEV convert from a high to a flat endothelial morphology following ligation of the afferent lymphatics (Mebius *et al.*, 1991).

Our understanding of the actual process of adhesion to and migration through the endothelium has grown considerably since the mid-1980s mainly following studies investigating leukocyte adhesion under conditions of flow both *in vitro* and *in vivo* (Lawrence & Springer, 1991; Ley & Gaehtgens, 1991; Ley *et al.*, 1991; von Andrian *et al.*, 1991). It has become apparent that the way in which leukocytes overcome the shear forces associated with blood flow is through a series of co-ordinated events mediated by specific adhesion molecules. For exam-ple, it was observed that some of the leukocytes come into brief contact with the endothelial ligands, slow their movement and start rolling gently. Some cells then disengage and are carried on by the flow, whereas others come to a complete halt. These latter cells change shape, acquiring a flattened morphology and, within a few minutes, actively migrate between the endothelial cells. The cascade of molecular events that regulate these processes has been clarified by a number of studies. These have given rise to a consensus model of four sequential steps: (i) tethering/rolling, (ii) triggering/activation, (iii) strong adhesion, and (iv) transendothelial migration (Butcher, 1991; Adams & Shaw, 1994; Springer, 1994). These four phases, shown schematically in Fig. 8.1, will now be described in more detail.

Tethering/rolling

The first step, tethering/rolling, is transient, activation independent and mediated by inducible or constitutively expressed selectin molecules and their cognate oligosaccharide ligands (Table 8.1). The selectin family (CD62) consists of three similar single-chain membrane glycoproteins (L-selectin, E-selectin and P-selectin) each of which comprises a Ca^{2+}-dependent amino terminal lectin domain, a proximal epidermal growth factor-like motif and a series of complement regulatory protein-like units of approximately 60 amino acid residues each (Bevilacqua & Nelson, 1993; Lasky, 1995a). L-selectin is constitutively expressed by the majority of neutrophils and monocytes and by approximately half of the lymphocytes. E-selectin is expressed only by endothelial cells, mainly following activation by, for example, endotoxin, IL-1 or TNFα. Its expression requires *de novo* mRNA and protein synthesis and it is maximally expressed at 4 to 6 hours, with a decline to baseline level by 24 hours. P-selectin is found in synthesized form in the α granules of platelets and the Weibel–Palade bodies of the endothelium. P-selectin is rapidly mobilized, both in platelets and endothelial cells, to the cell surface after stimulation by several mediators including thrombin, histamine and terminal complement components (Bevilacqua & Nelson, 1993; Lasky, 1995a).

Selectins are long molecules, which makes them ideally designed to protrude from the cell surface and to interact with appropriate receptors in conditions of flow (Lasky, 1992). All selectins appear to bind to sialylated and fucosylated carbohydrate determinants on their counter-receptors. E-selectin and P-selectin recognize carbohydrate structures closely related to the tetrasaccharide sialyl Lewis[x] and its isomer sialyl Lewis[a] (Lasky, 1995a). In addition, P-selectin binds to a heavily glycosylated 120 kDa glycoprotein named P-selectin glycoprotein ligand 1 (PSGL-1). This is a member of the sialomucin family of adhesion proteins, which contain numerous O-linked carbohydrate side-chains that are attached to serine- and threonine-rich domains (Lasky, 1995b). Two other important members of this family function as ligands for L-selectin: glycosylation-dependent cell adhesion molecule-1 (GlyCAM-1) and CD34. GlyCAM-1 is highly expressed by peripheral lymph node HEV and, for this reason, it is believed to act as an addressin molecule for lymphocyte homing to peripheral lymph nodes (see below). Protein sequence analysis revealed that GlyCAM-1 does not contain a transmembrane anchoring motif, which suggests that either it binds indirectly to the luminal surface of HEV or that it functions as a soluble molecule. In contrast, CD34 contains a classical transmembrane domain that stabilizes the molecule within the endothelial membrane. Another important difference is that CD34 is globally expressed at various endothelial sites. However, the glycosy-

Table 8.1. *Selectins and their ligands in leukocyte–endothelial interactions*

Endothelial distribution	Endothelial receptor/ligand	Leukocyte receptor/ligand	Leukocyte distribution
HEV, activated endothelium	GlyCAM-1, CD34	L-selectin/CD62L	Lymphocyte subset, monocytes, neutrophils, eosinophils
Endothelial Weibel–Palade granules, platelet α granules	P-selectin/ CD62PP	P-selectin glycoprotein ligand 1 (PSGL-1), sialyl Lewis[x/a]	Neutrophils, monocytes, lymphocyte subset, natural killer cells
Activated endothelium	E-selectin/CD62E	Sialyl Lewis [x/a]	Neutrophils, monocytes, eosinophils, basophils, lymphocyte subset, natural killer cells

lation of CD34 differs according to the tissue in which it is expressed. Notably, the CD34 expressed by the HEV of peripheral lymph nodes contains the sulphated carbohydrate ligand for L-selectin while the CD34 expressed at other sites does not contain this unique oligosaccharide (Baumhueter *et al.*, 1994). Therefore, it is likely that the binding specificity of sialomucin is dependent on the types of carbohydrate modification that occur during its transit through the secretory pathway to the cell surface. The rigid rod-like structure of these molecules, however, is likely to produce the extended matrix upon which the various oligosaccharide ligands are presented above the cellular glycocalyx. Here they will be recognized by selectin molecules expressed on specific microvillar cell surface projections of leukocytes flowing nearby. This interaction, although not very strong, is sufficient to slow down the leukocytes, make them roll on the endothelium and facilitate their sampling the local microenvironment for the presence of migratory signals such as inflammatory products. If these are present, the adhesion cascade will be triggered to proceed towards the subsequent steps. If not, the transient nature of selectin binding allows leukocytes to disengage and to be carried on by the flow.

The functional role of selectin molecules *in vivo* is further illustrated by selective gene deletion in animals. Lymphocytes from L-selectin-deficient mice do not bind to peripheral lymph node HEV and show a significant defect in their rolling and migration capacity (Arbones *et al.*, 1994; Tedder, Steeber & Pizcueta, 1995). In E- and P-selectin double knock-out animals, leukocytes are virtually unable to extravasate from the circulation (Frenette *et al.*, 1996). As a consequence inflammatory/immune responses, including delayed-type hypersensitivity, are grossly impaired (Staite *et al.*, 1996). A human disease called leukocyte adhesion deficiency 2 (LAD-2) illustrates the importance of the carbohydrate ligands to which selectin molecules bind (Etzioni *et al.*, 1993). In this condition, an unknown metabolic defect results in a complete lack of fucose production, which, in turn, leads to the absence of surface-expressed fucosylated selectin ligands. Neutrophils from these patients are unable to bind to immobilized E-selectin *in vitro*, and, not surprisingly, these patients cannot mount an appropriate inflammatory response to external pathogens.

Triggering/activation

The second step, triggering/activation is necessary for the activation of integrin molecules. This leads to an increase in their avidity, which renders them capable of mediating the third phase: strong leukocyte–endothelial adhesion. Several chemotactic factors have been described as having triggering/activating properties, including bacterial wall components and complement products (Table 8.2). The most important molecules, however, appear to be a series of chemoattractant cytokines (chemokines) of which more than 40 have been described (Schall & Bacon, 1994; Baggiolini *et al.*, 1997). Chemokines (CKs) are small-molecular-weight molecules (68 to 120 amino acid residues in size) that share structural similarities, including four conserved cysteine residues, which form disulphide bonds in the tertiary structure of the proteins. The majority can be incorporated into two large subfamilies: C-X-C (where X is any amino acid) and C-C chemokines, according to whether an intervening residue spaces the first two cysteines in the motif or they remain adjacent. A third subfamily, which so far has only one member, lymphotactin, has been described (Kennedy *et al.* 1995). Lymphotactin has a high degree of homology with the other two subfamilies but lacks the first and third cysteine. Finally, a fourth molecule (fractalkine), characterized by an interposition of three amino acids between the first two cysteines (C-X$_3$-C), has recently been added to the list (Bazan *et al.*, 1997). Interestingly, unlike other CK types, the polypeptide chain of fractalkine is predicted to be part of a target 373 amino acid residue protein with a CK domain and an extended mucin-like stalk. This would allow one end of the molecule to anchor to the surface of the endothelium while the other end, carrying on its top the CK motif, would protrude deeply in the vascular lumen. Similarly, it has been suggested that other CKs can be immobilized in a solid phase on the endothelial surface

Table 8.2 *Leukocyte chemoattractants*

Chemoattractant	Origin	Responding cells
Classical chemoattractants		Monocytes, neutrophils,
N-formyl peptides	Bacterial protein processing	eosinophils, basophils
C5a	Complement activation	Monocytes, neutrophils, eosinophils, basophils
Leukotriene B4	Arachidonate metabolism	Monocytes, neutrophils
Platelet-activating factor	Phosphatidylcholine metabolism	Monocytes, neutrophils, eosinophils
C-X-C chemokines SDF-1, IL-8; GROα, GROβ, GROγ; NAP-2; ENA-78; GCP2; PF4, Ip10; Mig; CKα1; CKα2	T lymphocytes, monocytes, endothelial cells, fibroblasts, keratinocytes, chondrocytes, mesothelial cells	Neutrophils, basophils, fibroblasts
C-C chemokines MCP -1, -2, -3, -4; eotaxin; MIP-1α, MIP-1β; I–309; CK β4, β6, β7, β8, β9, β11, β12, β13; RANTES; HCC-1, -2, -3; TARC	T lymphocytes, monocytes, fibroblasts, endothelial cells, smooth muscle cells, platelets, mast cells	Monocytes, T lymphocyte subpopulation, eosinophils, basophils

via electrostatic interactions with negatively charged proteoglycans and CD44 molecules expressed by endothelial cells (Tanaka *et al.*, 1993a; Tanaka, Adams & Shaw, 1993b). This hypothesis provides a valid model of how, *in vivo*, a high concentration of chemotactic factors is maintained at the luminal surface of blood vessels adjacent to areas of inflammation, preventing them from being washed away by the flow.

CK are thought to mediate their effects via interactions with seven membrane-spanning domain receptors (CKR) that form a distinct group of structurally related proteins within the superfamily of receptors that signal through heterotrimeric GTP-binding proteins (Kelvin *et al.*, 1993; Neote *et al.*, 1993; Premack & Schall, 1996). CKR also have two conserved cysteines (one in the amino terminal domain and the other in the third extracellular loop), which are assumed to form a disulphide bond critical for the conformation of the lig-and-binding pocket. Engagement of CKR results in activation of phospholipases,

Table 8.3 *Ligand selectivity of chemokine (CK) receptors*

Receptors	New nomenclature	Old nomenclature	Ligands
C-X-C family	CXCR1	IL-8R1 (type A)	IL-8
	CXCR2	IL-8R2 (type B)	IL-8, GROα, GROβ, GROγ, NAP2, ENA78, GCP-2
	CXCR3	IP10/MigR	IP10, Mig
	CXCR4	LESTR, HUMSTR	SDF-1
C-C family	CCR1	RANTES, MIP-1αR	RANTES, MIP-1α, MCP-2, MCP-3
	CCR2a/b	MCP-1RA/B	MCP-1, MCP-2, MCP-3, MCP-4
	CCR3	EotaxinR, C-C CKR3	Eotaxin, RANTES, MCP-3, MCP-4
	CCR4	C-C CKR4	RANTES, MIP-1α, MCP-1
	CCR5	C-C CKR5	RANTES, MIP-1α, MIP-1β

with downstream generation of inositol triphosphate and intracellular mobilization of Ca^{2+} and of small GTP-binding proteins such as the Ras, Rac and Rho families. The Rho family, in particular, seems to be instrumental in relaying the signal from the CKR to cell-surface integrins (Laudanna, Campbell & Butcher, 1996). For each CK class several CKR have been identified (Table 8.3) (Premack & Schall, 1996; Baggiolini *et al.*, 1997). The majority of CKR interact with more than one CK (shared specificity within class), except CXCR1 and CXCR4, which are specific for IL-8 and SDF-1, respectively.

Besides the functions described, the interaction of CKs with their receptors appears to serve another very important role, which is the selective chemo-attraction of different leukocyte populations. It is well established that the C-X-C family act mainly on neutrophils while C-C members attract principally lymphocytes, monocytes, eosinophils and natural killer cells (Schall & Bacon, 1994; Schall *et al.* 1993b). Lymphotactin is uniquely specific for lymphocytes (Kennedy *et al.*, 1995) while, within the C-C family, eotaxin specifically attracts eosinophils (Kitaura *et al.*, 1996). CK selectivity is partially owing to a quantitative and/or qualitative variation of CKR expression by the responsive cells. For example, eotaxin specificity is strengthened by the high expression of the eotaxin receptor (CCR3) by eosinophils (Ponath *et al.*, 1996). Therefore, the combination of varied CK production and differential receptor expression may play an important role in regulating the diversity of leukocyte migration (see below). The report that, at least *in vitro*, some C-C CK (RANTES, MIP-1α, MIP-1β, MCP-1) favour chemoattraction, and transendothelial migration of specific lymphocyte subsets lends support to this hypothesis (Schall *et al.*, 1993a; Roth, Carr & Springer, 1995). Another factor to bear in mind is that, in response to inflammatory stimuli, several chemoattractant molecules are produced by the endothelial cells themselves (Table 8.2), which, therefore, actively contribute to recruiting leukocytes at sites of inflammation (Huber *et al.*, 1991; Zimmerman, Prescott & McIntyre, 1992).

Strong adhesion

The third stage is strong adhesion of the leukocytes. During this step leukocytes stop rolling and firmly adhere to the vascular endothelium before transmigrating between the endothelial cells. The third phase is primarily mediated by activated β_2 and α_4 integrins (Hogg & Landis, 1993; Hogg *et al.*, 1993; Springer, 1994) and their counter-receptors belonging to the immunoglobulin superfamily: ICAM-1, ICAM-2, VCAM-1 and MADCAM-1 (Table 8.4). Integrins are a large family of heterodimeric glycoproteins formed by two non-covalently linked subunits, a larger α chain (120–180 kDa) and smaller β chain (90–110 kDa). Both subunits are integral membrane proteins with a small carboxy terminal cytoplasmic domain and a large amino-terminal extracellular domain. At present there are at least 20 α chains and eight β chains, which can be found in many but not all of the possible combinations (Larson & Springer, 1990; Ruoslahti, 1991; Hynes, 1992). The heterodimeric structure of β_2 integrins comprises an α chain linked to a common β chain (Table 8.4). Three members belong to this subfamily: LFA-1 ($\alpha_L\beta_2$; CD11a/CD18), Mac-1 ($\alpha_M\beta_2$; CD11b/CD18), and p150,95 ($\alpha_X\beta_2$; CD11c/CD18). LFA-1 is present constitutively on the surface of virtually all circulating leukocytes while Mac-1 and p150,95 have a more limited distribution on neutrophils, monocytes and natural killer cells. Apart from their key role in mediating adhesion to endothelium, β_2 integrins are also involved in most immune functions requiring homo- and heterotypic cell contact. In comparison to the β_2 integrins, α_4 integrins have a common α chain associated with a variable β chain (Table 8.4). The $\alpha_4\beta_1$ molecule belongs to the β_1 integrin subfamily. This group is also known as VLA molecules and its main function is to act as receptors for extracellular matrix components (see below). However, in contrast to other members of this family, $\alpha_4\beta_1$ integrins can also mediate binding to the endothelial ligand VCAM-1(see below). Therefore, $\alpha_4\beta_1$ integrin can, through different binding sites, mediate leukocyte interactions with both the endothelium

Table 8.4. *Integrins and their ligands in leukocyte–endothelial interactions*

Subunit	Alternative name	Distribution	Ligand
β2-integrins			
$\alpha_L\beta_2$	LFA-1, CD11a/CD18	B and T lymphocytes, monocytes, neutrophils	ICAM-1, ICAM-2, ICAM-3
$\alpha_m\beta_2$	Mac-1, CR3, CD11b/CD18	Monocytes, neutrophils, natural killer cells	ICAM-1, iC3b, fibrinogen, factor X
$\alpha_x\beta_2$	p150,95, CD11c/CD18	Monocytes, neutrophils, natural killer cells	iC3b, fibrinogen
α4-Integrins			
$\alpha_4\beta_1$	VLA-4, CD49d/CD29	B and T lymphocytes, monocytes, neural crest-derived cells, fibroblasts, muscle cells	VCAM-1, fibronectin
$\alpha_4\beta_7$	LPAM-1, CD49d/CD	B and T lymphocyte subpopulations	MadCAM-1, VCAM-1, fibronectin

cells and the extracellular matrix (Pulido *et al.*, 1991; Masumoto & Hemler, 1993; Humphries *et al.*, 1995). This can facilitate not only the process of cell extravasation but also cell orientation and migration within the tissues. The α_4 integrin chain can also associate with the β_7 chain to form $\alpha_4\beta_7$ which, besides mediating adhesion to VCAM-1 and fibronectin, is involved in lymphocyte homing to mucosal associated lymphoid tissue and, for this reason, will be discussed below (Andrew *et al.*, 1994).

The immunoglobulin supergene family is a large group of cell membrane glycoproteins that are typified by a common structure similar in its domain organization to immunoglobulins. Their structure consists of a single chain that contains a series of C_2-like heavy chain immunoglobulin domains of approximately 100–110 amino acid residues. ICAM-1 (CD54) is a glycosylated cell surface protein, of about 90 kDa, containing five tandem extracellular immunoglobulin-like domains (Simmons, 1995; Etzioni, 1996). In contrast to LFA-1, which is restricted to leukocytes, ICAM-1 is expressed on a variety of other cell types including thymic epithelial cells, fibroblasts, epidermal keratinocytes and endothelial cells. On resting endothelium, ICAM-1 is present only at a low level, but its expression is rapidly upregulated following stimulation by several inflammatory mediators such as lipopolysaccharide, IFN-γ, IL-1 and TNFα. Enhanced surface expression of ICAM-1 is first seen at 4 hours, is usually maximal at 24 hours and can persist for up to 48 hours or longer (Dustin, Staunton & Springer,

1988). In contrast to ICAM-1, ICAM-2 has only two immunoglobulin-like domains, which show a 35% homology with the two amino terminal domains of ICAM-1 (Staunton, Dustin & Springer 1989). Furthermore, ICAM-2 is highly expressed on resting endothelium and cannot be upregulated by inflammatory mediators. Therefore, it would appear that ICAM-1 has a more prominent role in activation-dependent adhesion and migration, while ICAM-2 is likely to be more important in regulating basal physiological cell migration and cyto-adhesiveness. A third ICAM (ICAM-3) is also a ligand for LFA-1 but is not expressed by endothelial cells and will be not discussed further.

VCAM-1 has a molecular weight of approximately 110 000 and consists of six or seven extracellular immunoglobulin-like domains generated by alternative splicing of the same gene located on chromosome 1 (Cybulsky *et al.*, 1991a,b). Both forms are fully functional and, as is the case for ICAM-1 (Staunton *et al.*, 1990), only the first two domains are required for its adhesion function (Osborn *et al.*, 1994). VCAM-1 is not expressed on resting endothelial cells but is upregulated with the same kinetics as ICAM-1 after cytokine or endotoxin stimulation of the endothelium. This suggests that VCAM-1 is important in regulating cell migration in response to inflammation. Support for this hypothesis came from several studies, which confirmed the notable contribution of VLA-4-dependent pathways in lymphocyte adhesion and migration in inflammatory conditions (Elices *et al.*, 1993; Yang *et al.*, 1993; Rabb *et al.*, 1994). However, since the expression of VCAM-1 in the synovium has been shown to be confined mainly to the synovial lining and is expressed only weakly by the endothelium (Morales-Ducret *et al.*, 1992; Wilkinson *et al.*, 1993), some doubts have been expressed as to the real importance of the VLA-4/VCAM-1 interaction in leukocyte extravasation to the joint. The report of the presence of the CS-1 peptide of fibronectin on the luminal surface of synovial endothelial cells has prompted the attractive proposal that, in such an environment, the preferred ligand for VLA-4 could be the CS-1 fibronectin peptide rather than VCAM-1 (van Dinther-Janssen *et al.*, 1993; Elices *et al.*, 1994). The other important member of the immunoglobulin superfamily is the mucosal cell adhesion molecule 1 (MAdCAM-1). MAdCAM-1 is a hybrid molecule composed of three immunoglobulin-like domains and a mucin-like region interposed between domains 2 and 3 (Briskin *et al.*, 1993; Sampaio *et al.*, 1995). Given its predominant expression on the intestinal endothelium and in mucosal-associated lymphoid tissue (MALT), hence its name, MAdCAM-1 is instrumental in lymphocyte homing to mucosal organs and will be discussed in greater detail below.

As mentioned above, integrin activation is an essential component in the increased molecular adhesiveness that allows leukocytes to bind strongly to endothelial ligands and overcome the hydrodynamic shear forces in the circulation. Integrin-binding avidity has been shown to be rapidly modulated (within seconds) by divalent cations, such as Mn^{2+}, N-formylated peptide and chemokines (Dransfield et al., 1992; Hogg & Landis, 1993). The mechanism by which this occurs is not completely clear, but surface redistribution leading to integrin clustering and/or conformational changes in the tertiary molecular structure are thought to be the most important (Kornberg et al., 1992; Hogg & Landis, 1993; Hogg et al., 1993). Conformational changes in LFA-1 and Mac-1 are suggested by studies using monoclonal antibodies (mAbs) that react with these integrins after cellular activation but not in resting conditions (Diamond & Springer, 1993; Landis, Bennett & Hogg, 1993). For example, saturation binding studies have shown that, following neutrophil activation with chemoattractants, 10% of surface Mac-1 molecules express an activation epitope. Furthermore, blockade of this epitope inhibits neutrophil binding to purified ICAM-1 (Diamond & Springer, 1993). Finally, measurements of the affinity of cell surface LFA-1 for soluble monomeric ICAM-1 have directly demonstrated an increase of approximately 200-fold in a subpopulation of LFA-1 molecules after cellular activation (Lollo et al., 1993). The rapid ability to modulate the adhesion/de-adhesion integrin status is a crucial mechanism to prevent random adhesion in the bloodstream, to respond swiftly to microenvironmental signals and to facilitate the process of diapedesis (see below).

As for the selectins, much information on the importance of β_2 and α_4 integrins is gained from selective gene deletion experiments in animals (Sharpe, 1995; Arroyo et al., 1996; Shier et al., 1996) and from the human syndrome of leukocyte adhesion deficiency 1 (LAD-1) (Anderson & Springer, 1987; Fischer et al., 1988). This condition is caused by a mutation in the gene of the common β_2 subunit, which leads to deficient expression of mature integrins on the cell surface. Neutrophils from these patients fail to migrate in response to chemoattractants and are unable to bind to and cross the endothelium at sites of infection. Patients suffer from recurrent bacterial infections that are often fatal in childhood. Of course, the severity of the syndrome is also influenced by the fact that integrin molecules function as accessory molecules in leukocyte interactions with other cells such as antigen-presenting cells, stromal cells or infected cells and are, therefore, important for many other immune functions including antigen, presentation/response and cytotoxicity (Harlan, 1993).

Transendothelial migration

Of the four steps involved in leukocyte extravasation, transendothelial migration is the least characterized. To complete the process of transendothelial migration, or diapedesis, leukocytes that are strongly attached to the endothelium have to crawl between the endothelial cells and cross the basal membrane. Initiation of cell locomotion involves a directional protrusion of the leading edge, presumably via actin polymerization, to form a lamellipodium, which attaches to the substratum. The adhesive strength at the cell front must be sufficient to generate force and traction to pull the cell forward. In contrast, the adhesive strength at the cell rear must be weaker to allow the cell to detach and retract forward. Although our understanding of the molecular mechanisms governing these processes is limited, activated integrins seem to play an important role (Hogg & Landis, 1993; Springer, 1994). Integrins connect the external substratum with the cytoskeleton. The integrin cytoplasmic domain, at least *in vitro*, has been shown to associate with structural proteins present in focal adhesion such as talin and α-actin (Pavalko *et al.*, 1991; Otey, Pavalko & Burridge, 1990). The integrin–receptor complex serves not only as a structural link but also as a signalling unit, since, in addition to the above structural proteins, regulatory proteins such as focal adhesion kinase (FAK) are found in association with it (Kornberg *et al.*, 1992; Parsons *et al.*, 1994). Furthermore, phospholipase Cγ (PLCγ) and phosphoinositide (PI) 3-kinase also appear to associate with integrins as a necessary interaction for motogenesis (Clark & Brugge, 1995). Finally, the Rho subfamily is also involved in the signalling cascade that leads to the formation of lamellipodia, focal adhesion and stress fibres (Hotchin & Hall, 1996; Tapon & Hall, 1997). In addition, regulation of Rho is implicated in adhesive release, as when Rho is inactivated the actin cytoskeleton collapses and the cells adopt a rounded morphology (Miura *et al.*, 1993). Even less is known concerning the mechanisms involved in crossing the basal membrane; however, surface-associated proteases seem to be important.

In conclusion, although there are still more questions than answers, some progress has been made in defining the relevant molecules that regulate this last process of cell extravasation.

Diversity of leukocyte migration: specific mechanisms

The mechanisms discussed up to now apply generally to all leukocytes. However, the migration of various leukocyte populations is not a random process but has been fine tuned to allow for diversity and specialization in response to different conditions. These include, among others, the stage and type of inflammation, the prevalent pattern of cytokines/chemokines produced in various tissues and the state of lymphocyte differentiation (Pitzalis, 1993). It is well known, for example, that during an acute inflammatory response neutrophils are the prevalent cells, while during the chronic phase mononuclear cells predominate. In allergic reactions or in responses to parasites, by comparison, eosinophils come prominently into play. This is mainly a result of the increased production of IL-5, which stimulates eosinophil differentiation in the bone marrow and, as discussed above, of the local production of eotaxin, which favours eosinophil extravasation into the allergic tissues (Rothenberg *et al.*, 1996). Finally the state of leukocyte differentiation can greatly influence their trafficking pattern. The most striking example is the different recirculatory pattern shown by naive/resting (CD45RA+) versus memory/activated (CD45R0+) lymphocyte populations. Naive lymphocytes recirculate mainly through secondary lymphoid organs (peripheral lymph nodes, Peyer's patches, tonsils and spleen), where they are primed to various antigens drained from different tissues. Memory/activated lymphocytes, although capable of accessing lymphoid organs, primarily recirculate to peripheral inflamed tissues, where they can exert their effector function (Mackay *et al.*, 1992a). Evidence for this dichotomy *in vivo* comes from animal work demonstrating that immunoblasts from the gut and skin, as well as from peripheral lymph nodes, preferentially home to the same type of tissue from which they were isolated (Gowans & Knight, 1964; Rose, Parrott & Bruce, 1978; Issekutz, Chin & Hay, 1982; Mackay *et al.*, 1992b). However, in humans the evidence is mainly indirect. *In vitro* studies, using a lymphocyte-binding assay with frozen tissue sections, have demonstrated a differential ability of various lymphoblastoid lines to bind to peripheral lymph node tissue and synovial microvascular endothelium (Jalkanen *et al.*, 1986). Using the same assay, it has been also shown that T cell lines derived from peripheral lymph node, gut and synovium preferentially adhere to homotypic tissue sections (Salmi *et al.*, 1992). On the basis of these and many other studies, it has been proposed that entry into different tissue sites is regulated by specific receptor/counter-receptor pairs of adhesion molecules expressed by migrating lymphocytes and by the microvascular endothelium of a given organ. The lymphocyte-associated molecules, bearing the organ selective interaction with the microvascular endothelium, are termed homing receptors (HR), while the cognate microvascular endothelial ligands are defined as vascular addressins (VA) (Butcher, 1992; Picker, 1992; Butcher & Picker, 1996).

The first characterized example of HR–VA interaction was the HR expressed by lymphocytes homing to peripheral lymph nodes. This HR, initially defined in the mouse by the mAb MEL-14 (Gallatin, Weissman & Butcher, 1983) and in human by the DREG series of mAbs (Kishimoto, Jutila & Butcher, 1990), which recognizes L-selectin, specifically mediates binding to endothelial VA of the peripheral lymph nodes (Imai *et al.*, 1991). The carbohydrate-based VA in the peripheral lymph nodes was initially identified in mice using the mAb MECA-79 (Streeter, Rouse & Butcher, 1988b). This was subsequently found to be the equivalent of human GlyCAM-1 (Michie *et al.*, 1993). Another mAb from the MECA-series (MECA-367) (Streeter *et al.*, 1988a) was instrumental in identifying the mucosa-associated VA. While MECA-79 differentially stains and blocks the adhesive function of VA in peripheral lymph nodes, MECA-367 shows the converse pattern of reactivity, staining the microvascular endothelium of Peyer's patches. This led to the definition of a second pair of HR/VA molecules in which the $\alpha_4\beta_7$ integrin was shown to selectively bind to mucosal VA, now called MAdCAM-1 (Berlin *et al.*, 1993; Briskin *et al.*, 1993). The functional role of L-selectin and $\alpha_4\beta_7$ integrin in mediating specific lymphocyte homing has been recently demonstrated by specific gene ablation in mice. As expected, L-selectin knock-out mice have a severe reduction in the size of their peripheral lymph nodes (Arbones *et al.*, 1994) while β_7 integrin-deficient animals show an underdeveloped MALT (Wagner *et al.*, 1996). Lymphocytes derived from these animals display a decreased capacity to bind to peripheral lymph nodes and mucosal HEV, respectively. Moreover, in humans, a particular type of non-Hodgkin's lymphoma characterized by multifocal infiltration of the intestinal tract (malignant lymphomatous polyposis) expresses $\alpha_4\beta_7$ integrin, unlike the nodal variety of the disease (Pals *et al.*, 1994). This suggests that HR are involved not only in normal lymphocyte recirculation but also in determining the pattern of dissemination of malignant cells. Further support for this hypothesis comes from the fact that, in cutaneous T cell lymphoma, most lymphocytes infiltrating the skin express the cutaneous lymphocyte antigen (CLA) (Picker *et al.*, 1990). CLA is a cell-surface glycosylated protein that contains a CD15 (Lewis[x]) carbohydrate backbone and binds strongly to E-selectin (Koszik *et al.*, 1994). This has led to the proposal of CLA and E-selectin as the HR-VA specific for the skin (Picker *et al.*, 1990; Berg *et al.*, 1991; Picker, 1992).

Although other homing specificities to organs such as the lung (Picker *et al.*, 1994) and the synovium (Jalkanen *et al.*, 1986) have been described, the idea of selective migration to different peripheral tissues remains controversial. Whereas there is little doubt of the critical importance of HR–VA adhesive interactions, it has become clear that the molecular control of lymphocyte homing is a flexible process that can adapt to different pathophysiological situations. For example, while selective lymphocyte homing is of major importance during the 'basal patrolling' of various organs, it becomes much less so during acute inflammation. For instance, in basal conditions, the traffic of memory cells through lymph nodes is low while this increases dramatically in those lymph nodes draining an inflammatory focus (reactive lymphadenopathy) (Mackay, Marston & Dudler, 1992a). It has also been recognized that a model postulating that a single tissue specificity depends on a single homing receptor–addressin molecule interaction is too simplistic (Picker, 1994; Butcher & Picker, 1996). Some HR, for example, facilitate lymphocyte adhesion to more than one tissue and some of the proposed 'specific' VA molecules have a widespread distribution in different organs (Picker, 1994; Butcher & Picker, 1996). For example, as mentioned above, it has been suggested that the accumulation of memory T cells to the skin is dependent on the interaction of CLA with E-selectin (Picker *et al.*, 1990; Berg *et al.*, 1991). However, E-selectin is highly expressed on the MVE of various inflamed tissues, including the skin and synovium in psoriatic arthritis, but CLA-positive lymphocytes are found only in the skin and not the joint (Pitzalis *et al.*, 1996). Therefore, the expression of E-selectin *per se* is not sufficient to favour the migration of CLA-positive cells to tissues other than the skin. Conversely, a single molecule found mainly on one tissue can bind more than one subset of T cells. For example, a variant of the gut addressin MAdCAM-1, when expressing a carbohydrate determinant that ligates L-selectin, binds both $\alpha_4\beta_7$-positive/L-selectin-positive (naive) and $\alpha_4\beta_7$-positive/L-selectin-negative (memory) lymphocytes (Sampaio *et al.*, 1995). Therefore, it is likely that the extravasation of different lymphocyte subsets into various tissues is the result of the interaction of multiple adhesion molecule pairs acting in combination, 'telephone area code model' (Springer, 1994). Quantitative as well as qualitative differences in the expression of HR/VA molecules also appear to be important (Butcher & Picker, 1996).

In addition, it is now clear that the original description of the multistep model as a hierarchical process, in which each step was mediated in sequence by different adhesion molecules, was too inflexible. Subsequent studies have, in fact, demonstrated that the same molecule can be involved in more than one step of the adhesion cascade and that some adhesion proteins can be equally involved in general migration and organ-specific homing. For example, α_4 integrins can mediate both secondary and primary adhesion, as indicated by the fact that $\alpha_4\beta_1$ and $\alpha_4\beta_7$ integrins can mediate both firm adhesion and tethering/rolling to purified VCAM-1 and MAdCAM-1, respectively, under conditions of flow (Alon *et al.*, 1995; Berlin *et al.*, 1995). L-selectin, however, is involved in primary adhesion as well as in naive lymphocyte homing to peripheral lymph nodes. Moreover, it is also apparent that selective leukocyte extravasation is dependent not only on ligand–receptor adhesive interactions but also on specific activation signals. For example, it would appear that GlyCAM-1 mediates the migration of naive lymphocytes to the peripheral lymph nodes, not only because of its preferential expression on HEV in that tissue and its interaction with L-selectin, but also because of its capacity to activate CD45 RA lymphocytes specifically (Hwang *et al.*, 1996). Finally, the capacity of CKs to activate selectively different leukocyte populations can further contribute to the development of migration specificity and diversity. In summary, therefore, evolution has allowed provisions for a combinatorial adhesion and signalling system in which general mechanisms of migration integrate and overlap with organ-specific homing, depending on the various requirements associated with different pathophysiological situations.

Mechanisms of cell orientation, migration and retention within tissues

Once recruited into tissues, leukocytes follow different fates. Neutrophils tend to die while mononuclear cells may return to the circulation via the lymphatics or may be retained within the tissue, where they tend to segregate into specialized microenvironments. The best example of this 'microenviromental homing' is represented by the specific localization of B and T cells in particular areas of lymphoid tissue. In chronic inflammatory lesions, such as the RA synovium, mononuclear cells can be found either in a diffuse distribution, scattered throughout the synovium, or in large focal aggregates, constituting follicle-like structures similar to those found in lymphoid organs. The molecular mechanisms controlling cell locomotion and retention within tissues are complex, once again, and not completely understood. However, adhesion to extracellular matrix constituents such as collagen, proteoglycans, laminin and fibronectin plays a major part. Lymphocytes interact with the extracellular matrix by means of specific adhesion receptors mainly belonging to the β_1 integrin subfamily (also known as VLA molecules). Each VLA integrin has been shown to mediate adhesion to at least one of the three major extracellular matrix glycoproteins. In addition, each ligand is recognized by multiple VLA integrins. Lymphocytes adhere to fibronectin mainly via VLA-4 and VLA-5 integrin receptors, which recognize two different binding sites on the fibronectin molecule. VLA-4 binds to the third connecting segment (IIICS) region (Wayner *et al.*, 1989; Mould *et al.*, 1990), whilst VLA-5 recognizes the key short peptide sequence RGDS within the central cell-binding domain (Pierschbacher, Hayman & Ruoslahti, 1985; Ruoslahti & Pierschbacher, 1987). The collagen receptor has been identified as VLA-1, VLA-2 and VLA-3. Interestingly, VLA-1 and VLA-2 are not present on resting T cells, but they are expressed after long-term activation *in vitro* and in approximately 60% of synovial T cell in RA. The VLA-6 integrin, which was first identified as a laminin receptor on platelets, has recently also been shown to be the laminin receptor on lymphocytes. As a result, the extracellular matrix can provide the supporting physical environment in which lymphocytes can come into close contact with other cells such as antigen-presenting cells for the initiation of the immune response. Furthermore, proteins in the extracellular matrix have multiple adhesive domains that facilitate, in return, a multiplicity of interactions between cells and the matrix; these provide co-stimulatory signals for the amplification of such responses (Matsuyama *et al.*, 1989; Shimizu *et al.*, 1990; Yamada *et al.*, 1991).

In addition to these general mechanisms, specific mechanisms must exist to provide directionality and selective interactions with specialized stromal cells such as the follicular dendritic cells of B cell follicles and the interdigitating cells of T cell zones. In this respect, chemotactic factors and hapoptactic signals are thought to be important. In chemotaxis, cells migrate in the direction of the highest concentration of a chemoattractant (typically a soluble molecule). In hapoptaxis, cells move toward the region of highest adhesiveness (increased expression of adhesion ligands). Several of the molecules already discussed appear to be important in providing spatial orientation signals. CK and CKR may play a critical role in microenvironmental homing, as suggested by the lack of germinal centre formation in BLR-1 (CKR homologue)-deficient animals, which arises because of the inability of B cells from these animals to migrate from the T cell to the B cell areas (Forster *et al.*, 1996). Cytokines also seem important. For example, focal lymphoid aggregate formation in inflamed tissues appears to be dependent on the local production of TNFα as suggested by the fact that TNFα-deficient animals lack proper germinal centres (Pasparakis *et al.*, 1996). By comparison, transgenic animals overexpressing the human TNFα gene have increased formation of focal lymphoid aggregates and develop a chronic arthritis very similar to RA (Keffer *et al.*, 1991). In summary, cell migration and retention within the tissues is probably regulated by overlapping and combinatorially determined adhesion and activation signals in a similar manner to that seen in the events that control cell extravasation from the blood into the tissues.

Adhesion mechanisms as therapeutic targets

Studies in the 1990s have illustrated the paramount importance of adhesion mechanisms in the pathogenesis of inflammation. Not surprisingly, therefore, there has been a great deal of interest in targeting these mechanisms to treat inflammatory conditions such as rheumatic diseases. Moreover, it has become clear that some of the commonly used therapeutic agents in rheumatology have the capacity of modulating these mechanisms. For example, corticosteroids are known to induce leukocytosis and a concomitant decrease in leukocytes in the RA synovium by mobilizing the marginated pool and inhibiting the migration of leukocytes to the joint (Smith *et al.*, 1988; Youssef *et al.*, 1996). Studies *in vitro* have confirmed that corticosteroids can directly inhibit the expression of endothelial (E-selectin and ICAM-1) and leukocyte (LFA-1 and CD2) adhesion molecules (Cronstein *et al.*, 1992; Pitzalis *et al.*, 1997). Methotrexate has been shown to decrease *in vivo* leukocyte adhesion and migration in rat mesenteric venules

(Asako, Wolf & Granger, 1993). This effect is related to the ability of methotrexate to enhance adenosine release, which in turn inhibits the production of the superoxide normally responsible for increasing leukocyte adhesion to endothelial cells (Cronstein *et al.*, 1991). Sulphasalazine, but not sulphapyridine (inactive moiety), has been shown to inhibit the activation-dependent upregulation of CD11b/CD18 by granulocytes and monocytes but not from lymphocytes (Greenfield *et al.*, 1993). Gold treatment decreases the expression of E-selectin by synovial endothelial cells in patients with RA (Corkill *et al.*, 1991). Finally, in patients with psoriasis, cyclosporin A has been shown to reduce dramatically the number of T cells infiltrating the skin and the expression of ICAM-1 on keratinocytes, although, interestingly, not on endothelial cells (Horrocks *et al.*, 1991).

In addition to the 'old drugs', new therapeutic modalities specifically designed to modulate adhesion mechanisms have been developed. The therapeutic potential of mAbs against adhesion molecules has been demonstrated in a variety of animal models, including allograft rejection, cardiac reperfusion injury and experimental autoimmune encephalomyelitis (Isobe *et al.*, 1992; Ma *et al.*, 1992; Yednock *et al.*, 1992). As far as arthritis is concerned, blocking either the LFA-1 or the VLA-4 pathways has been shown to inhibit disease in animals (Jasin *et al.*, 1992; Barbadillo *et al.*, 1995). As a result of these studies, a trial using anti-ICAM-1 mAb has been conducted in RA (Kavanaugh *et al.*, 1994). The patients showed a transient improvement that correlated with the development of a peripheral blood lymphocytosis, suggesting that inhibition of lymphocyte migration into inflammatory sites was occurring. However, the therapeutic effect could also have occurred by inhibiting other adhesion-dependent immune functions in which ICAM-1 plays a major role. Other attempts to block ICAM-1 have been made using soluble and recombinant ICAM-1 constructs (Martin *et al.*, 1993). A new and very exiting therapeutic modality, presented by W. R. Shanahan at the Fourth Symposium on Immunotherapy in Cyprus (May, 1997), is the usage of an ICAM-1 antisense oligodeoxynucleotide product. This preparation hybridizes with a 20 base sequence of the 3'-untranslated region of human ICAM-1 mRNA and inhibits ICAM-1 expression *in vivo* as well as *in vitro*. The drug was shown to prolong cardiac allograft survival and to inhibit dextran sulphate-induced colitis and collagen-induced arthritis in mice. The results of a double-blind placebo-controlled trial in patients with steroid-dependent Crohn's disease were also very encouraging. Despite a very short half-life of approximately 60 minutes, the drug produced a significant steroid-sparing effect and durable remission (mean approximately 5 months) in 47% of the patients. Other ways of modulating cell adhesion involve the use of selectin blockers. Several animal studies have demonstrated the efficacy of this therapeutic modality either using mAbs or blocking oligosaccharides (Mulligan *et al.*, 1993; Nelson *et al.*, 1993; Buerke *et al.*, 1994; Ward & Mulligan, 1994).

However, although therapies designed to block general mechanisms of adhesion might be feasible and effective in acute inflammation or during flares, their usage in chronic diseases requires some caution. In these conditions, the prolonged adhesion blockade, which is likely to be required, may lead to unacceptable side effects similar to those seen in the leukocyte adhesion deficiency syndromes. The alternative strategy would be to target molecules responsible for selective leukocyte migration, for example the inhibition of eotaxin in allergic inflammation. Blocking molecules involved in specific homing may also be a fruitful option. For example, the blockade of the $\alpha_4\beta_7$ integrin has been very effective in an animal model of inflammatory bowel disease (Hesterberg *et al.*, 1996). The discovery of joint-specific mechanisms of migration might open this therapeutic avenue for the treatment of rheumatic diseases.

References

Adams, D.H. & Shaw, S. (1994). Leucocyte–endothelial interactions and regulation of leucocyte migration. [See comments] [Review]. *Lancet*, 343: 831–836.

Alon, R., Kassner, P.D., Carr, M.W., Finger, E.B., Hemler, M.E. & Springer, T.A. (1995). The integrin VLA-4 supports tethering and rolling in flow on VCAM-1. *J. Cell Biol.* 128: 1243–1253.

Anderson, A.O. & Anderson, N.D. (1976). Lymphocyte emigration from high endothelial venules in rat lymph nodes. *Immunology* 31: 731–748.

Anderson, D.C. & Springer, T.A. (1987). Leukocyte adhesion deficiency: an inherited defect in the Mac-1, LFA-1, and p150,95 glycoproteins. *Annu. Rev. Med.* 38: 175–194.

Andrew, D.P., Berlin, C., Honda, S., Yoshino, T., Hamann, A., Holzmann, B. & Butcher, E.C. (1994). Distinct but overlapping epitopes are involved in alpha 4 beta 7-mediated adhesion to vascular cell adhesion molecule-1, mucosal addressin-1, fibronectin, and lymphocyte aggregation. *J. Immunol.* 153: 3847–3861.

Arbones, M.L., Ord, D.C., Ley, K., Ratech, H., Maynard-Curry, C., Otten, G., Capon, D.J. & Tedder, T.F. (1994). Lymphocyte homing and leukocyte rolling and migration are impaired in L-selectin-deficient mice. *Immunity* 1: 247–260.

Arroyo, A.G., Yang, J.T., Rayburn, H. & Hynes, R.O. (1996). Differential requirements for alpha4 integrins during fetal and adult hematopoiesis. *Cell* 85: 997–1008.

Asako, H., Wolf, R.E. & Granger, D.N. (1993). Leukocyte adherence in rat mesenteric venules: effects of adenosine and methotrexate. *Gastroenterology* 104: 31–37.

Baggiolini, M., Dewald, B. & Moser, B. (1997). Human chemokines: an update. *Annu. Rev. Immunol.* 15:675–705.

Barbadillo, C., G-Arroyo, A., Salas, C., Mulero, J., Sanchez-Madrid, F. & Andreu, J.L. (1995). Anti-integrin immunotherapy in rheumatoid arthritis: protective effect of anti-alpha 4 antibody in adjuvant arthritis. [Review] *Springer Sem. Immunopathol.* 16: 427–436.

Baumhueter, S., Dybdal, N., Kyle, C. & Lasky, L.A. (1994). Global vascular expression of murine CD34, a sialomucin-like endothelial ligand for L-selectin. *Blood* 84: 2554–2565.

Bazan, J.F., Bacon, K.B., Hardiman, G., Wang, W., Soo, K., Rossi, D., Greaves, D.R., Zlotnik, A. & Schall, T.J. (1997). A new class of membrane-bound chemokine with a CX_3C motif. *Nature* 385: 640–644.

Berg, E.L., Yoshino, T., Rott, L.S., Robinson, M.K., Warnock, R.A., Kishimoto, T.K. & Butcher, E.C. (1991). The cutaneous lymphocyte antigen is a skin lymphocyte homing receptor for the vascular lectin endothelial cell-leukocyte adhesion molecule 1. *J. Exp. Med.* 174: 1461–1466.

Berlin, C., Berg, E.L., Briskin, M.J., Andrew, D.P., Kilshaw, P.J., Holzmann, B., Hamann, A. & Butcher, E.C. (1993). Alpha 4 beta 7 integrin mediates lymphocyte binding to the mucosal vascular addressin MAdCAM-1. *Cell* 74: 185–195.

Berlin, C., Bargatze, R.F., Campbell, J.J., von Andrian, U.H., Szabo, M.C., Hasslen, S.R., Nelson, R.D., Berg, E.L., Erlandsen, S.L. & Butcher, E.C. (1995). Alpha 4 integrins mediate lymphocyte attachment and rolling under physiologic flow. *Cell* 80: 413–422.

Bevilacqua, M.P. & Nelson, R.M. (1993). Selectins. [Review] *J. Clin. Invest.* 91: 379–387.

Briskin, M.J., McEvoy, L.M. & Butcher, E.C. (1993). MAdCAM-1 has homology to immunoglobulin and mucin-like adhesion receptors and to IgA1. *Nature* 363: 461–464.

Buerke, M., Weyrich, A.S., Zheng, Z., Gaeta, F.C., Forrest, M.J. & Lefer, A.M. (1994). Sialyl Lewis[x]-containing oligosaccharide attenuates myocardial reperfusion injury in cats. *J. Clin. Invest.* 93: 1140–1148.

Butcher, E.C. (1991). Leukocyte–endothelial cell recognition: three (or more) steps to specificity and diversity. [Review] *Cell* 67: 1033–1036.

Butcher, E.C. (1992). Leukocyte–endothelial cell adhesion as an active, multi-step process: a combinatorial mechanism for specificity and diversity in leukocyte targeting. [Review] *Adv. Exp. Med. Biol.* 323: 181–194.

Butcher, E.C & Picker, L.J. (1996). Lymphocyte homing and homeostasis. [Review] *Science* 272: 60–66.

Clark, E.A. & Brugge, J.S. (1995). Integrins and signal transduction pathways: the road taken. [Review] *Science* 268: 233–239.

Corkill, M.M., Kirkham, B.W., Haskard, D.O., Barbatis, C., Gibson, T. & Panayi, G.S. (1991). Gold treatment of rheumatoid arthritis decreases synovial expression of the endothelial leukocyte adhesion receptor ELAM-1. *J. Rheum.* 18: 1453–1460.

Cronstein, B.N., Eberle, M.A., Gruber, H.E. & Levin, R.I. (1991). Methotrexate inhibits neutrophil function by stimulating adenosine release from connective tissue cells. *Proc. Natl. Acad. Sci., USA* 88: 2441–2445.

Cronstein, B.N., Kimmel, S.C., Levin, R.I., Martiniuk, F. & Weissmann, G. (1992). A mechanism for the antiinflammatory effects of corticosteroids: the glucocorticoid receptor regulates leukocyte adhesion to endothelial cells and expression of endothelial-leukocyte adhesion molecule 1 and intercellular adhesion molecule 1. *Proc. Natl. Acad. Sci., USA* 89: 9991–9995.

Cybulsky, M.I., Fries, J.W., Williams, A.J., Sultan, P., Davis, V.M., Gimbrone, M.A.J. & Collins, T. (1991a). Alternative splicing of human VCAM-1 in activated vascular endothelium. *Am. J. Pathol.* 138: 815–820.

Cybulsky, M.I., Fries, J.W., Williams, A.J., Sultan, P., Eddy, R., Byers, M., Shows, T., Gimbrone, M.A., Jr & Collins, T. (1991b). Gene structure, chromosomal location, and basis for alternative mRNA splicing of the human VCAM1 gene. *Proc. Natl. Acad. Sci., USA* 88: 7859–7863.

174   *C. Pitzalis*

Diamond, M.S. & Springer, T.A. (1993). A subpopulation of Mac-1 (CD11b/CD18) molecules mediates neutrophil adhesion to ICAM-1 and fibrinogen. *J. Cell Biol.* 120: 545–556.

Dransfield, I., Cabanas, C., Craig, A. & Hogg, N. (1992). Divalent cation regulation of the function of the leukocyte integrin LFA-1. *J. Cell Biol.* 116: 219–226.

Dustin, M.L., Staunton, D.E. & Springer, T.A. (1988). Supergene families meet in the immune system. [Review] *Immunol. Today* 9: 213–215.

Elices, M.J., Tamraz, S., Tollefson, V. & Vollger, L.W. (1993). The integrin VLA-4 mediates leukocyte recruitment to skin inflammatory sites in vivo. *Clin. Exp. Rheum.* 11 (Suppl. 8): S77–S80.

Elices, M.J., Tsai, V., Strahl, D., Goel, A.S., Tollefson, V., Arrhenius, T., Gaeta, F.C., Fikes, J.D. & Firestein, G.S. (1994). Expression and functional significance of alternatively spliced CS1 fibronectin in rheumatoid arthritis microvasculature. *J. Clin. Invest.* 93: 405–416.

Etzioni, A. (1996). Adhesion molecules in leukocyte endothelial interaction. [Review] *Adv. Exp. Med. Biol.* 408: 151–157.

Etzioni, A., Harlan, J.M., Pollack, S., Phillips, L.M. & Gershoni-Baruch, R. (1993). Leukocyte adhesion deficiency (LAD) II: a new adhesion defect due to absence of sialyl Lewis X, the ligand for selectins. *Immunodeficiency* 4: 307–308.

Fischer, A., Lisowska-Grospierre, B., Anderson, D.C. & Springer, T.A. (1988). Leukocyte adhesion deficiency: molecular basis and functional consequences. [Review] *Immunodefici. Rev.* 1: 39–54.

Forster, R., Mattis, A.E., Kremmer, E., Wolf, E., Brem, G. & Lipp, M. (1996). A putative chemokine receptor, BLR1, directs B cell migration to defined lymphoid organs and specific anatomic compartments of the spleen. *Cell* 87: 1037–1047.

Freemont, A.J. (1988). Functional and biosynthetic changes in endothelial cells of vessels in chronically inflamed tissues: evidence for endothelial control of lymphocyte entry into diseased tissues. *J. Pathol.* 155: 225–230.

Freemont, A.J., Jones, C.J., Bromley, M. & Andrews, P. (1983). Changes in vascular endothelium related to lymphocyte collections in diseased synovia. *Arthritis Rheum.* 26: 1427–1433.

Frenette, P.S., Mayadas, T.N., Rayburn, H., Hynes, R.O. & Wagner, D.D. (1996). Double knockout highlights value of endothelial selectins. *Immunol. Today* 17: 205.

Gallatin, W.M., Weissman, I.L. & Butcher, E.C. (1983). A cell-surface molecule involved in organ-specific homing of lymphocytes. *Nature* 304: 30–34.

Gowans, J.L. & Knight, E.J. (1964). The route of recirculation of lymphocytes in the rat. *Proc. R. Soc. Lond., Biol. Sci.* 159: 257.

Greenfield, S.M., Hamblin, A.S., Shakoor, Z.S., Teare, J.P. & Punchard, N.A. (1993). Inhibition of leucocyte adhesion molecule upregulation by tumor necrosis factor alpha: a novel mechanism of action of sulphasalazine. *Gut* 34: 252–256.

Harlan, J.M. (1993). Leukocyte adhesion deficiency syndrome: insights into the molecular basis of leukocyte emigration. [Review] *Clin. Immunol. Immunopathol.* 67: S16–S24.

Hesterberg, P.E., Winsor-Hines, D., Briskin, M.J., Soler-Ferran, D., Merrill, C., Mackay, C.R., Newman, W. & Ringler, D.J. (1996). Rapid resolution of chronic colitis in the cotton-top tamarin with an antibody to a gut-homing integrin alpha 4 beta 7. *Gastroenterology* 111: 1373–1380.

Hogg, N. & Landis, R.C. (1993). Adhesion molecules in cell interactions. [Review] *Curr. Opin. Immunol.* 5: 383–390.

Hogg, N., Harvey, J., Cabanas, C. & Landis, R.C. (1993). Control of leukocyte integrin activation. [Review] *Am. Rev. Resp. Dis.* 148: S55–S59.

Horrocks, C., Duncan, J.I., Oliver, A.M. & Thomson, A.W. (1991). Adhesion molecule expression in psoriatic skin lesions and the influence of cyclosporin A. *Clin. Exp. Immunol.* 84: 157–162.

Hotchin, N.A. & Hall, A. (1996). Regulation of the actin cytoskeleton, integrins and cell growth by the Rho family of small GTPases. [Review] *Cancer Surv.* 27: 311–322.

Huber, A.R., Kunkel, S.L., Todd, R.F. & Weiss, S.J. (1991). Regulation of transendothelial neutrophil migration by endogenous interleukin-8. *Science* 254: 99–102.

Humphries, M.J., Sheridan, J., Mould, A.P. & Newham, P. (1995). Mechanisms of VCAM-1 and fibronectin binding to integrin alpha 4 beta 1: implications for integrin function and rational drug design. [Review] *Ciba Found. Symp.* 189: 177–191; discussion 191–199.

Hwang, S.T., Singer, M.S., Giblin, P.A., Yednock, T.A., Bacon, K.B., Simon, S.I. & Rosen, S.D. (1996). GlyCAM-1, a physiologic ligand for L-selectin, activates beta 2 integrins on naive peripheral lymphocytes. *J. Exp. Med.* 184: 1343–1348.

Hynes, R.O. (1992). Integrins: versatility, modulation, and signaling in cell adhesion. [Review] *Cell* 69: 11–25.

Imai, Y., Singer, M.S., Fennie, C., Lasky, L.A. & Rosen, S.D. (1991). Identification of a carbohydrate-based endothelial ligand for a lymphocyte homing receptor. *J. Cell Biol.* 113: 1213–1221.

Isobe, M., Yagita, H., Okumura, K. & Ihara, A. (1992). Specific acceptance of cardiac allograft after treatment with antibodies to ICAM-1 and LFA-1. *Science* 255: 1125–1127.

Issekutz, T.B., Chin, W. & Hay, J.B. (1982). The characterization of lymphocytes migrating through chronically inflamed tissues. *Immunology* 46: 59–66.

Jalkanen, S., Steere, A.C., Fox, R.I. & Butcher, E.C. (1986). A distinct endothelial cell recognition system that controls lymphocyte traffic into inflamed synovium. *Science* 233: 556–558.

Jasin, H.E., Lightfoot, E., Davis, L.S., Rothlein, R., Faanes, R.B. & Lipsky, P.E. (1992). Amelioration of antigen-induced arthritis in rabbits treated with mono-clonal antibodies to leukocyte adhesion molecules. *Arthritis Rheum.* 35: 541–549.

Kavanaugh, A.F., Davis, L.S., Nichols, L.A., Norris, S.H., Rothlein, R. & Lipsky, P.E. (1994). Treatment of refractory rheumatoid arthritis with a monoclonal antibody to intercellular adhesion molecule 1. *Arthritis Rheum.* 37: 992–999.

Keffer, J., Probert, L., Cazlaris, H., Georgopoulos, S., Kaslaris, E., Kioussis, D. & Kollias, G. (1991). Transgenic mice expressing human tumour necrosis factor: a predictive genetic model of arthritis. *EMBO J.* 10: 4025–4031.

Kelvin, D.J., Michiel, D.F., Johnston, J.A., Lloyd, A.R., Sprenger, H., Oppenheim, J.J. & Wang, J.M. (1993). Chemokines and serpentines: the molecular biology of chemokine receptors. [Review] *J. Leukocyte Biol.* 54: 604–612.

Kennedy, J., Kelner, G.S., Kleyensteuber, S., Schall, T.J., Weiss, M.C., Yssel, H., Schneider, P.V., Cocks, B.G., Bacon, K.B. & Zlotnik, A. (1995). Molecular cloning and functional characterization of human lymphotactin. *J. Immunol.* 155: 203–209.

Kishimoto, T.K., Jutila, M.A. & Butcher, E.C. (1990). Identification of a human peripheral lymph node homing receptor: a rapidly down-regulated adhesion molecule. *Proc. Natl. Acad. Sci., USA* 87: 2244–2248.

Kitaura, M., Nakajima, T., Imai, T., Harada, S., Combadiere, C., Tiffany, H.L.,

Murphy, P.M. & Yoshie, O. (1996). Molecular cloning of human eotaxin, an eosinophil-selective CC chemokine, and identification of a specific eosinophil eotaxin receptor, CC chemokine receptor 3. *J. Biol. Chem.* 271: 7725–7730.

Kornberg, L., Earp, H.S., Parsons, J.T., Schaller, M. & Juliano, R.L. (1992). Cell adhesion or integrin clustering increases phosphorylation of a focal adhesion-associated tyrosine kinase. *J. Biol. Chem.* 267: 23 439–23 442.

Koszik, F., Strunk, D., Simonitsch, I., Picker, L.J., Stingl, G. & Payer, E. (1994). Expression of monoclonal antibody HECA-452-defined E-selectin ligands on Langerhans cells in normal and diseased skin. *J. Invest. Dermatol.* 102: 773–780.

Landis, R.C., Bennett, R.I. & Hogg, N. (1993). A novel LFA-1 activation epitope maps to the I domain. *J. Cell Biol.* 120: 1519–1527.

Larson, R.S. & Springer, T.A. (1990). Structure and function of leukocyte integrins. [Review] *Immunol. Rev.* 114: 181–217.

Lasky, L.A. (1992). Selectins: interpreters of cell-specific carbohydrate information during inflammation. [Review] *Science* 258: 964–969.

Lasky, L.A. (1995a). Selectin–carbohydrate interactions and the initiation of the inflammatory response. [Review] *Annu. Rev. Biochem.* 64: 113–139.

Lasky, L.A. (1995b). Sialomucins in inflammation and hematopoiesis. *Adv. Exp. Med. Biol.* 376: 259.

Laudanna, C., Campbell, J.J. & Butcher, E.C. (1996). Role of Rho in chemoattractant-activated leukocyte adhesion through integrins. *Science* 271: 981–983.

Lawrence, M.B. & Springer, T.A. (1991). Leukocytes roll on a selectin at physiologic flow rates: distinction from and prerequisite for adhesion through integrins. *Cell* 65: 859–873.

Ley, K. & Gaehtgens, P. (1991). Endothelial, not hemodynamic, differences are responsible for preferential leukocyte rolling in rat mesenteric venules. *Circ. Res.* 69: 1034–1041.

Ley, K., Gaehtgens, P., Fennie, C., Singer, M.S., Lasky, L.A. & Rosen, S.D. (1991). Lectin-like cell adhesion molecule 1 mediates leukocyte rolling in mesenteric venules in vivo. *Blood* 77: 2553–2555.

Lollo, B.A., Chan, K.W., Hanson, E.M., Moy, V.T. & Brian, A.A. (1993). Direct evidence for two affinity states for lymphocyte function-associated antigen 1 on activated T cells [published erratum appears in *J. Biol. Chem.* (1994) 269, 10 184]. *J. Biol. Chem.* 268: 21 693–21 700.

Ma, X.L., Lefer, D.J., Lefer, A.M. & Rothlein, R. (1992). Coronary endothelial and cardiac protective effects of a monoclonal antibody to intercellular adhesion molecule-1 in myocardial ischemia and reperfusion. *Circulation* 86: 937–946.

Mackay, C.R., Marston, W. & Dudler, L. (1992a). Altered patterns of T cell migration through lymph nodes and skin following antigen challenge. *Eur. J. Immunol.* 22: 2205–2210.

Mackay, C.R., Marston, W.L., Dudler, L., Spertini, O., Tedder, T.F. & Hein, W.R. (1992b). Tissue-specific migration pathways by phenotypically distinct subpopulations of memory T cells. *Eur. J. Immunol.* 22: 887–895.

Marchesi, V.T. & Gowans, J.L. (1964). The migration of lymphocytes through the endothelium of venules in lymph nodes. *Proc. R. Soc. Lond., Biol. Sci.* 159: 283.

Martin, S., Casasnovas, J.M., Staunton, D.E. & Springer, T.A. (1993). Efficient neutralization and disruption of rhinovirus by chimeric ICAM-1/immunoglobulin molecules. *J. Virol.* 67: 3561–3568.

Masumoto, A. & Hemler, M.E. (1993). Multiple activation states of VLA-4. Mechanistic differences between adhesion to CS1/fibronectin and to vascular cell adhesion molecule-1. *J. Biol. Chem.* 268: 228–234.

Matsuyama, T., Yamada, A., Kay, J., Yamada, K.M., Akiyama, S.K. & Schlossman, S.F. (1989). Activation of CD4 cells by fibronectin and anti-CD3 antibody. A synergistic effect mediated by the VLA-5 fibronectin receptor complex. *J. Exp. Med.* 170: 1133–1148.

Mebius, R.E., Streeter, P.R., Breve, J., Duijvestijn, A.M. & Kraal, G. (1991). The influence of afferent lymphatic vessel interruption on vascular addressin expression. *J. Cell Biol.* 115: 85–95.

Michie, S.A., Streeter, P.R., Bolt, P.A., Butcher, E.C. & Picker, L.J. (1993). The human peripheral lymph node vascular addressin. An inducible endothelial antigen involved in lymphocyte homing. *Am. J. Pathol.* 143: 1688–1698.

Miura, Y., Kikuchi, A., Musha, T., Kuroda, S., Yaku, H., Sasaki, T. & Takai, Y. (1993). Regulation of morphology by rho p21 and its inhibitory GDP/GTP exchange protein (rho GDI) in Swiss 3T3 cells. *J. Biol. Chem.* 268: 510–515.

Morales-Ducret, J., Wayner, E., Elices, M.J., Alvaro-Gracia, J.M. & Zvaifler, N.J. (1992). Alpha 4/beta 1 integrin (VLA-4) ligands in arthritis. Vascular cell adhesion molecule-1 expression in synovium and on fibroblast-like synoviocytes. *J. Immunol.* 149: 1424–1431.

Mould, A.P., Wheldon, L.A., Komoriya, A., Wayner, E.A., Yamada, K.M. & Humphries, M.J. (1990). Affinity chromatographic isolation of the melanoma adhesion receptor for the IIICS region of fibronectin and its identification as the integrin alpha 4 beta 1. *J. Biol. Chem.* 265: 4020–4024.

Mulligan, M.S., Paulson, J.C., de Frees, S., Zheng, Z.L., Lowe, J.B. & Ward, P.A. (1993). Protective effects of oligosaccharides in P-selectin-dependent lung injury. *Nature* 364: 149–151.

Nelson, R.M., Cecconi, O., Roberts, W.G., Aruffo, A., Linhardt, R.J. & Bevilacqua, M.P. (1993). Heparin oligosaccharides bind L- and P-selectin and inhibit acute inflammation. *Blood* 82: 3253–3258.

Neote, K., DiGregorio, D., Mak, J.Y., Horuk, R. & Schall, T.J. (1993). Molecular cloning, functional expression, and signaling characteristics of a C-C chemokine receptor. *Cell* 72: 415–425.

Osborn, L., Vassallo, C., Browning, B.G., Tizard, R., Haskard, D.O., Benjamin, C.D. & Kirchhausen, T. (1994). Arrangement of domains, and amino acid residues required for binding of vascular cell adhesion molecule-1 to its counter-receptor VLA-4 (alpha 4 beta 1). *J. Cell Biol.* 124: 601–608.

Otey, C.A., Pavalko, F.M. & Burridge, K. (1990). An interaction between alpha-actinin and the beta 1 integrin subunit in vitro. *J. Cell Biol.* 111: 721–729.

Pals, S.T., Drillenburg, P., Dragosics, B., Lazarovits, A.I. & Radaszkiewicz, T. (1994). Expression of the mucosal homing receptor alpha 4 beta 7 in malignant lymphomatous polyposis of the intestine. *Gastroenterology* 107: 1519–1523.

Parsons, J.T., Schaller, M.D., Hildebrand, J., Leu, T.H., Richardson, A. & Otey, C. (1994). Focal adhesion kinase: structure and signalling. [Review] *J. Cell Sci.* 18(Suppl.): 109–113.

Pasparakis, M., Alexopoulou, L., Episkopou, V. & Kollias, G. (1996). Immune and inflammatory responses in TNF alpha-deficient mice: a critical requirement for TNF alpha in the formation of primary B cell follicles, follicular dendritic cell networks and germinal centers, and in the maturation of the humoral immune response [see comments]. *J. Exp. Med.* 184: 1397–1411.

Pavalko, F.M., Otey, C.A., Simon, K.O. & Burridge, K. (1991). Alpha-actinin: a direct link between actin and integrins. [Review] *Biochem. Soc. Trans.* 19: 1065–1069.

Picker, L.J. (1992). Mechanisms of lymphocyte homing. [Review] *Curr. Opin. Immunol.* 4: 277–286.

Picker, L.J. (1994). Control of lymphocyte homing. [Review] *Curr. Opin. Immunol.* 6: 394–406.

Picker, L.J., Michie, S.A., Rott, L.S. & Butcher, E.C. (1990). A unique phenotype of skin-associated lymphocytes in humans. Preferential expression of the HECA-452 epitope by benign and malignant T cells at cutaneous sites. *Am. J. Pathol.* 136: 1053–1068.

Picker, L.J., Martin, R.J., Trumble, A., Newman, L.S., Collins, P.A., Bergstresser, P.R. & Leung, D.Y. (1994). Differential expression of lymphocyte homing receptors by human memory/effector T cells in pulmonary versus cutaneous immune effector sites. *Eur. J. Immunol.* 24: 1269–1277.

Pierschbacher, M.D., Hayman, E.G. & Ruoslahti, E. (1985). The cell attachment determinant in fibronectin. [Review] *J. Cell. Biochem.* 28: 115–126.

Pitzalis, C. (1993). Adhesion and migration of inflammatory cells. [Review] *Clin. Exp. Rheum.* 11 (Suppl. 8): 71–76.

Pitzalis, C., Cauli, A., Pipitone, N., Smith, C., Barker, J., Marchesoni, A., Yanni, G. & Panayi, G. (1996). Cutaneous lymphocyte antigen-positive T lymphocytes preferentially migrate to the skin but not to the joint in psoriatic arthritis. *Arthritis Rheum.* 39: 137–145.

Pitzalis, C., Pipitone, N., Bajocchi, G., Hall, M., Goulding, N., Lee, A., Kingsley, G., Lanchbury, J. & Panayi, G. (1997). Corticosteroids inhibit lymphocyte binding to endothelium and intercellular adhesion: an additional mechanism for their anti-inflammatory and immunosuppressive effect. *J. Immunol.* 10: 5007–5016.

Ponath, P.D., Qin, S., Post, T.W., Wang, J., Wu, L., Gerard, N.P., Newman, W., Gerard, C. & Mackay, C.R. (1996). Molecular cloning and characterization of a human eotaxin receptor expressed selectively on eosinophils. [See comments] *J. Exp. Med.* 183: 2437–2448.

Premack, B.A. & Schall, T.J. (1996). Chemokine receptors: gateways to inflammation and infection. [Review] *Nature Med.* 2: 1174–1178.

Pulido, R., Elices, M.J., Campanero, M.R., Osborn, L., Schiffer, S., Garcia-Pardo, A., Lobb, R., Hemler, M.E. & Sanchez-Madrid, F. (1991). Functional evidence for three distinct and independently inhibitable adhesion activities mediated by the human integrin VLA-4. Correlation with distinct alpha 4 epitopes. *J. Biol. Chem.* 266: 10 241–10 245.

Rabb, H.A., Olivenstein, R., Issekutz, T.B., Renzi, P.M. & Martin, J.G. (1994). The role of the leukocyte adhesion molecules VLA-4, LFA-1, and Mac-1 in allergic airway responses in the rat. *Am. J. Resp. Crit. Care Med.* 149: 1186–1191.

Rose, M.L., Parrott, D.M.V. & Bruce, R.G. (1978). The accumulation of immunoblasts in extravascular tissues including mammary gland, peritoneal cavity, gut and skin. *Immunology* 35: 415–423.

Roth, S.J., Carr, M.W. & Springer, T.A. (1995). C-C chemokines, but not the C-X-C chemokines interleukin-8 and interferon-gamma inducible protein-10, stimulate transendothelial chemotaxis of T lymphocytes. *Eur. J. Immunol.* 25: 482–3488.

Rothenberg, M.E., Ownbey, R., Mehlhop, P.D., Loiselle, P.M., van de Rijn, M., Bonventre, J.V., Oettgen, H.C., Leder, P. & Luster, A.D. (1996). Eotaxin triggers eosinophil-selective chemotaxis and calcium flux via a distinct receptor and induces pulmonary eosinophilia in the presence of interleukin 5 in mice. *Mol. Med.* 2: 334–348.

Ruoslahti, E. (1991). Integrins. *J. Clin. Invest.* 87: 1–5.

Ruoslahti, E. & Pierschbacher, M.D. (1987). New perspectives in cell adhesion: RGD and integrins. [Review] *Science* 238: 491–497.

Salmi, M., Granfors, K., Leirisalo-Repo, M., Hamalainen, M., MacDermott, R., Havia,

T. & Jalkanen, S. (1992). Selective endothelial binding of interleukin-2-dependent human T-cell lines derived from different tissues. *Proc. Natl. Acad. Sci., USA* 89: 11 436–11 440.

Sampaio, S.O., Li, X., Takeuchi, M., Mei, C., Francke, U., Butcher, E.C. & Briskin, M.J. (1995). Organization, regulatory sequences, and alternatively spliced transcripts of the mucosal addressin cell adhesion molecule-1 (MAdCAM-1) gene. *J. Immunol.* 155: 2477–2486.

Schall, T.J. & Bacon, K.B. (1994). Chemokines, leukocyte trafficking, and inflammation. *Curr. Opin. Immunol.* 6: 865–873.

Schall, T.J., Bacon, K., Camp, R.D., Kaspari, J.W. & Goeddel, D.V. (1993a). Human macrophage inflammatory protein alpha (MIP-1 alpha) and MIP-1 beta chemokines attract distinct populations of lymphocytes. *J. Exp. Med.* 177: 1821–1826.

Schall, T.J., Mak, J.Y., DiGregorio, D. & Neote, K. (1993b). Receptor/ligand interactions in the C-C chemokine family. [Review] *Adv. Exp. Med. Biol.* 351: 29–37.

Sharpe, A.H. (1995). Analysis of lymphocyte costimulation in vivo using transgenic and 'knockout' mice. [Review] *Curr. Opin. Immunol.* 7: 389–395.

Shier, P., Otulakowski, G., Ngo, K., Panakos, J., Chourmouzis, E., Christjansen, L., Lau, C.Y. & Fung-Leung, W.P. (1996). Impaired immune responses toward alloantigens and tumor cells but normal thymic selection in mice deficient in the beta2 integrin leukocyte function-associated antigen-1. *J. Immunol.* 157: 5375–5386.

Shimizu, Y., van Seventer, G.A., Horgan, K.J. & Shaw, S. (1990). Costimulation of proliferative responses of resting CD4+ T cells by the interaction of VLA-4 and VLA-5 with fibronectin or VLA-6 with laminin. *J. Immunol.* 145: 59–67.

Simmons, D.L. (1995). The role of ICAM expression in immunity and disease. [Review] *Cancer Surv.* 24: 141–155.

Smith, M.D., Ahern, M.J., Brooks, P.M. & Roberts-Thomson, P.J. (1988). The clinical and immunological effects of pulse methylprednisolone therapy in rheumatoid arthritis. III. Effects on immune and inflammatory indices in synovial fluid. *J. Rheum.* 15: 238–241.

Smith, M.E. & Ford, W.L. (1983). The recirculating lymphocyte pool of the rat: a systematic description of the migratory behaviour of recirculating lymphocytes. *Immunology* 49: 83–94.

Springer, T.A. (1994). Traffic signals for lymphocyte recirculation and leukocyte emigration: the multistep paradigm. [Review] *Cell* 76: 301–314.

Staite, N.D., Justen, J.M., Sly, L.M., Beaudet, A.L. & Bullard, D.C. (1996). Inhibition of delayed-type contact hypersensitivity in mice deficient in both E-selectin and P-selectin. *Blood* 88: 2973–2979.

Staunton, D.E., Dustin, M.L. & Springer, T.A. (1989). Functional cloning of ICAM-2, a cell adhesion ligand for LFA-1 homologous to ICAM-1. *Nature* 339: 61–64.

Staunton, D.E., Dustin, M.L., Erickson, H.P. & Springer, T.A. (1990). The arrangement of the immunoglobulin-like domains of ICAM-1 and the binding sites for LFA-1 and rhinovirus. [Published errata appear in *Cell* (1990) 61, 1157 and (1991), following 1311.] *Cell* 61: 243–254.

Streeter, P.R., Berg, E.L., Rouse, B.T., Bargatze, R.F. & Butcher, E.C. (1988a). A tissue-specific endothelial cell molecule involved in lymphocyte homing. *Nature* 331: 41–46.

Streeter, P.R., Rouse, B.T. & Butcher, E.C. (1988b). Immunohistologic and functional characterization of a vascular addressin involved in lymphocyte homing into peripheral lymph nodes. *J. Cell Biol.* 107: 1853–1862.

Tanaka, Y., Adams, D.H., Hubscher, S., Hirano, H., Siebenlist, U. & Shaw, S. (1993a). T-cell adhesion induced by proteoglycan-immobilized cytokine MIP-1 beta. [See comments] *Nature* 361: 79–82.

Tanaka, Y., Adams, D.H. & Shaw, S. (1993b). Proteoglycans on endothelial cells present adhesion-inducing cytokines to leukocytes. [Review] *Immunol. Today* 14: 111–115.

Tapon, N. & Hall, A. (1997). Rho, Rac and Cdc42 GTPases regulate the organization of the actin cytoskeleton. [Review] *Curr. Opin. Cell Biol.* 9: 86–92.

Tedder, T.F., Steeber, D.A. & Pizcueta, P. (1995). L-selectin-deficient mice have impaired leukocyte recruitment into inflammatory sites. *J. Exp. Med.* 181: 2259–2264.

van Dinther-Janssen, A.C., Pals, S.T., Scheper, R., Breedveld, F. & Meijer, C.J. (1990). Dendritic cells and high endothelial venules in the rheumatoid synovial membrane. *J. Rheum.* 17: 17.

van Dinther-Janssen, A.C., Pals, S.T., Scheper, R.J. & Meijer, C.J. (1993). Role of the CS1 adhesion motif of fibronectin in T cell adhesion to synovial membrane and peripheral lymph node endothelium. *Ann. Rheum. Dis.* 52: 672–676.

von Andrian, U.H., Chambers, J.D., McEvoy, L.M., Bargatze, R.F., Arfors, K.E. & Butcher, E.C. (1991). Two-step model of leukocyte–endothelial cell interaction in inflammation: distinct roles for LECAM-1 and the leukocyte beta 2 integrins in vivo. *Proc. Natl. Acad. Sci., USA* 88: 7538–7542.

Wagner, N., Lohler, J., Kunkel, E.J., Ley, K., Leung, E., Krissansen, G., Rajewsky, K. & Muller, W. (1996). Critical role for beta7 integrins in formation of the gut-associated lymphoid tissue. *Nature* 382: 366–370.

Ward, P.A. & Mulligan, M.S. (1994). Blocking of adhesion molecules in vivo as anti-inflammatory therapy. [Review] *Ther. Immunol.* 1: 165–171.

Wayner, E.A., Garcia-Pardo, A., Humphries, M.J., McDonald, J.A. & Carter, W.G. (1989). Identification and characterization of the T lymphocyte adhesion receptor for an alternative cell attachment domain (CS-1) in plasma fibronectin. *J. Cell Biol.* 109: 1321–1330.

Wilkinson, L.S., Edwards, J.C., Poston, R.N. & Haskard, D.O. (1993). Expression of vascular cell adhesion molecule-1 in normal and inflamed synovium. *Lab. Invest.* 68: 82–88.

Yamada, A., Nikaido, T., Nojima, Y., Schlossman, S.F. & Morimoto, C. (1991). Activation of human CD4 T lymphocytes. Interaction of fibronectin with VLA-5 receptor on CD4 cells induces the AP-1 transcription factor. *J. Immunol.* 146: 53–56.

Yang, X.D., Karin, N., Tisch, R., Steinman, L. & McDevitt, H.O. (1993). Inhibition of insulitis and prevention of diabetes in nonobese diabetic mice by blocking L-selectin and very late antigen 4 adhesion receptors. *Proc. Natl. Acad. Sci., USA* 90: 10 94–10 498.

Yanni, G., Whelan, A., Feighery, C., Fitzgerald, O. & Bresnihan, B. (1993). Morphometric analysis of synovial membrane blood vessels in rheumatoid arthritis: associations with the immunohistologic features, synovial fluid cytokine levels and the clinical course. *J. Rheum.* 20: 634–638.

Yednock, T.A., Cannon, C., Fritz, L.C., Sanchez-Madrid, F., Steinman, L. & Karin N. (1992). Prevention of experimental autoimmune encephalomyelitis by antibodies against alpha 4 beta 1 integrin. *Nature* 356: 63–66.

Youssef, P.P., Cormack, J., Evill, C.A., Peter, D.T., Roberts-Thomson, P.J., Ahern, M.J. & Smith, M.D. (1996). Neutrophil trafficking into inflamed joints in patients

with rheumatoid arthritis, and the effects of methylprednisolone. *Arthritis Rheum.*
39: 216–225.

Zimmerman, G.A., Prescott, S.M. & McIntyre, T.M. (1992). Endothelial cell interactions with granulocytes: tethering and signaling molecules. [Review] *Immunol. Today* 13: 93–100.

9

Regulation of apoptosis in the rheumatic disorders

J. MCNALLY, A. K. VAISHNAW and K. B. ELKON

Introduction

Apoptosis is the name used to describe the morphology of cells that die by a variety of insults as well as during normal physiological processes such as embryogenesis and metamorphosis (Kerr, Wyllie & Currie, 1972). The characteristic features of apoptosis include membrane ruffling, cytoplasmic and organelle contraction, nuclear condensation and DNA cleavage. The resulting cellular fragments or apoptotic bodies, are subject to rapid ingestion by neighbouring cells and resident tissue phagocytes. Cell death associated with apoptosis, programmed cell death, has been contrasted with necrotic cell death, which occurs as the result of external damage and is characterized by cell expansion and apparently random disintegration of cellular constituents. More recently, apoptosis and necrosis have been shown not to be two entirely different modes of death but rather the consequence of the nature and strength of the inductive stimulus coupled with the availability of energy sources such as ATP (Leist *et al.*, 1997). A detailed description of apoptosis and its relevance to biomedical science is beyond the scope of this review and the reader is referred to a series of reviews in *Science*, 10 March, 1995 and 28 August, 1998.

Biochemical regulation of apoptosis

There are two aspects of apoptotic death that are of particular relevance to immune responses.

1. Apoptotic death is non-inflammatory. Cell fragments are phagocytosed by neighbouring cells and/or professional phagocytes and degraded. Most evidence indicates that phagocytes are not activated following ingestion of these bodies (Savill *et al.*, 1993). The receptors and ligands responsible for uptake of apoptotic cells in mammalian cells are not yet defined.

2.   Apoptosis occurs through ordered biochemical pathways, and because of this is often referred to as programmed cell death (PCD). The pathways are regulated by a variety of stimuli related to immune cell function. These biochemical pathways have been intensely studied in the 1990s. They are schematically illustrated in Figs. 9.1–9.3 and discussed below.

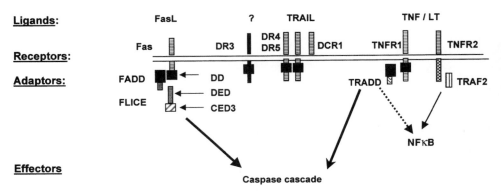

Fig. 9.1. Cell death pathways: inducers and early signal transduction pathways of the major known apoptosis pathways. Interaction of the ligand with the receptor causes receptor clustering and recruitment of the adaptor molecules. These, in turn, facilitate enzymatic activity of the caspases. Note that TNFα may induce a death signal through TRADD or stimulate cell activation through the NFκB pathway. These pathways are modulated by the Bcl-2 family of proteins (see Figs. 9.2 and 9.3) and by other downstream signal transduction pathways (see text). Dissolution of the cell is orchestrated by caspases and nucleases. DD, death domain; DED, death effector domain; CED3, *C. elegans* 3 homologous domain.

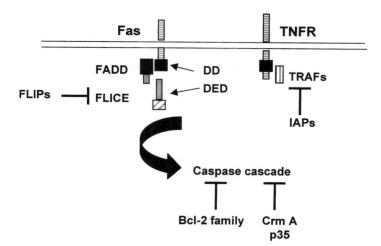

Fig. 9.2. Inhibitors of apoptosis. Endogenous and virus-encoded (Crm A, p35) inhibitors of apoptosis block the biochemical pathway at different stages. See text for discussion and references.

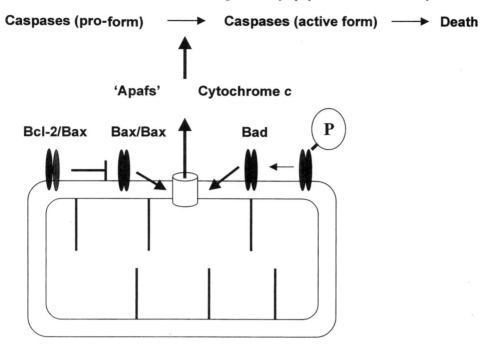

Caspases (pro-form) ⟶ **Caspases (active form)** ⟶ **Death**

'Apafs' Cytochrome c

Bcl-2/Bax Bax/Bax Bad P

Fig. 9.3. Mechanisms of apoptosis regulation by the Bcl family. Most of the Bcl family are located at the outer mitochondrial membrane. Unapposed, proteins such as Bcl-2 and Bcl-X$_L$ promote cell survival whereas Bax and Bad promote cell death. Bcl-2 and Bcl-X$_L$ may act by forming heterodimers with the Bax or Bad and preventing the latter molecules from forming pores in the membrane (left side of figure). Pore formation is thought to allow the release of Apafs (apoptotic protease activating factors), which include cytochrome *c*. Another way in which survival is regulated is through phosphorylation of Bad (see right side of figure), which, in turn, results in the dissociation of Bad from Bcl-2/Bcl-X$_L$.

Induction and early signal transduction

Fas ligand (FasL) and TNFα are the prototypic inducers of apoptosis (Nagata & Golstein, 1995). These ligands induce clustering of their cognate receptors (Fas, TNFR1 or TNFR2), which leads to recruitment of the early signal transducing molecules (Fig. 9.1) (reviewed in Fraser & Evan, 1996). TNFα may induce either cell death or activation depending on cell type, the receptor (TNFR1 or TNFR2) engaged and the action of intracellular regulators. While FasL and TNFα are the best characterized, a number of other apoptotic ligands (TRAIL (APO-2L) and AIM-2) and receptors (DR3 (also called APO-3/TRAMP/wsl-1/LARD), DR4 and DR5) have recently been identified. The receptors share a domain of 60–80 amino acid residues in the intracytoplasmic portion of the protein, called the 'death domain'. TRAIL is the ligand for DR4, DR5 and DcR1, a 'decoy receptor' that shares the same ligand binding as DR4 and DR5 but lacks a cyto-plasmic signalling domain (see Gura, 1997) (Fig. 9.1). Since the roles of the newly described receptors have not yet been studied in rheumatic diseases, they will not be considered further in this review.

Fas and TNFR belong to a superfamily of molecules that now includes almost 20 members. The majority of the family members (e.g. CD40, OX-40, CD30, 4-1BB) promote cell survival. The complex interplay between different members of this family are exemplified by CD40 and Fas. Whereas activation of B cells by CD40 upregulates Fas expression and enhances susceptibility of B cells to Fas-mediated apoptosis, co-ligation of the B cell receptor inhibits apoptosis (Elkon & Marshak-Rothstein, 1996).

Intracellular regulators

Regulators of different stages of the apoptotic pathway have been identified and are shown schematically in Fig. 9.2. FLIPs (FLICE inhibitory proteins) regulate the most proximal part of the apoptotic pathway by competing for binding of FADD and FLICE (caspase 8) (Irmler et al., 1997). Crm A and p35 are virus-encoded products that inhibit the function of specific caspases. IAPs (inhibitors of apoptosis) are thought to bind to TRAFs (Uren et al., 1996) – although the precise way in which they promote cell survival remains to be determined.

Mitochondria have become a major focus for studies of apoptosis regulation. Kroemer, Zamzami & Susin (1997) have proposed that opening of mitochondrial megachannels associated with a 'permeability transition' (PT) is a necessary step for the release of soluble factor(s) required for the execution of apoptosis. Bcl-2 family members (Reed, 1994) are localized to the mitochondrial and nuclear membranes. Bcl-2 and Bcl-X_L are prototypic cell survival proteins whereas Bax and Bad induce cell death. These molecules are thought to regulate cell fate by differential pairing (Oltvai & Korsmeyer, 1994; Yin, Oltvai & Korsmeyer, 1994). For example, heterodimers of Bax and Bcl-2 repress cell death, whereas if most Bax protein is in a homodimeric form, apoptosis is induced (Fig. 9.3, left side). Since the Bcl-2 family share sequence and structural homology to bacterial pore-forming proteins (Muchmore et al., 1996), one scenario is that induction of pores by Bax homodimers allows the leakage of cytochrome c and Apafs (apoptotic protease-activating factors) from the mitochondria (Golstein, 1997). Very recently, another regulatory pathway influencing Bcl pairing has been described (Franke & Cantley, 1997). Survival signals activate a PI_3-kinase/Akt signalling cascade leading to phosphorylation of Bad (Fig. 9.3, right side). Phosphorylation of Bad results in dissociation of this molecule from Bcl-2 or Bcl-X_L, allowing homodimers to suppress release of Apafs.

In lymphocytes, many survival signals are thought to act via modulation of expression of Bcl-2 family members; for example, CD28 co-stimulation of T cells or IL-4 stimulation of B cells enhance expression of the anti-apoptotic protein Bcl-X_L.

Proteolytic cascade

The major family of proteases involved in apoptosis of mammalian cells comprises cysteine proteases (previously called the ICE family, now renamed caspases: cysteine aspartate-specific proteases) that are homologous of the *C. elegans* CED-3 (Fraser & Evan, 1996). The first protease identified was an ICE (interleukin-1β-converting enzyme) homologue, a cysteine protease that cleaves pro-IL-1β. More recently, a number of ICE homologues, caspases 2–9, have been identified (Alnemri *et al.*, 1996). Caspases are cysteine-dependent proteases that have an unusual substrate specificity for peptidyl sequences with a P1 aspartate residue. They can be grouped into ICE-like (caspases 1, 4 and 5) and CED-3-like (caspases 3, 6, 7, 8, 9 and 10) proteases based on sequence similarity and their relative susceptibility to the tetrapeptide inhibitors zYVAD and DEVD-fmk, respectively. Most evidence suggests that, analogous to the clotting and complement pathways, many caspases activate each other in a cascade that leads to amplification of the death signal. The exact sequence of events in this cascade remain to be determined, although recent *in vitro* studies indicate that FLICE (Fig. 9.1) is able to process/activate all known ICE/CED-3-like caspases (Margolin *et al.*, 1997). Transcriptional alterations in caspase levels have been detected under some circumstances but by far the most important mode of caspase regulation is post-translational and occurs by protein–protein interaction and proteolytic cleavage (reviewed in Kumar, 1995). All of the caspases are expressed constitutively as proenzymes that are cleaved to generate two subunits of ~ 20 and 10 kDa; these combine to form the catalytically active $\alpha_2\beta_2$ tetramer. The specificity of caspases for aspartate residues is similar to that of granzyme B, one of the proteolytic enzymes released by cytotoxic T cells, suggesting that similar substrates are cleaved by quite different inducers of apoptosis.

Apoptosis modifiers

Susceptibility to apoptosis is affected by the stage of ontogeny and the activation of the cell. Pro-proliferative cytokines such as IL-4, L-7 and IL-15 that signal through the common γ chain of the IL-2 receptor are generally anti-apoptotic for T (Akbar *et al.*, 1996) and B (Elkon & Marshak-Rothstein, 1996) cells and are associated with upregulation of Bcl-2 and/or Bcl-X_L. Cytokines such as

IL-2 and IL-10 play more complex roles that can promote or inhibit apoptosis. Other signal transduction pathways impact on the final decision of the cell, including ceramide, the balance between the stress kinases (JNK and p38) and MAP kinases, and the *Ras* pathway of cellular activation.

Viruses regulate apoptosis

Viruses have often been implicated as aetiological agents in autoimmune diseases, including Sjögren's syndrome (see below). A number of viruses express apoptotic inhibitory proteins (reviewed in Thompson, 1995) and it is, therefore, worth considering their role in disease in this context. Two examples discussed are Epstein–Barr Virus (EBV) and herpesviruses, which produce v-FLIPs (see also Fig. 9.2). EBV expresses a number of anti-apoptotic proteins: LMP1, a transmembrane protein, recruits TRAF-like molecules and results in NFκB activation, cell proliferation and induction of Bcl-2. EBV also expresses a homologue of Bcl-2 (BHRF1) as well as a homologue of IL-10; these homologues protect human B cells from apoptosis. EBV, therefore, employs a number of anti-apoptotic strategies that may lead to persistent viral infection. Viruses of the γ herpesviruses family and molluscipoxvirus express viral homologues of FLIP, an endogenous protein known to inhibit Fas-mediated apoptosis of naive lymphocytes. The viral inhibitors of apoptosis (v-FLIPs) act as FLICE antagonists (Fig. 9.2) and are thought to block the early signalling events of several other death receptors (DR-3, DR-4 and TNFR1).

Apoptosis in the immune system

Cell turnover

Cells of the immune system include T and B lymphocytes, monocytes, dendritic cells, natural killer cells and neutrophils. The enormous (billions) daily production of these cells is balanced by their removal. There is abundant evidence that these cells die by apoptosis and are removed by non-inflammatory mechanisms. A potential explanation for this observation in T cells could be that a Kruppel-like zinc finger transcription factor, lung Kruppel-like factor (LKLF), is transcribed in resting cells and maintains their viability (Kuo, Veselits & Leiden, 1997).

Central tolerance

Deletion of high-affinity, self-reactive lymphocytes in the thymus is one of the cardinal mechanisms that helps to avoid autoimmunity. Immature T (thymocytes) and B (early B cells in the bone marrow) lymphocytes are more sensitive to ligation of their antigen receptors than are mature lymphocytes, ensuring that the high-affinity cells are deleted. Although very large numbers of these immature lymphocytes die by apoptosis, the precise signalling pathways have not yet been defined. Abnormalities that influence thresholds for apoptosis may have major impact on susceptibility to autoimmunity (see below).

Peripheral tolerance

Since T cells are positively selected on self MHC (perhaps + peptide) in the thymus, T cells react with low affinity to self MHC. Recent studies, in fact, suggest that this interaction is necessary for the short-term survival of T cells in the peripheral immune system (Benoist & Mathis, 1997). Autoreactivity is generally avoided by the induction of anergy when the T cell receptor (TCR) is engaged but CD28, the major co-receptor, is not (Schwartz, 1996). However, at sites of inflammation, co-receptor ligands such as B7–1 and B7–2 are highly expressed by antigen-presenting cells. Furthermore, these cells present self-peptides in the MHC grooves. This situation provides a potent setting for the initiation of autoimmune responses. It is counteracted by the removal of potentially autoreactive cells by activation-induced cell death (AICD).

Antigen-specific T cell activation and proliferation is associated with upregulation of Fas and FasL and, after several days, acquired susceptibility to FasL–Fas mediated apoptosis. Since Fas and FasL may be expressed on the same cell, activated clones may die by fratricide or suicide (Nagata & Golstein, 1995). The Fas pathway is probably one of many pathways to terminate T cell proliferation. AICD, therefore, limits unwanted expansion of T cell clones reacting against foreign antigens beyond the course of infection, as well as of clones that cross-react with self-antigens or have been activated by autoantigens during an inflammatory event.

Autoreactive B cell clones are subject to several levels of regulation (Nossal, 1996). To generate high-affinity IgG antibodies, B cells also require at least two signals: one generated through the B cell receptor and others derived from T cells (CD40L and cytokines). B cells that chronically encounter low levels of antigen downregulate their antigen-receptor signalling apparatus such that autoantigen recognition does not lead to clonal activation and proliferation (Goodnow, 1992). These anergized clones are rendered susceptible to FasL-mediated apoptosis in lymph nodes by a mechanism involving CD40-mediated upregulation of Fas on the B cell (Rathmell *et al.*, 1996).

Apoptosis regulation in autoimmune disorders

Defects in apoptosis are a cause of systemic autoimmunity

SLE is a systemic autoimmune disease characterized by the presence of auto-antibodies directed against a range of intracellular nucleoprotein targets. The role of lymphocyte apoptosis in both central and peripheral tolerance has suggested that self-reactivity may result from abnormal regulation of apoptosis (Fig. 9.4*a*).

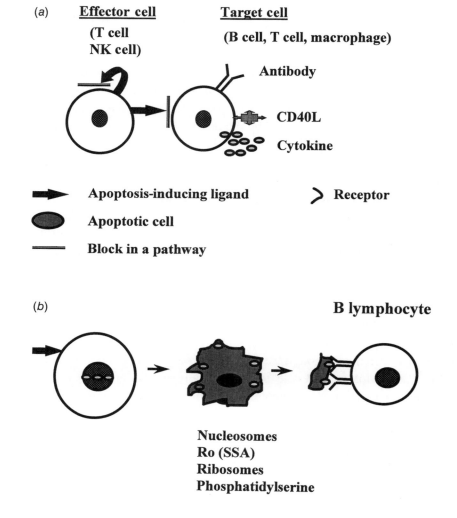

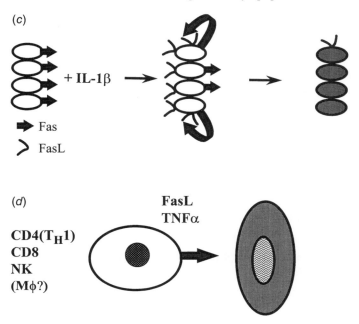

(c)

+ IL-1β →

➡ Fas

❯ FasL

(d)

CD4(T$_H$1)
CD8
NK
(Mφ?)

FasL
TNFα

Fig. 9.4. Possible role of apoptotic pathways in autoimmune disorders. (*a*) Defects in apoptotic pathways promote the survival of potentially autoreactive, proinflammatory cells. The defect may arise through failure of a suicide mechanism, as shown on the left, or a failure to 'murder' activated target cells of the T, B or macrophage lineages (right). Failure to eliminate activated cells can result in prolonged effector functions such as CD40L 'help' to B cells, inappropriate survival of primed autoantibody-producing B cells or cytokine release by macrophages. (*b*) Apoptosis as a source of immunogens. In view of the prominence of nucleosomes and negatively charged phospholipids as antigens in diseases such as SLE, it has been speculated that highly accelerated rates and/or abnormal sites or abnormal processing of apoptotic cells could lead to autoantibody production. (*c*) Organ suicide. Cytokines could provoke the destruction of cells by turning on a cell death pathway. It has been reported that thyrocytes constitutively express FasL and that IL1-β induces the expression of Fas resulting in apoptotic death of the gland (Giordano *et al.*, 1997). A similar co-expression of Fas and FasL, coupled with high expression of Bax, but not Bcl–2, in acini, may account for loss of glandular tissue in Sjögren's syndrome (Kong *et al.*, 1997) and, possibly, in insulin-dependent diabetes mellitus (Chervonsky *et al.*, 1997). (*d*) Tissue injury in organ-specific autoimmune diseases. As shown in (*a*), defects in apoptosis may allow persistence of activated effector cells. The effector cell may be resistant to apoptosis but can itself induce tissue injury by apoptosis of specialized cells within the organ or by proinflammatory effects (*b*). Examples may include graft-versus-host disease, multiple sclerosis and, possibly, RA and Sjögren's syndrome. Most organ-specific autoimmune diseases show evidence of fragmented DNA at sites of tissue injury. This is not always proportional to the degree of inflammation, as macrophages are remarkably efficient at ingesting apoptotic cells.

Murine models of autoimmunity

Three different mouse models of lupus-like autoimmunity with lymphadenopathy and mutations in Fas or FasL have been described (reviewed in Nagata &
Golstein, 1995). The severity of the lymphadenopathy and autoimmunity varies
among the strains, which either fail to express Fas (MRL*lpr/lpr*), produce a dysfunctional Fas molecule (CBA*lpr*^cg^/*lpr*^cg^) or a mutant FasL (C3H*gld/gld*).
Analysis of these mice has led to several important conclusions. All three strains
exhibit diminished Fas-mediated lymphocyte apoptosis, resulting in lymphocyte
accumulation and lymphadenopathy. Lymphocyte apoptosis is probably normal
in the thymus and bone marrow but clearly is abnormal in the periphery, resulting in the failure to delete autoreactive T and B cells (defective AICD) (Russell
et al., 1993; Singer & Abbas, 1994). The mutations amplify any pre-existing ten-
dency to autoimmunity, such as those that exist in the MRL (Watson *et al.*, 1992)
but not the C57BL/6 strains.

Other lupus-prone strains have also been reported to have abnormalities in
apoptosis. In these cases, the mutations probably interfere with the threshold
required for apoptosis induction rather than defects in apoptosis receptors *per se*.
In motheaten mice, deficiency of SHP-1 (PTP1c), a phosphatase that downreg-
ulates antigen receptor-mediated signalling in T and B cells and macrophages,
leads to enhanced survival of autoreactive lymphocytes, autoantibody formation
and an aggressive multisystem autoimmune syndrome (Tsui *et al.*, 1993; Pani *et
al.*, 1995). NZB mice have reduced B cell apoptosis induced by cross-linking of
surface IgM receptors (Kozono, Kotzin & Holers, 1996), suggesting that a defect
in B cell signalling may explain the survival of autoreactive B cells.

The idea that defects in apoptosis induce systemic autoimmune disease is
strongly supported by transgenic and knock-out studies in mice, as illustrated in
the following examples. Bcl-2 transgenic mice with B cell-specific overexpression of Bcl–2 produced anti-DNA, anti-Sm autoantibodies and developed
glomerulonephritis (Strasser *et al.*, 1991). IL-2 and IL-2 receptor knock-out mice
developed lymphoproliferation, polyclonal T and B cell activation and evidence
of systemic autoimmunity, with anti-red cell and anti-colon antibodies (Sadlack
et al., 1993; Suzuki *et al.*, 1995; Willerford *et al.*, 1995). Rather than the expected
immunodeficiency state, defects in the IL-2 pathway led to reduced sensitization
to Fas-mediated AICD (Fournel *et al.*, 1996). Widespread autoimmunity was
reported in CTLA-4-deficient mice, consistent with the observation that CTLA-
4 (the inhibitory homologue of the CD28 T cell co-stimulatory molecule) down-
regulates antigen-specific responses and may directly lead to T cell apoptosis
(Tivol *et al.*, 1995; Waterhouse *et al.*, 1995). Deficiency of Lyn, a *src* family
tyrosine kinase that is part of the B cell antigen-receptor signalling cascade, causes

impaired B cell apoptosis associated with anti-dsDNA antibodies and glomerulonephritis (Hibbs *et al.*, 1995; Nishizumi *et al.*, 1995).

Human lupus and related systemic syndromes

Inherited Fas deficiency in humans (Canale–Smith syndrome (Drappa *et al.*, 1996), ALPS (Fisher *et al.*, 1995) HLPS (Rieux-Laucat *et al.*, 1995)) is also associated with lymphadenopathy, hepatosplenomegaly and systemic autoimmunity: most commonly antibodies against red cells and platelets. As in *lpr* mice, the phenotype associated with human *fas* mutations depends upon predisposing background factors (genetic or environmental). Although there are obvious differences between SLE and the Canale–Smith syndrome, it should be noted that one SLE patient with a *fasL* mutation has been reported (Wu *et al.*, 1996) and we have recently encountered a young girl with a heterozygous *fas* mutation, autoantibodies and lupus-like disease involving the central nervous system and kidneys. A small subgroup of SLE patients may, therefore, have structural Fas or FasL defects. Perhaps the most interesting possibility is that, as in the mice, *fas* mutations amplify autoimmunity traits in the affected families.

Most patients with SLE do not appear to have a defect in Fas expression or function (Mysler *et al.*, 1994; Ohsako *et al.*, 1994). Soluble Fas (sFas), a secreted variant with the potential to block FasL, can be detected in the serum of 10–50% of SLE patients. The levels of sFas, however, are only twice those of normals and similar findings have been observed in many other systemic autoimmune disorders (Mountz *et al.*, 1995). Detailed studies of FasL function and soluble FasL (sFasL) are yet to be published. One study has reported reduced anti-CD3-mediated T cell apoptosis in T cell lines derived from SLE patients (Kovacs *et al.*, 1996).

Observations in murine models of systemic autoimmunity and in the Canale–Smith syndrome suggest that regulation of lymphocyte apoptosis is crucial to the maintenance of peripheral tolerance. The only pathway that has been extensively analysed in human lupus so far is Fas/FasL. Other cell death molecules have now been identified (see the machinery of apoptosis, above) and it will be important to consider alternative pathways that contribute to the elimination of activated T and B cells. For example, TNFα is a potent inducer of apoptosis and some RA patients treated with anti-TNFα antibodies develop anti-dsDNA antibodies, which disappeared on cessation of treatment (Elliot *et al.*, 1993).

Apart from its role in immune tolerance, apoptosis may play a direct role in antigen selection and, possibly, even the autoimmune response in SLE (Fig. 9.4*b*). It has recently been shown that the translocation of nuclear antigens to near the surface of ultraviolet-irradiated keratinocytes (LeFeber *et al.*, 1984; Golan *et al.*, 1992) can be explained by apoptosis (Casciola-Rosen, Anhalt & Rosen, 1994). Membrane alterations during apoptosis cause externalization of phosphatidyl-serine, of potential importance in the generation of anti-phospholipid antibodies. Furthermore, SLE patients frequently have lymphopenia and accelerated AICD *in vitro* (Emlen, Niebur & Kadera, 1994). On the basis of these findings, it has been suggested that apoptotic bodies contain biochemically modified self-antigens, which could be immunogenic (Casciola-Rosen *et al.*, 1994). However, Tan and colleagues (Casiano *et al.*, 1996) have demonstrated that a minority of lupus autoantigens are cleaved during apoptosis, and, conversely, many proteins that are not common antigens in SLE *are* cleaved.

In preliminary studies, Mevorach, Zhou & Elkon (1996) reported that large amounts of apoptotic material administered by the intravenous route can, albeit transiently, induce the production of certain autoantibodies in mice. In most individuals, however, extensive apoptosis occurs in the central lymphoid organs without evidence of autoimmunity, so an understanding of the qualitative and quantitative aspects of apoptosis, as well as the disposal mechanisms of apoptotic bodies may be informative.

Rheumatoid arthritis

In RA, an abnormal accumulation of inflammatory cells in the synovium leads to pannus formation and destruction of cartilage and bone. The mechanism responsible for synovial hyperplasia is not well understood and may result from an increase in the number of and/or reduced apoptosis of synoviocytes and infiltrating cells. Although evidence of apoptosis has been detected in RA synoviocytes (Firestein, Yeo & Zvaifler, 1995; Nakajima *et al.*, 1995), it has been suggested that the extent of synoviocyte apoptosis *in vivo* is inadequate to counteract ongoing proliferation. This imbalance may be explained by the production of cytokines such as $TGF\beta_1$ and IL-1β, which favour synoviocyte proliferation and inhibit susceptibility to apoptosis (Kawakami *et al.*, 1996; Tsuboi *et al.*, 1996). These and other signals could reduce apoptosis of synoviocytes, possibly through increased expression of the Bcl-2 family of proteins (Firestein *et al.*, 1995; Sugiyami *et al.*, 1996). TNFα is a pleiotropic cytokine that appears to be acting as a proinflammatory molecule in the RA synovium (Paleolog *et al.*, 1996). Since TNFα most likely signals through TNFR2 (see Fig. 9.1), NFκB is activated, which, in turn, inhibits apoptosis (Beg & Baltimore, 1996). Alternatively, inflammatory changes such as oxidation may result in upregulation (Sugiyami *et al.*, 1996) and mutations (Firestein *et al.*, 1996) of the p53 protein. It remains to be determined whether there is a loss of function of this important growth suppressor.

Synoviocytes can be triggered to undergo apoptosis via a Fas-mediated pathway. Whereas anti-Fas-mediated apoptosis of synoviocytes from patients with and osteoarthritis was equivalent *in vitro* (Firestein *et al.*, 1995; Nakajima *et al.*, 1995), an increase in sFas has been detected in RA synovial fluid (Hasunuma *et al.*, 1997). At present it is unclear whether sFas is functional and whether sFasL is also produced in the joint.

The inflammatory infiltrate in RA comprises T cells, plasma cells, macrophages and neutrophils. Despite expression of Fas and detection of FasL mRNA (Sumida *et al.*, 1997a) in infiltrating T cells, *in situ* observations of synovial lymphoid aggregates suggest low levels of apoptosis ((Firestein *et al.*, 1995; Sugiyami *et al.*, 1996). This may be because of high Bcl-2 expression by the T cells (Firestein *et al.*, 1995; Sugiyami *et al.*, 1996) or the production of an anti-apoptotic factor(s) by stromal cells (Salmon *et al.*, 1997). Of interest, Sumida *et al.* (1997a) report that there are two distinct T cell populations in the rheumatoid synovium, one susceptible to Fas-mediated apoptosis and the other resistant. Fas-sensitive T cell clones had conserved amino acid residues in the CDR3 domain of their T cell receptor, consistent with an *in situ* antigen-driven response. The same group has reported that local administration of an anti-Fas mAb to HTLV-1 *tax* transgenic mice (a mouse model of RA) led to an improvement in arthritis within 48 hours which was sustained for 2 weeks (Fujisawa *et al.*, 1996). Immunohistochemistry showed that 35% of synovial fibroblasts, 75% of mononuclear cells and some of the infiltrating neutrophils underwent apoptosis. It will be important to determine whether the induction of apoptosis in the rheumatoid joint can be used to therapeutic advantage.

Neutrophils isolated from RA joints spontaneously undergo programmed cell death *in vitro* with the same kinetics as those from peripheral blood (Bell *et al.*, 1995) and evidence of phagocytosis by macrophages has been reported (Savill *et al.*, 1989; Jones *et al.*, 1993). It is unknown whether macrophage phagocytosis of apoptotic neutrophils is sufficient to remove all of these cells and whether there are any pathological consequences of this process.

Sjögren's syndrome

Sjögren's syndrome is associated with intense lymphocytic infiltration and destruction of the salivary and lacrimal glands. Several reports have implicated apoptosis in the glandular destruction, and the high expression of the pro-apoptotic Bax protein in acini (Krajewski *et al.*, 1994; Kong *et al.*, 1996) suggests that they may be especially vulnerable to induction of apoptosis.

Acinar destruction may occur secondary to abnormal co-expression of Fas and FasL on the epithelial cells. Talal and co-workers have reported that whereas Fas is only expressed on ductal epithelium and FasL is not expressed in normal glands both molecules are expressed on the acini and ducts in Sjögren's syndrome (Kong *et al.*, 1997). This abnormal co-expression could lead to apoptosis by a suicidal mechanism (Fig. 9.4*c*). In Hashimoto's thyroiditis, a similar mechanism, triggered by IL-1β, has been proposed (Giordano *et al.*, 1997). IL-1β leads to upregulation of Fas, engagement of constitutively expressed FasL and apoptosis of thyrocytes.

Since the majority of infiltrating mononuclear cells are CD4[+], and FasL mRNA has been detected in lesional tissue (Sumida *et al.*, 1997b), an alternative mechanism of glandular injury has been proposed (Matsumura *et al.*, 1996; Sumida *et al.*, 1997b). In this model (Fig. 9.4*d*), cytotoxic T cells infiltrating the salivary glands induce apoptosis of the acinii.

Although Kong *et al.* (1997) have detected increased expression of Bcl-2 in the infiltrating mononuclear cells by immunohistochemistry, 40% of the T cells isolated from the glands of patients with Sjögren's syndrome are susceptible to Fas-mediated death *in vitro* (Sumida *et al.*, 1997b). The susceptibility of those T cells with more conserved TCR amino acid motifs to anti-Fas-mediated apoptosis led the authors to suggest that the anti-Fas-sensitive cells are the activated, effector T cell population. In addition to the acini and T cells, it will be important to examine the susceptibility of B cells to apoptosis since the 'pseudolymphomas' that occur in Sjögren's syndrome are derived from B lymphocytes.

Conclusions

Human diseases can be classified in terms of life and death problems of specialized cells (Carson & Ribeiro, 1993; Thompson, 1995). In this context, many autoimmune rheumatic diseases are characterized by immune cell infiltration resulting in the destruction of local specialized cells. Other autoimmune diseases are associated with inflammatory infiltrates and the accumulation of cells that fail to die. The first phase of investigative studies in these human diseases has focused on the necessary baseline information regarding which cells show the hallmarks of apoptosis and which cells express high levels of inducers or inhibitors of apoptosis. These studies, however, provide limited understanding of apoptosis regulation *in vivo*. Fortunately, in many cases, it has been possible to obtain cells from diseased tissues and examine their effector status and susceptibility to apoptosis *in vitro*. These functional studies, coupled with phenotypic or other markers of pathogenic effector cells, are necessary to distinguish whether the effectors are sensitive or resistant to apoptosis. This crucial distinction has important therapeutic implications.

In view of the major role of cytokines in mediating inflammation, it will also be important to integrate the results of the studies on apoptosis with known abnormalities of cytokine production in each disease. For example, cytokines that promote proliferation (see above) are often associated with expression of survival molecules such as Bcl-2 and Bcl-X$_L$ and will be expected to block many apoptotic pathways. Therefore, high Bcl-2/Bcl-X$_L$ expression and relative resistance to apoptosis induction should not be interpreted as a primary abnormality of an apoptotic programme under these circumstances. Removal of cells from their *in vivo* milieu may artefactually effect their survival through cytokine/growth factor withdrawal.

The elucidation of the biochemical pathways and specific proteins that regulate apoptosis provide a remarkable opportunity to manipulate the life and death decisions of the cell. For example, terapeptide inhibitors can selectively block different caspases and arrest apoptosis (Rodriguez *et al.*, 1996). Alternatively, agonists of apoptosis such as FasL, TNF-α and even soluble autoantigens (Critchfield *et al.*, 1994) can be harnessed to destroy autoreactive cells or cells that have escaped from the normal regulation of cell death programme. The basic understanding and therapeutic manipulation of apoptosis will have far reaching implications for the future health of patients with rheumatic disease.

References

Akbar, A.N., Borthwick, N.J., Wickremasinghe, R.G. *et al.* (1996). Interleukin-2 receptor common gamma-chain signaling cytokines regulate activated T cell apoptosis in response to growth factor withdrawal: selective induction of anti-apoptotic (*bcl-2, bcl-xL*) but not pro-apoptotic (*bax, bcl-xS*) gene expression. *Eur. J. Immunol.* 26: 294–299.

Alnemri, E.S., Livingstone, D.J., Nicholson, D.W. *et al.* (1996). Human ICE/CED3 protease nomenclature. *Cell* 87: 171.

Beg, A.A. & Baltimore, D. (1996). An essential role for NF-κB in preventing TNF-α-induced cell death. *Science* 274: 782–784.

Bell, A.L., Magill, M.K., McKane, R. & Irvine, A.E. (1995). Human blood and synovial fluid neutrophils cultured in vitro undergo programmed cell death which is promoted by the addition of synovial fluid. *Ann. Rheum. Dis.* 54: 910–915.

Benoist, C. & Mathis, D. (1997). Selection for survival? *Science* 276: 2000–2001.

Carson, D.A. & Ribeiro, J.R. (1993). Apoptosis and disease. *Lancet* 341: 1251–1254.

Casciola-Rosen, L.A., Anhalt, G. & Rosen, A. (1994). Autoantigens targeted in systemic lupus erythematosus are clustered in two populations of surface structures on apoptotic keratinocytes. *J. Exp. Med.* 179: 1317–1330.

Casiano, C.A., Martin, S.J., Green, D.R. & Tan., E.M. (1996). Selective cleavage of nuclear autoantigens during CD95 (Fas/APO-1)-mediated T cell apoptosis. *J. Exp. Med.* 184: 765–770.

Chervonsky, A.V., Wang, Y., Wong, S.F. *et al.* (1997). The role of Fas in autoimmune diabetes. *Cell* 89: 17–24.

Critchfield, J.M., Racke, M.K.J., Zuniga-Pflucker, C. *et al.* (1994). T cell deletion in high antigen dose therapy of autoimmune encephalomyelitis. *Science* 263: 1139–1143.

Drappa, J., Vaishnaw, A.K., Sullivan, K.E., Chu, J.L. & Elkon, K.B. (1996). The Canale Smith syndrome: an inherited autoimmune disorder associated with defective lymphocyte apoptosis and mutations in the Fas gene. *N. Engl. J. Med.* 335: 1643–1649.

Elkon, K.B. & Marshak-Rothstein, A. (1996). B cells in systemic autoimmune disease: recent insights from Fas-deficient mice and men. *Curr. Opin. Immunol.* 8: 852–59.

Elliott, M.J., Maini, R.N., Feldmann, M. *et al.* (1993). Treatment of rheumatoid arthritis with chimeric monoclonal antibodies to tumor necrosis factor. *Arthritis Rheum.* 36: 1681–1690.

Emlen, W., Niebur, J.-A. & Kadera, R. (1994). Accelerated *in vitro* apoptosis of lymphocytes from patients with systemic lupus erythematosus. *J. Immunol.* 152: 3685–3692.

Firestein, G.S., Yeo, M. & Zvaifler, N.J. (1995). Apoptosis in rheumatoid arthritis synovium. *J. Clin. Invest.* 96: 1631–1638.

Firestein, G.S., Nguyen, K., Aupperle, K.R., Yeo, M. & Zvaifler, N.J. (1996). Apoptosis in rheumatoid arthritis II. p53 overexpression in rheumatoid arthritis synovium. *Am. J. Pathol.* 149: 2143–2151.

Fisher, G.H., Rosenberg, F.J., Straus, S.E. *et al.* (1995). Dominant interfering Fas gene mutations impair apoptosis in a human lymphoproliferative syndrome. *Cell* 81: 935–946.

Fournel, S., Genestier, L., Robinet, E., Flacher, M. & Revillard, J.-P. (1996). Human T cells require IL-2 but not G1/S transition to acquire susceptibility to Fas-mediated apoptosis. *J. Immunol.* 157: 4309–4315.

Franke, T.F. & Cantley, L.C. (1997). A bad kinase makes good. *Nature* 390: 116–117.

Fraser, A. & Evan, G. (1996). A license to kill. *Cell* 85: 781–784.

Fujisawa, K., Asahara, H., Okamoto, K. *et al.* (1996). Therapeutic effect of the anti-Fas antibody on arthritis in HTLV-1 tax transgenic mice. *J. Clin. Invest.* 98: 271–278.

Giordano, C., Stassi, G., de Maria, R. *et al.* (1997). Potential involvement of Fas and its ligand in the pathogenesis of Hashimoto's thyroiditis. *Science* 275: 960–963.

Golan, T.D., Elkon, K.B., Gharavi, A.E. & Krueger, J.G. (1992). Enhanced membrane binding of autoantibodies to cultured keratinocytes of SLE patients after UVB/UVA irradiation. *J. Clin. Invest.* 90: 1067–1076.

Golstein, P. (1997). Controlling cell death. *Science* 275: 1081–1082.

Goodnow, C.C. (1992). Transgenic mice and analysis of B cell tolerance. *Annu. Rev. Immunol.* 10: 489–518.

Gura, T. (1997). How TRAIL kills cancer cells, but not normal cells. *Science* 277: 768.

Hasunuma, T., Kayagaki, N., Asahara, H. *et al.* (1997). Accumulation of soluble Fas in inflamed joints of patients with rheumatoid arthritis. *Arthritis Rheum.* 40: 80–86.

Hibbs, M.L., Tarlinton, D.M., Armes, J. *et al.* (1995). Multiple defects in the immune system of *lyn*-deficient mice, culminating in autoimmune disease. *Cell* 83: 301–311.

Irmler, M., Thome, M., Hahne, M., Schneider, P. *et al.* (1997). Inhibition of death receptor signals by cellular FLIP. *Nature* 388: 190–195.

Jones, S.T.M., Denton, J., Holt, P.J.L. & Freemont, A.J. (1993). Possible clearance of effect polymorphonuclear leucocytes from synovial fluid by cytophagocytic mononuclear cells: implications for pathogenesis and chronicity in inflammatory arthritis. *Ann. Rheum. Dis.* 52: 121–126.

Kawakami, A., Eguchi, K., Matsuoka, N. *et al.* (1996). Inhibition of Fas antigen-mediated apoptosis of rheumatoid synovial cells in vitro by transforming growth factor 1. *Arthritis Rheum.* 39: 1267–1276.

Kerr, J.F.R., Wyllie, A.H. & Currie, A.R. (1972). Apoptosis: a basic biological phenomenon with wide-ranging implications in tissue kinetics. *Br. J. Cancer* 26: 239–257.

Kong, L., Ogawa, N., Masago, R., Talal, N. & Dang, H. (1996). Bcl-2 family in salivary gland from Sjogren's syndrome: Bax may be involved in the destruction of SS salivary glandular epithelium. *Arthritis Rheum.* 39: S89.

Kong, L., Ogawa, N., Nakabayashi, T. *et al.* (1997). Fas and Fas ligand expression in the salivary glands of patients with primary Sjogren's syndrome. *Arthritis Rheum.* 40: 87–97.

Kovacs, B., Vassilopoulos, D., Vogelgesang, S.A. & Tsokos, G.C. (1996). Defective CD3-mediated cell death in activated T cells from patients with systemic lupus erythematosus: role of decreased intracellular TNF-alpha. *Clin. Immunol. Immunopathol.* 81: 293–302.

Kozono, Y., Kotzin, B.L. & Holers, V.M. (1996). Resting B cells from New Zealand Black mice demonstrate a defect in apoptosis induction following surface IgM ligation. *J. Immunol.* 156: 4498–4503.

Krajewski, S., Krajewska, M., Shabaik, A., Miyashita, T., Wang, H.G. & Reed, J.C. (1994). Immunohistochemical determination of in vivo distribution of Bax, a dominant inhibitor of Bcl-2. *Am. J. Pathol.* 145: 1323–1336.

Kroemer, G., Zamzami, N. & Susin, S.A. (1997). Mitochondrial control of apoptosis [Review]. *Immunol. Today* 18: 44–51.

Kumar, S. (1995). ICE-like proteases in apoptosis. *TIBS* 20: 198–202.

Kuo, C.T., Veselits, M.L. & Leiden, J.M. (1997). LKLF: a transcriptional regulator of single-positive T cell quiescence and survival. *Science* 277: 1986–1990.

LeFeber, W.P., Norris, D.A., Ryan, S.R. *et al.* (1984). Ultraviolet light induces binding of antibodies to selected nuclear antigens on cultured human keratinocytes. *J. Clin. Invest.* 74: 1545–1551.

Leist, M., Single, B., Castoldi, A.F., Kuhnle, S. &. Nicotera. P. (1997). Intracellular adenosine triphosphate (ATP) concentration: a switch in the decision between apoptosis and necrosis. *J. Exp. Med.* 185: 1481–1486.

Margolin, N., Raybuck, S.A., Wilson, K.P. *et al.* (1997). Substrate and inhibitor specificity of interleukin-1-converting enyzme and related caspases. *J. Biol. Chem.* 272: 7223–7228.

Matsumura, R., Kagami, M., Tomioka, H. *et al.* (1996). Expression of ductal Fas antigen in sialoadenitis of Sjogren's syndrome. *Clin. Exp. Rheum.* 14: 309–311.

Mevorach, D., Zhou, J.-L., Song, X. & Elkon K.B. (1998). Systemic exposure to irradiated apoptotic cells induces autoantibody production *J. Exp. Med.* 188: 387–393.

Mountz, J.D., Pierson, M.C., Zhou, T. *et al.* (1995). Fas expression in patients with autoimmune disease. *Arthritis Rheum.* 38: 127.

Muchmore, S.W., Sattler, M., Liang, H. *et al.* (1996). X-ray and NMR structure of human Bcl-xL, an inhibitor of programmed cell death. *Nature* 381: 335–341.

Mysler, E., Bini, P., Drappa, J., Ramos, P., Friedman, S.M., Krammer, P.H. & Elkon, K.B. (1994). The APO-1/Fas protein in human systemic lupus erythematosus. *J. Clin. Invest.* 93: 1029–1034.

Nagata, S. & Golstein, P. (1995). The Fas death factor. *Science* 267: 1449–1456.

Nakajima, T., Aono, H., Hasunuma, T. *et al.* (1995). Apoptosis and functional Fas antigen in rheumatoid arthritis synoviocytes. *Arthritis Rheum.* 38: 485–491.

Nishizumi, H., Taniuchi, I., Yamanashi, Y. *et al.* (1995). Impaired proliferation of peripheral B cells and indication of autoimmune disease in *lyn*-deficient mice. *Immunity* 3: 549–560.

Nossal, G.J.V. (1996). Clonal anergy of B cells: a flexible, reversible, and quantitative concept. *J. Exp. Med.* 183: 1953–1956.

Ohsako, S., Hara, M., Harigai, M., Fukusawa, C. & Kashiwazaki, S. (1994). Expression and function of Fas antigen and Bcl–2 in human systemic lupus erythematosus lymphocytes. *Clin. Immunol. Immunopathol.* 73: 109–114.

Oltvai, Z.N. & Korsmeyer, S.J. (1994). Checkpoints of dueling dimers foil death wishes. *Cell* 79: 189–192.

Paleolog, E.M., Hunt, M., Elliot, M.J., Feldmann, M., Maini, R. & Woody, J.N. (1996). Deactivation of vascular endothelium by monoclonal anti-tumor necrosis factor α antibody in rheumatoid arthritis. *Arthritis Rheum.* 39: 1082–1091.

Pani, G., Kozlowski, M., Cambier, J.C., Mills, G.B. & Siminovitch, K.A. (1995). Identification of the tyrosine phosphatase PTP1C as a B cell antigen receptor-associated protein involved in the regulation of B cell signaling. *J. Exp. Med.* 181: 2077–2084.

Rathmell, J.C., Townsend, S.E., Xu, J.C., Flavell, R.A. & Goodnow, C.C. (1996). Expansion or elimination of B cells in vivo: dual roles for CD40- and Fas (CD95)-ligands modulated by the B cell antigen receptor. *Cell* 57: 319–329.

Reed, J.C. (1994). Bcl–2 and the regulation of programmed cell death. *J. Cell. Biol.* 124: 1–6.

Rieux-Laucat, F., le Deist, F., Hivroz, C. *et al.* (1995). Mutations in Fas associated with human lymphoproliferative syndrome and autoimmunity. *Science* 268: 1347–1349.

Rodriguez, I., Matsuura, K., Ody, C., Nagata, S. & Vassalli, P. (1996). Systemic injection of a tripeptide inhibits the intracellular activation of CPP32-like proteases in vivo and fully protects mice against Fas-mediated fulminant liver destruction and death. *J. Exp. Med.* 184: 2067–2072.

Russell, J.H., Rush, B., Weaver, C. & Wang, R. (1993). Mature T cells of autoimmune *lpr/lpr* mice have a defect in antigen-stimulated suicide. *Proc. Natl. Acad. Sci., USA* 90: 4409–4413.

Sadlack, B., Merz, H., Schorle, H., Schimpl, H., Feller, A.C. & Horak, I. (1993). Ulcerative colitis-like disease in mice with a disrupted interleukin-2 gene. *Cell* 75: 253–261.

Salmon, M., Scheel-Toellner, D., Huissoon, A.P. *et al.* (1997). Inhibition of T cell apoptosis in the rheumatoid synovium. *J. Clin. Invest.* 99: 439–446.

Savill, J.S., Wyllie, A.H., Henson, J.E., Walport, M.J., Henson, P.M. & Haslett, C. (1989). Macrophage phagocytosis of aging neutrophils in inflammation. Programmed cell death in the neutrophil leads to its recognition by macrophages. *J. Clin. Invest.* 83: 865–875.

Savill, J., Fadok, V., Henson, P. & Haslett, C. (1993). Phagocyte recognition of cells undergoing apoptosis. *Immunol. Today* 14: 131–136.

Schwartz, R.H. (1996). Models of T cell anergy: is there a common molecular mechanism? *J. Exp. Med.* 184: 1–8.

Singer, G.G. & Abbas, A.K. (1994). The Fas antigen is involved in peripheral but not thymic deletion of T lymphocytes in T cell receptor transgenic mice. *Immunity* 1: 365–371.

Strasser, A., Whittingham, S., Vaux, D.L. *et al.* (1991). Enforced Bc1–2 expression in B-lymphoid cells prolongs antibody responses and elicits autoimmune disease. *Proc. Natl. Acad. Sci., USA* 88: 8661–8665.

Sugiyama, M., Tsukazaki, T., Yonekura, A., Matsuzaki, S., Yamashita, S. & Iwasaki, K. (1996). Localization of apoptosis and expression of apoptosis-related proteins in the synovium of patients with rheumatoid arthritis. *Ann. Rheum. Dis.* 55: 442–449.

Sumida, T., Minh Hoa, T.T., Asahara, H., Hasunuma, T. & Nishioka, K. (1997a). T cell receptor of Fas-sensitive T cells in rheumatoid synovium. *J. Immunol.* 158: 1965–1970.

Sumida, T., Matsumoto, I., Murata, H. *et al.* (1997b). TCR in Fas-sensitive T cells from labial salivary glands of patients with Sjogren's syndrome. *J. Immunol.* 158: 1020–1025.

Suzuki, H., Kundig, T.M., Furlonger, C. *et al.* (1995). Deregulated T cell activation and autoimmunity in mice lacking interleukin-2 receptor. *Science* 268: 1472–1476.

Thompson, C.B. (1995). Apoptosis in the pathogenesis and treatment of disease. *Science* 267: 1456–1462.

Tivol, E.A., Borriello, F., Schweitzer, A.N., Lynch, W.P., Bluestone, J.A. & Sharpe A.H. (1995). Loss of CTLA-4 leads to massive lymphoproliferation and fatal multiorgan tissue destruction, revealing a critical negative regulatory role of CTLA-4. *Immunity* 3: 541–547.

Tsuboi, M., Eguchi, K., Kawakami, A. *et al.* (1996). Fas antigen expression on synovial cells was downregulated by interleukin 1. *Biochem. Biophys. Res. Commun.* 218: 280–285.

Tsui, H.W., Siminovitch, K.A., de Souza, L. & Tsui, F.W.L. (1993). Motheaten and viable motheaten mice have mutations in the haematopoietic cell phosphatase gene. *Nature Genetics* 4: 124–129.

Uren, A.G., Pakusch, M., Hawkins, C.J., Puls, K.L. & Vaux, D.L. (1996). Cloning and expression of apoptosis inhibitory protein homologs that function to inhibit apoptosis and/or bind tumor necrosis factor receptor-associated factors. *Proc. Natl. Acad. Sci., USA* 93: 4974–4978.

Waterhouse, P., Penninger, J.M., Timms, E. *et al.* (1995). Lymphoproliferative disorders with early lethality in mice deficient in CTLA-4. *Science* 270: 985–988.

Watson, M.L., Rao, J.K., Gilkeson, G.S. *et al.* (1992). Genetic analysis of MRL-*lpr* mice: Relationship of the Fas apoptosis gene to disease manifestations and renal disease-modifying loci. *J. Exp. Med.* 176: 1645–1656.

Willerford, D.M., Chen, J., Ferry, J.A., Davidson, L., Ma, A. & Alt, F.W. (1995). Interleukin-2 receptor α chain regulates the size and content of the peripheral lymphoid compartment. *Immunity* 3: 521–530.

Wu, J., Wilson, J., He, J., Xiang, L., Schur, P.H. & Mountz, J.D. (1996). Fas ligand mutation in a patient with systemic lupus erythematosus and lymphoproliferative disease. *J. Clin. Invest.* 98: 1107–1113.

Yin, X.M., Oltvai, Z.N. & Korsmeyer, S.J. (1994). BH1 and BH2 domains of Bcl-2 are required for inhibition of apoptosis and heterodimerization with Bax. *Nature* 369: 321–323.

10

The role of monokines in arthritis

W. B. VAN DEN BERG and F. A. J. VAN DE LOO

Introduction

Rheumatoid arthritis (RA) is generally considered an autoimmune disease, with its main manifestation a chronic inflammatory process in the synovial tissues of multiple joints and concomitant local destruction of cartilage and bone. RA synovial fluid is predominantly enriched with neutrophils, whereas the most abundant cells in the synovial tissue are macrophages and T cells, with foci of plasma cells and variable degrees of fibroblast proliferation. Another characteristic feature is the considerable thickening of the synovial lining layer, comprising macrophage-like type A cells and fibroblast-like type B cells. A major site of cartilage and bone destruction originates from overgrowth of activated synovial tissue at the margins, the so-called pannus tissue, although cartilage destruction away from overgrowth is noted as well. A key ongoing issue of debate in this destructive process is whether it is mainly linked to the inflammatory infiltrate in the synovial tissue or whether autonomous activation of synovial tissue fibroblasts and macrophages is a major event. There is at least suggestive evidence from transfer studies in SCID mice that RA synovial tissue cells are potentially destructive and may cause substantial cartilage damage in the absence of T cells. Apart from mechanism of the destructive process, there is also a longstanding debate on chronic synovitis: is it a dominant T cell-dependent immune inflammation or does it reflect perpetuated activation of synovial fibroblasts and macrophages, with secondary but minor involvement of T cells. Arguments for the latter hypothesis are based on the detection of an abundance of macrophage-derived cytokines (monokines) in the RA synovial tissue and the relative paucity of T cell factors (Firestein & Zvaifler, 1990; Firestein, Alvaro-Garcia & Maki, 1990). However, low amounts of T_H1-derived cytokines such as IFN-γ and IL-2 may be sufficient to maintain T cell-driven synovitis, since similar difficulties were encountered in detecting T cell cytokines in proven, T cell-dependent delayed-type hypersensitivity reactions. There is no doubt that arthritis in animal models is more chronic and more destructive in the presence of T cell reactivity, either directed against retained antigens in joint tissues or cartilage-specific autoantigens such as collagen type II and proteoglycans. However, in the absence of a defined autoantigen in RA, antigen-specific immunomodulation is not a therapeutic option. In this chapter, we will focus on the role of the monokines IL-1, TNF, IL-6, IL-10, IL-12 and IL-15 in arthritic processes, with an emphasis on findings in animal models as well as human RA and identification of potential therapeutic targets.

Pathogenesis of arthritis

A central problem in chronic arthritis is the nature of the stimuli that drive the synovial inflammation. Theoretically, this may be provided by persistant exogenous stimuli such as bacteria or viruses that localize to joint tissues, either causing direct activation of synovial macrophages and fibroblasts or driving this pathway through T cell triggering. In addition, cartilage autoantigens may be involved, initiating the process or playing a major part at later stages as a consequence of marked tissue destruction and autoantigen release in the presence of loss of tolerance. Articular cartilage must somehow be involved, retaining exogenous antigens, releasing autoantigens or amplifying the synovial activation, since it is a long recognized finding in RA that arthritis wanes in a particular joint when the cartilage is fully destroyed or removed at joint replacement. A final option emerged from careful analysis of RA synovial cells, which demonstrate tumour-like behaviour upon culture *in vitro* and do not need additional stimuli to continue to mediator release and proliferation for several cell passages. Whether this transformed phenotype is cause or consequence of the chronic synovitis remains to be established.

As a reflection of T cell-driven or direct activation of macrophages and fibroblasts, large amounts of cytokines, chemokines and enzymes are produced. Proinflammatory cytokines and chemokines will then amplify the synovitis through stimulation of neighbouring cells, upregulation of adhesion molecule expression on endothelial cells, facilitating influx of more leukocytes from the blood and promoting enzyme release, which contributes to cartilage damage. Cytokines detected in vast amounts include TNFα, IL-1, GM-CSF and other growth factors, IL-6 and, more recently, IL-15 (Firestein *et al.*, 1990; Feldmann, Brennan & Maini, 1996). In addition, two modulatory cytokines are also abundant, IL-10 and TGFβ, which possess immunoregulatory as well as anti-inflammatory activity, inhibiting IL-1/TNF production but also inducing enzyme inhibitors such as TIMP, the natural inhibitor of metalloproteinases (Fig. 10.1). IL-4 is virtually absent in the RA synovium, in line with T_H1 dominance.

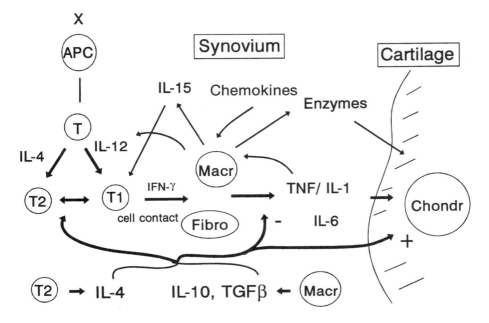

Fig. 10.1. Interplay of cytokines in the synovial tissue. The regulatory cytokines IL-4, IL-10 and TGFβ may interfere at various levels, their actions including skewing of T cell balances, inhibition of cytokine production by macrophages (Macr) and synovial fibroblasts (Fibro), and direct protective effects on the chondrocytes (Chondr) in the articular cartilage. APC, antigen-presenting cell.

Cytokine hierarchy, dominant role of TNF/IL-1

Given the vast abundance of a whole range of inflammatory mediators in the RA synovial tissue, it is encouraging to note that there seems to be substantial hierarchy. Evidence has emerged that TNF and IL-1 function as so-called master cytokines, orchestrating the synovitis (Arend & Dayer, 1995; Feldmann *et al.*, 1996). IL-1 and TNF protein were detected in the synovial fluid and in the synovial tissue; these mediators have been demonstrated at the mRNA level by Nothern blotting and *in situ* hybridization. Immunolocalization has identified predominant expression in macrophages. In addition, culture studies of synovial membranes or isolated cells further confirmed the enhanced production in RA synovia of these cytokines and it was claimed that TNF drives most of the IL-1 production (Feldmann *et al.*, 1996). It has to be noted that the synovial tissue is usually obtained at joint replacement surgery, at late stages of the disease. Samples from early stages are now becoming available through arthroscopic biopsies or blind small needle biopsies. Although some studies confirm the earlier findings, TNF and IL-1 are not always found and uncoupled mRNA expression of these cytokines may occur as well (Deleuran, 1996; Tak *et al.*, 1997; Wagner *et al.*, 1997). It is our impression from recent analysis of multiple biopsies that large variations exist among differing areas in the arthritic synovial tissue and clearly also among RA patients. TNF and IL-1 are not always seen in such samples.

Clinical trials with TNF/IL-1 inhibitors

Apart from detection of the presence of a cytokine, their roles can only be validated *in vivo*, by using specific antagonists such as neutralizing antibodies, soluble receptors or, in the case of IL-1, a natural inhibitor, IL-1ra. First studies done with the Centocor cA2 anti-TNF antibody led to rapid improvement in all RA patients studied (Elliott *et al.*, 1993) and the magnitude of the clinical response and reduction in CRP was reproduced in a randomized, double-blind, multicentre placebo-controlled trial. Subsequent studies with other anti-TNF antibodies and engineered soluble TNF receptors linked to the Fc portion of IgG confirmed the prominent role of TNF in RA, although the degree of suppression was variable. Second and third injections were often less efficacious, and precise use and limitations in individual patients must await further development. First studies into the mechanism of action of anti-TNF therapy points to reduction of expression of vascular adhesion molecules and lower cell numbers in the synovial tissue (Paleolog *et al.*, 1996). Recent X-ray analysis of a 6-month follow-up study did not provide evidence for protection against ongoing joint destruction (unpublished observations) and it is tempting to speculate that TNF is mainly involved in symptomatic aspects and pain in RA and less so in the joint destructive process. This would fit with a more dominant role of IL-1 in the latter process, which has emerged from studies in experimental arthritis models (see below).

Clinical trials with anti-IL-1 therapy are less well advanced, probably because of several factors, including the dogma that TNF blocking will eliminate most of the IL-1 effect, as well, the absence of eminent humanized anti-IL-1 antibodies, problems encountered with proper, scavenging soluble IL-1 receptors (sIL-1R) and the poor pharmacokinetics of IL-1 receptor antagonist (IL-1ra). When soluble IL-1 receptor was administered daily for 28 days and significant improvement was noted. Later on it became apparent that two types of IL-1 receptor exist (Collota *et al.*, 1993), the type I being the signalling receptor and the type II being a decoy receptor, having a function in scavenging. Unfortunately, the type I receptor was used in the clinical studies; it has poor affinity for IL-1β and high affinity for IL-1ra, in this respect interfering with the natural inhibitors. Recent studies with sustained dosing of IL-1ra yielded promising results. The impact on clinical parameters was less impressive compared with the anti-TNF data, but the treatment appeared to reduce joint erosions (Breshnihan *et al.*, 1996; Campion *et al.*, 1996). Given the huge dosages needed to control experimental arthritis with IL-1Ra, it is possible that optimal dosing has simply not been achieved yet. However, the relatively minor effect on joint inflammation but consistent effect on joint destruction fits with observations of IL-1 blocking in certain animal models of arthritis (see below).

Studies in animal models

While no animal model of arthritis fully mimics human RA, such models can be used to study certain aspects of the disease and comparison of findings in various models may provide insight into general pathogenic mechanisms. Further belief in an initiating role of TNF in arthritis has emerged from elegant studies in TNF transgenic mice. Overexpression of human TNF leads to chronic, erosive arthritis, and the disease can be prevented with anti-human TNF antibodies (Keffer *et al.*, 1991). It is not yet understood why arthritis is the major pathology in this mouse. Interestingly, the arthritis was completely abolished upon treatment with antibodies to the IL-1R, excluding the direct action of TNF. This is in line with the major arthritogenic potential of IL-1 (Probert *et al.*, 1995) and fits with earlier studies of direct injections of cytokines into knee joints of mice or rabbits. These studies showed major synovitis and characteristic cartilage damage with IL-1, either alone or in combination with TNF, whereas single injections of TNF alone were only marginally effective (Henderson & Pettipher, 1989; van de Loo & van den Berg, 1990).

Although the above data illustrate the potency of TNF and IL-1, it remains to be proved that these cytokines are also of crucial importance in established models of arthritis. The model most widely studied is the autoimmune collagen-induced arthritis (CIA) in mice, which is based on immunization with foreign collagen type II(CII) in genetically susceptible mice, mainly DBA/1j or B10RIII mice. The arthritis expression is dependent on a mixture of anti-collagen type II antibodies and anti-CII $T_H 1$ cells, and arthritis expression can be facilitated by injection of TNF/IL-1 or generation of non-specific inflammatory events with concomitant cytokine release at the time of expected onset (Killar & Dunn, 1989; Joosten, Helsen & van den Berg, 1994). When anti-TNF antibodies or other TNF inhibitors are given before or shortly after onset of disease, marked amelioration of arthritis was demonstrated by various groups (Williams, Feldmann & Maini, 1992; Wooley *et al.*, 1993). We have recently compared the efficacy of TNF and IL-1 blocking in this model, including a kinetic study starting anti-cytokine treatment at day 0, 3 or 7 after onset of arthritis. It confirmed that TNF blocking is mainly effective in early stages and less so at established disease, whereas the

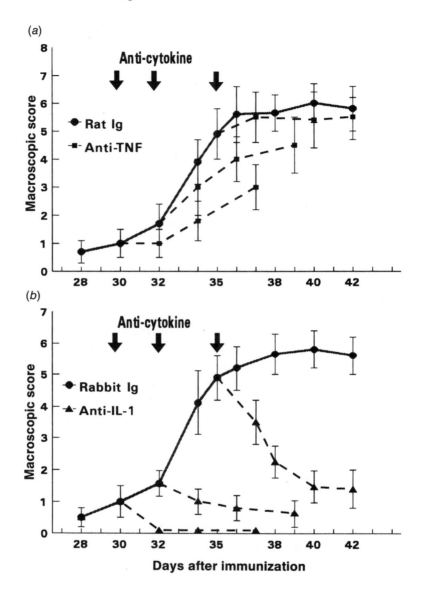

Fig. 10.2. Treatment of collagen-induced arthritis with anti-TNFα (*a*) or anti-IL-1α,β (*b*). A single injection of antibodies was given intraperitoneally, at various time points after disease onset (arrows). Rat anti-TNFα was marginally effective at late stages. In contrast, combinations of anti-IL-1α/anti-IL-1β showed prevention at the beginnning and impressive reduction when given in fully established disease (Joosten *et al.*, 1996).

suppressive effect of IL-1 elimination was more pronounced and also still prominent in established disease (Fig. 10.2). The role of IL-1 was substantiated with IL-1Ra treatment, which, however, appeared only effective when supplied with osmotic minipumps and high, sustained dosing (van den Berg *et al.*, 1994; Joosten *et al.*, 1996). Recently, we also showed efficacy of local IL-1Ra gene transfer in the knee joint of mice with CIA (Bakker *et al.*, 1997). The strong IL-1 dependence of this model is further substantiated by reduced expression in IL-1β converting enzyme (ICE) knock-out mice and efficacy of ICE inhibitors in CIA in normal mice (Ku *et al.*, 1996). Moreover, full prevention of CIA is seen in IL-1β knock-out mice (unpublished observations). Similar approaches using immune-driven models in TNF-deficient mice are hampered by the fact that these mice show major developmental abnormalities in lymphoid tissue organization and generation of immune responses (Pasparakis *et al.*, 1996). An elegant alternative is provided by the recent studies in TNF-receptor 1 (TNFR1)-deficient mice, crossed to DBA/1. Upon immunization with CII, these mice developed CIA with a low incidence and in a milder form. However, once a joint was afflicted, the arthritis progressed in that joint to the same end stage as observed in the wild-type mice (Mori *et al.*, 1996). This again argues that TNF is important at onset but that progression is TNF independent. It could also suggest that anti-TNF treatment in RA patients may be beneficial, when the chronicity of the disease is, in fact, based on repeated flares, with each flare displaying TNF dependency.

In earlier studies in the mouse, it was shown that a chronic synovitis can be caused to flare with tiny amounts of antigen, when the joint displays local hyperreactivity by retained T cells in the chronic infiltrate (Lens *et al.*, 1986). Anti-IL-1 treatment appeared effective in these flares (van de Loo *et al.*, 1995a). However, such a joint is also highly sensitive to flares induced by cytokines such as TNF or IL-1 and, in fact, it suggests that any non-specific inflammatory insult, with concomitant release of such proinflammatory cytokines, may exacerbate a chronic arthritis through reactivation of retained macrophages (van de Loo, Arntz & van den Berg, 1992a).

In other models of arthritis we have analysed the relative impact of TNFα and IL-1 in inflammation and cartilage destruction. In a simple passive immune complex model in mice, we found strong IL-1 dependence (van Lent *et al.*, 1994), in line with the observations in the collagen arthritis and perhaps suggesting that collagen arthritis is to a large extent an immune complex-driven disease. In murine antigen-induced arthritis (a model based on a T cell-driven reaction to locally injected and retained antigen in the knee joint of preimmunized animals, the initial inflammation (i.e. joint swelling and early cell influx) was barely dependent on TNF and IL-1, suggesting substantial overkill by other inflammatory mediators. However, late cellular infiltrate in the synovium and cartilage destruction was markedly reduced with anti-IL-1 treatment, showing high IL-1 dependence of these aspects of inflammation. In subsequent studies in non-immune arthritis, induced with zymosan or streptococcal cell wall (SCW) fragments, the IL-1 dependence of cartilage destruction was further substantiated (van de Loo *et al.*, 1992b; 1995b). Although IL-1 is not always the dominant cytokine in early joint swelling, cell influx and enzymatic proteoglycan degradation of cartilage, in all models tested so far it is the pivotal cytokine in cartilage proteoglycan synthesis inhibition. Normalization of this function by IL-1 neutralization always results in markedly reduced cartilage damage in late stages of the disease.

The TNF–IL-1 cascade

Returning to the issue of a TNF–IL-1 cytokine cascade in arthritis, we have carefully analysed the relative role of TNF and IL-1 in arthritis induced with SCW, allowing for proper measurement of inflammation, cartilage destruction and TNF/IL-1 levels in the inflamed synovium. In this model, we see pronounced uncoupling of joint swelling and cartilage proteoglycan synthesis inhibition. When TNF was blocked, using either anti-TNF antibodies or TNF binding protein (TNFbp: an engineered soluble receptor from Amgen), marked reduction in joint swelling was found, whereas inhibition of chondrocyte proteoglycan synthesis remained unchanged. In sharp contrast, IL-1 blocking with neutralizing antibodies or IL-1ra did not reduce joint swelling but fully normalized the chondrocyte synthetic function (Fig. 10.3). Intriguingly, TNF blocking *in vivo* did not reduce IL-1 levels in the arthritic synovial tissue. These findings indicate that TNF and IL-1 have separate functions. Moreover, a stringent TNF–IL-1 cascade is not seen in this model, and, in fact, potential uncoupling was already suggested by the greater impact of anti-IL-1 treatment compared with anti-TNF treatment in CIA. Potential uncoupling was further supported by unabated IL-1 production in SCW-induced arthritis in TNF-deficient mice. Swelling was much reduced but late arthritis was still prominent (unpublished observations). Although the triggering process in the human synovial tissue of RA patients may be different to that in SCW-induced arthritis or CIA, the claim that TNF is the key therapeutic target must be treated cautiously, especially with respect to the pivotal role of IL-1 in amplifying late synovial infiltrate and cartilage destruction.

A final remark should be made regarding the role of soluble TNF versus membrane-bound TNF. Although aspects of CIA and SCW-induced arthritis could be blocked with TNF inhibitors, pointing to TNF involvement, it appeared difficult to detect substantial levels of TNF in tissue washouts apart from the first hours after induction of arthritis. Recently, it was shown that arthritis could also

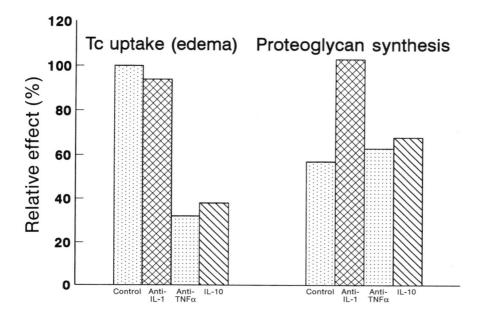

Fig. 10.3. Differential effect of anti-TNFα and anti-IL-1α,β on joint swelling and inhibition of chondrocyte proteoglycan synthesis in the early stage (day 2) of SCW-induced arthritis. The latter in the articular cartilage is only normalized with anti-IL-1. IL-10 displays an activity pattern similar to anti-TNFα treatment, consistent with dominant suppression of TNFα levels. Similar TNF/IL-1 specific results were obtained using TNF-binding proteins and IL-1ra as scavenging molecules (data not shown).

be induced by transgenic overexpression of transmembrane TNF (Georgopoulos, Plows & Kollias, 1996), elegantly demonstrating that soluble TNF is not needed to get full expression of arthritis. First studies with SCW-induced arthritis in TNF-deficient mice, 'knocked in' with transmembrane TNF (in collaboration with the group of George Kollias do suggest restoration of the arthritis. It remains to be seen whether anti-TNF treatment with antibodies or binding proteins is sufficiently effective in such mice.

Role of IL-6

IL-6 is a glycosylated polypeptide of around 26 kDa mainly produced by monocytes, T cells and fibroblasts. It belongs to a family of proteins with overlapping functions: leukemia inhibitory factor (LIF), oncostatin-M, ciliary neurotrophic factor and IL-11. The IL-6 receptor consists of two subunits: the α chain, with the IL-6 binding site (gp80) and the signal-transducing β chain (gp130). The gp130 receptor is shared by all members of the IL-6 family (Kishimoto, Akira & Taga, 1992). Both TNF and IL-1 can induce IL-6 in numerous cell types, and of the growing list of cytokines found in RA synovial fluid the concentration of IL-6 is high, many times greater than IL-1 and TNF levels (Houssiau, 1995). The levels of IL-6 in paired samples of synovial fluid and blood correlated in patients with RA. The higher levels found in synovial fluid of affected joints makes a plasma IL-6 flow into these joints unlikely, pointing to local production as the main source. In rats and mice, increased serum IL-6 activity followed closely the kinetics of development of collagen-induced and adjuvant arthritis (Sugita *et al.*, 1993). Indeed, human synovial tissue and the articular chondrocytes can produce huge amounts of IL-6 (Guerne *et al.*, 1989; Guerne, Carson & Lotz, 1990), and IL-1 and TNF synergistically increase the production of IL-6 in both tissues (Guerne *et al.*, 1990) The expression of mRNA and protein in the inflamed RA synovium showed that IL-6 was detected in cells present in lymphocyte-rich aggregates, and these cells were often in contact with CD14+ tissue macrophages (Wood *et al.*, 1992). It was shown that CD13+ synoviocytes can be stimulated to produce IL-6 by macrophages via CD14-mediated cell–cell contact (Chomarat *et al*, 1995a). In RA patients, the synoviocytes also expressed mRNA and protein of the other members of the IL-6-family, IL-11 and LIF. Oncostatin M was, however, exclusively expressed in the synovial tissue macrophages (Okamoto *et al.*, 1997). The physiological relevance of this discrepancy has to be elucidated.

Although IL-6 levels reflect the local inflammatory activity, radiological changes in the joint did not correlate with IL-6 (van Leeuwen *et al.*, 1995). However, IL-6 has recently been detected in complex with the shed form of the IL-6 receptor (sIL-6R; pg80) and, in contrast to IL-6, the local levels of IL-6/sIL-6R complex did correlate with the radiographic grades of joint destruction in patients with RA (Kotake *et al.*, 1996). Both sIL-6R and 'neutralizing' anti-IL-6 antibodies can chaperone circulating IL-6, and in high-IL-6 producers, monomeric immune complexes are formed, causing accumulation of IL-6 and preserving its bioactivity (May *et al.*, 1993). In the open study of Wendling, Racadot & Wijdenes (1993), murine anti-human IL-6 mAb treatment of patients with RA markedly improved ESR (eosinophil sedimentation rate) and the Ritchie's articular index. Indeed this treatment raised the serum IL-6 levels, suggesting a dominant carrier instead of scavenging function for the antibodies, resulting in enhanced IL-6 activity and, thus, supporting a beneficial role of IL-6 under these conditions. The recent development of IL-6R mutants with clean antagonistic activity (Romani *et al.*, 1997) will provide new tools to study the role of IL-6 in human diseases.

The general impression generated by all of the activities linked to IL-6 is that this molecule may have inflammatory as well as protective activity in the RA process (Fig. 10.4). A prominent activity, associated with its former name BSF-2 (B cell stimulatory factor) is stimulation of antibody production. Marked reduction in antibody levels was found after T cell-dependent antigen exposure in IL-6-deficient mice, whereas the T cell-independent IgM responses were not reduced. This suggests that IL-6 might have a prominent role in autoimmune rheumatoid factor (RF) production, as far as it reflects a T cell-dependent triggering. Although the role of RF is still not clear, its presence correlates with more severe and more destructive disease. A second aspect of proinflammatory activity is linked to its role in the bone marrow. IL-6, either injected or transgenically expressed in mice, resulted in increased numbers of megakaryocytes in bone marrow (Ishibashi *et al.*, 1989). Enhanced maturation of macrophages and granulocytes and subsequent influx in inflamed joints might contribute to severity. It is also claimed that IL-6 can induce chemokines. Intriguingly, endothelial cells do express gp130 but lack the IL-6R. It was elegantly shown that IL-6 alone was ineffective but that IL-6 together with sIL-6R clearly induced chemokines (Romani *et al.*, 1997). The relevance for leukocyte traffic of this IL-6 activity remains to be seen, since in the same study IL-1 and TNFα were shown to be much more potent inducers. A final activity to be mentioned is the stimulating role of IL-6 in bone resorption. IL-6 is produced by osteoblasts and exerts its activity through osteoclasts. Oestrogen-induced bone loss is reduced in IL-6-deficient mice, but no information is yet available on bone loss in arthritis.

Apart from these potentially proinflammatory activities, there is no doubt that IL-6 also induces protective effects. Induction of acute-phase proteins in hepatocytes includes enzyme inhibitors such as α_1-antitrypsin. Recently, it was shown that soluble IL-1 receptor antagonist (sIL-1ra) is also an acute-phase protein and levels of both IL-6 and sIL-1ra paralleled the fever spikes in systemic juvenile chronic arthritis (Prieur, Roux-Lombard & Dayer, 1996; Gabay *et al.*, 1997). Moreover, IL-1 and TNF are potent inducers of IL-6; however, in marked contrast, IL-6 does not induce destructive proteases in macrophages or fibroblasts but instead upregulates inhibitors, including TIMP as well as IL-1ra and TNF soluble receptors (Ito *et al.*, 1992; Tilg *et al.*, 1994) This suggests that IL-6 is not a downstream mediator of TNF/IL-1 activity but more a protein exerting feedback control. Cartilage cells make large amounts of IL-6 upon stimulation with IL-1, but studies in IL-6-deficient mice excluded a cofactor role of IL-6 in the cartilage destructive activity of IL-1 (van de Loo *et al.*, 1997). In addition, there is ample evidence of the suppressive effect of IL-6 on IL-1 and TNF production.

Since it is difficult to block the high levels of IL-6 satisfactorily with

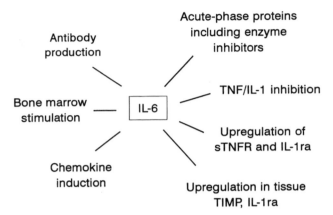

Fig. 10.4. Pleiotropic activity of IL-6, reflecting both inflammatory and protective actions.

antibodies or receptor blockers, the best approach in animal models is the use of IL-6-deficient mice. Given the role of IL-6 in antibody responses, immune models based on active immunization should be excluded and it comes as no surprise that CIA is markedly reduced in such a background, these mice displaying markedly lower anti-CII antibody levels. We have chosen to analyse non-immunologically mediated acute joint inflammation by intra-articular injection of zymosan in IL-6-deficient mice. No differences were observed in local mediator release of IL-1 or nitric oxide, or in systemic corticosterone concentrations compared with wildtype mice (van de Loo *et al.*, 1997). However, although the cellular infiltrate in the synovium was slightly reduced, cartilage destruction was higher, suggesting that IL-6 normally exerts a major protective role in cartilage damage.

IL-10 and TGFβ, regulation of arthritis

Additional cytokines with immunoregulatory and anti-inflammatory properties include IL-4, IL-10, IL-13 and TGFβ. These cytokines may derive from T_H2 cells or T3 cells (TGFβ), and their function in regulation of T_H1 responses and its consequence for chronic synovitis will be addressed elsewhere in this book. Apart from immunomodulation, these mediators also suppress IL-1 and TNF production and have a direct impact on the chondrocytes in the articular cartilage. Moreover, activated macrophages involved in control of inflammation will be an important source of IL-10 and TGFβ in the inflamed synovium. At the local level in the inflamed joint, this might be a more important contribution in regulation of the arthritis than T_H2 or T3 cells. T_H2 cells are virtually absent in RA synovia as is IL-4 (Deleuran, 1996; Feldmann *et al.*, 1996).

IL-10 is abundant in RA synovial tissue as detected by reverse transcriptase–polymerase chain reaction (RT–PCR) and immunostaining and also in supernatant of synovial cell cultures (Katsikis *et al.*, 1994). The endogenous IL-10 is functional, since neutralization enhanced the TNFα and IL-1 production in RA synovial cultures. However, the control is not maximal, since addition of recombinant IL-10 further inhibited TNF/IL-1 production. In similar studies with intact synovial tissue culture, it was found that exogenous IL-10 again inhibited IL-1β production, but IL-4 appeared more potent and also induced the inhibitor IL-1ra. IL-10 appears to upregulate soluble TNF receptors. The sensitivity to IL-10 regulation is dependent on the differentiation stage of the synovial cells (Chomarat, Banchereau & Miossec, 1995b; Dechanet *et al.*, 1995a), and in that sense the use of isolated cell cultures may give a skewed impression of *in vivo* events.

Studies in arthritis models demonstrated that systemic anti-IL-10 treatment shortly before onset of CIA markedly enhanced the expression and severity of the disease (Kasama *et al.*, 1995) and this is probably linked to increased expression of chemokines as well as enhanced IL-1/TNFα levels. We found that the best expression of CIA was achieved with a combination of anti-IL-10 and anti-IL-4 antibodies (Joosten *et al.*, 1997a). Moreover, suppression of established CIA was shown with IL-10 treatment (Walmsley *et al.*, 1996), but a much more pronounced suppression, including protection against cartilage destruction, was achieved with the combination of IL-10 and IL-4, although IL-4 alone was marginally effective (Joosten *et al.*, 1997a). RT–PCR revealed suppressed TNF/IL-1 levels and upregulated IL-1Ra/IL-1 balance in synovial tissue and arthritic cartilage. Further studies in SCW-induced arthritis confirmed that pronounced suppression of TNF as well as IL-1 was only achieved with the combination treatment. Again, IL-10 was a dominant endogenous regulator, since anti-IL-10 treatment prolonged the chronicity of the synovitis and enhanced the cartilage damage (Lubberts *et al.*, 1998).

Although IL-4/IL-10 treatment may seem an intriguing option compared with plain inhibition of TNF/IL-1, with additional upregulation of inhibitors, one should be aware of potential side effects. IL-10 is a potent B cell stimulator and is suggested to be involved in RF production in RA synovia (Dechanet *et al.*, 1995b). IL-4 has a positive effect on chondrocytes, preincubation reducing subsequent destructive effects of IL-1. However, IL-4 can also stimulate fibroblast proliferation and enzyme release, and analysis of safe dosing regimens needs proper attention.

TGFβ is perhaps even more pleiotropic, showing strong immunosuppressive activity but also chemotactic potential. When given systemically it reduced CIA, but when injected in a normal joint, it induced recruitment of leukocytes and stimulated local fibroblast proliferation, mimicking tissue fibrosis. When injected in an inflamed joint, it enhanced the cell mass in the synovial tissue yet counteracted the proteoglycan depletion in the articular cartilage, probably by stimulation of the chondrocyte proteoglycan synthesis and through its ability to inhibit production of metalloproteinases and to induce TIMP. This protective effect on the articular cartilage has been demonstrated by co-injection of TGFβ, both in an IL-1-driven arthritis (van Beuningen *et al.*, 1994a; Glansbeek *et al.*, 1997) and in zymosan-induced arthritis. In addition, TGFβ induced characteristic osteophytes at the joint margins, through its strong activation of periosteal cells and cartilage-inductive potential (van Beuningen *et al.*, 1994b). High levels of TGFβ are found in RA synovial fluid and expression in synovial tissue has been noted, but interpretation of its role is complicated by difficulties in discriminating between the inactive precursor form, complexed with LAP (latency associated peptide) and the active TGFβ.

In general, the destructive character of an arthritis probably depends more on the balance of proinflammatory and modulatory cytokines than on the actual levels of the former. Some models of arthritis are more aggressive than others, and it is tempting to speculate that this is linked to different cytokine balances, as a result of various arthritogenic stimuli or more T cell- or macrophage-driven pathogenesis. Progression of RA in various patients is also variable, perhaps related to different underlying processes or linked to differences in genetic regulation of proinflammatory and modulatory cytokines. There is no doubt that factors such as IL-10, IL-4 and TGFβ have a protective potential, controlling the impact of proinflammatory and destructive cytokines such as TNF and IL-1. However, given the risk of side effects, it seems more safe just to block the proinflammatory cytokines. Further studies are needed to examine whether protective effects and side effects of modulatory cytokines are seen at similar or different concentration ranges or whether they vary with differing routes of administration (including targeted gene transfer).

IL-12, unmasking or controlling autoimmune reactivity

IL-12 is a heterodimeric cytokine, mainly produced by activated macrophages. It stimulates the development of naive T cells into T_H1 cells and stimulates IFNγ secretion by such cells. Efficient stimuli to induce IL-12 in macrophages include lipopolysaccharides (LPS), bacteria and intracellular parasites, and this production is enhanced by IFNγ and suppressed by IL-4 and IL-10. In general, IL-12 is considered as a principal protective factor in bacterial infections, where it bridges innate resistance and antigen-specific immunity. However, IL-12 may unmask T_H1-dependent autoimmune reactions by its skewing of the T_H1/T_H2

ratios and may be a crucial intermediate in the often suggested link between bacterial infections and expression of autoimmune diseases. There are few data on production of IL-12 in RA synovial tissue, but in view of the predominance of T_H1 cells in this compartment, its involvement is not unlikely. First studies in murine CIA have shown that early treatment with IL-12 during immunization promotes severe arthritis in disease-prone DBA/1 mice; in fact, IL-12 can replace the mycobacterial adjuvant normally needed to induce anti-collagen type II autoimmunity (German *et al.*, 1995). However, IL-12 failed to promote CIA in C57B1 mice: it provoked CII-specific IFNγ-producing T cells but failed to induce the arthritogenic anti-CII-specific antibody subclasses needed to bind to cartilage surface and to initiate arthritis by release of cartilage-specific T cell epitopes (Szeliga *et al.*, 1996). Follow-up studies in DBA/1 mice showed that daily high-(1 μg) instead of low-dose IL-12 treatment suppressed CIA, and this was linked to reduced antibody responses (Hess *et al.*, 1996). It is now apparent that high IL-12 dosing has profound side effects on lymphoid organs and bone marrow. Apart from the role of IL-12 in skewing immune responses, we have studied the role of IL-12 at later stages of the development of arthritis. When IL-12 is given at the time of onset of CIA, it markedly enhanced disease expression and severity, whereas anti-IL-12 antibodies prevented spontaneous and LPS-triggered expression of CIA. This makes IL-12 a challenging therapeutic target. However, in established disease, anti-IL-12 treatment is poorly suppressive; in contrast, late daily IL-12 treatment (0.1 μg) significantly suppressed instead of enhanced CIA (Joosten *et al.*, 1997b). It was also apparent that IL-12 is a potent inducer of IL-10 production by macrophages and T cells *in vitro*, providing an important negative feedback mechanism that could prevent excessive activation and tissue pathology (Meyaard *et al.*, 1996). In fact, we did observe extremely high IFNγ and IL-10 levels after late IL-12 treatment, and the suppression of CIA by IL-12 could be abolished with concomitant anti-IL-10 antibody treatment (Joosten *et al.*, 1997b). This suggests that IL-12 promotes arthritis at the onset whereas it is a suppressive factor in late-stage disease. This bimodal activity will seriously complicate IL-12-directed therapy in human arthritis.

IL-15, an alternative to IL-2 in T cell stimulation

IL-15 is an IL-2 homologue that, in contrast to IL-2 itself, is abundantly present in RA synovia. Many cell types including macrophages and fibroblasts, with the notable exception of normal T cells, can produce IL-15, but the trigger inducing IL-15 production is not known. Its potent T cell-activating activity and the subsequent triggering of macrophage TNF production by these IL-15 activated T cells makes it a pivotal candidate in the RA process. IL-15 potently attracts memory T cells, and much of the T cell chemotactic activity present in RA synovial fluid appears to be attributable to IL-15 (McInnes *et al.*, 1996; 1997). The induction of macrophage TNF production by IL-15-activated T cells appeared to be dependent on cell–cell contact and was linked to CD69 expression. Interestingly, CD69 is also pivotal in the cell–cell interaction of T cells and synoviocytes, resulting in cartilage-degrading protease release (Lacraz *et al.*, 1994). This new pathway of T cell-driven TNF production sheds new light on the critical T cell involvement in the RA process, which was long debated because of low IL-2 and IFNγ levels. Future studies with anti-IL-15 antibodies in RA patients and animals models are needed to show the relevance of this cytokine, which may potentially be higher in the hierarchy than TNF/IL-1.

Final considerations

This discussion of the role of the various monokines in the arthritic process surveys recent developments and provides some insight into the contribution of the more recently discovered cytokines with the higher code numbers. Although some of these display intriguing activities, it might still be therapeutically attractive to focus on the straightforward, arthritogenic cytokines TNF and IL-1. Given the separate activities regarding inflammation and cartilage destruction and the clear evidence from experimental models that IL-1-driven processes may occur uncoupled from TNF, it may be advisable to go for combination therapy, perhaps also including a protease inhibitor to control for cytokine-independent enzyme activities in the synovial tissue. As a basic approach, we have, in recent studies, selectively eliminated the synovial lining macrophages from the murine knee joint, using local application of phagocytosable toxic liposomes, before arthritis induction. This treatment almost completely reduced the onset of arthritis in the joint but did not fully control the destructive process (van Lent *et al.*, 1996; van den Berg & van Lent, 1996). The synovial lining cells are highly reactive to TNF and IL-1 and are a major source of chemokines. However, our treatment probably also eliminated lining macrophages involved in production of controlling cytokines. It would appear that, in line with the various subsets of lymphocytes, there exists macrophage subset with more destructive or protective character. If such cells can be more properly defined, for instance with regard to CD markers, this may offer novel therapeutic targets in the near future.

This approach does not encompass arthritogenic antigens. If these exist in RA and are not different in every patient, they would provide an even better therapeutic target, provided that we could achieve in antigen-specific immunomodulation in established arthritis. At present, we are left with manipulation of key mediators. This might include the 'immunologic' approach of local generation of suppressive cytokines/monokines from T cell/macrophage origin, such as IL-4 and TGFβ by so-called bystander suppression. This refers to skewing towards protective T_H2 or T_H3 responses against endogenous proteins abundantly present in the inflamed joint, such as heat-shock proteins or cartilaginous components. Another intriguing variant might be the focused introduction of 'planted antigens' in the joint by direct injection, in the presence of a manipulated, protective T cell response against these proteins. Further knowledge is needed on the true protective character of mediators such as IL-4, IL-10, IL-13 and TGFβ in arthritis before such approaches can be safely applied to human arthritides.

References

Arend, W.P. & Dayer, J.M. (1995). Inhibition of the production and effects of IL-1 and TNFα in RA. *Arthritis Rheum.* 38: 151–160.

Bakker, A.C., Joosten, L.A.B., Arntz, O.J., Helsen, M.M.A., Bendele, A., van de Loo, F.A.J. & van den Berg, W.B. (1997). Prevention of murine collagen-induced arthritis in the knee and ipsilateral paw by local expression of human IL-Ira protein in the knee. *Arthritis Rheum.* 40: 893–900.

Breshnihan, B., on behalf of the collaborating investigators Lookabaugh, J., Witt, K. & Musikic, P. (1996). Treatment with recombinant human IL-Ira in RA: results of a randomized double blind, pacebo controlled multicenter trial. *Arthritis Rheum.* 39(Suppl. 9): S73.

Campion, G.V., Lebsack, M.E., Lookabaugh, J., Catalano, M. *et al.* (1996). Dose-range and dose-frequency study of recombinant human-IL-1ra in patients with rheumatoid arthritis. *Arthritis Rheum.* 39: 1092–1101.

Chomarat, P., Rissoan, M.C., Banchereau, J. & Miossec, P. (1995a). Contribution of IL-1, CD14, and CD13 in the increased IL-6 production induced by *in vitro* monocyte–synoviocyte interactions. *J. Immunol.* 155: 3645–3652.

Chomarat, P., Banchereau, J. & Miossec, P. (1995b). Differential effects of interleukins 10 and 4 on the production of IL-6 by blood and synovium monocytes in rheumatoid arthritis. *Arthritis Rheum.* 38: 1046–1054.

Collota, F., Re, F., Muzio, M., Bertini, R., Polentarutti, N., Sironi, M., Dower, S.K., Sims, J.E. & Montovani, A. (1993). IL-1 type II receptor: as a decoy target for IL-1 that is regulated by IL-4. *Science* 261: 472–474.

Dechanet, J., Rissoan, M.C., Banchereau, J. & Miossec, P. (1995a). IL-4, but not IL-10, regulates the production of inflammation mediators by rheumatoid synoviocytes. *Cytokine* 7: 176–183.

Dechanet, J., Merville, P., Durand, I., Banchereau, J. & Miossec, P. (1995b). The ability of synoviocytes to support terminal differentiation of activated B cells may explain plasma cell accumulation in rheumatoid synovium. *J. Clin. Invest.* 95: 456–463.

Deleuran, B. (1996). Cytokines in RA: localization in arthritic joint tissue and regulation in vitro. *Scand. J. Rheumatol.* 25(Suppl. 104), 1–38.

Elliott, M.J., Maini, R.N., Feldmann, M., Long-Fox, A., Charles, P., Katsikis, P., Brennan, F.M., Walker, J., Bijl, H., Ghrayeb, J. & Woody, J. (1993). Treatment of rheumatoid arthritis with chimeric monoclonal antibodies to TNFα. *Arthritis Rheum.* 36: 1681–1690.

Firestein, G.S. & Zvaifler, N.J. (1990). How important are T cells in chronic rheumatoid synovitis. *Arthritis Rheum.* 33: 768–773.

Firestein, G.S., Alvaro-Garcia, J.M. & Maki, R. (1990). Quantitative analysis of cytokine gene expression in RA. *J. Immunol.* 144: 3347–3353.

Feldmann, M., Brennan, F. & Maini, R.N. (1996). Role of cytokines in rheumatoid arthritis. *Annu. Rev. Immunol.* 14: 397–440.

Gabay, C., Smith, M.F., Eidlen, D. & Arend, W.P. (1997). Interleukin 1 receptor antagonist (IL-1Ra) is an acute-phase protein. *J. Clin. Invest.* 99: 2930–2940.

Georgopoulos, S., Plows, D. & Kollias, G. (1996). Transmembrane TNF is sufficient to induce localized tissue toxicity and chronic inflammatory arthritis in transgenic mice. *J. Inflam.* 46: 86–97.

German, T., Szeliga, J., Hess, H., Storkel, S., Podlaski, F.J., Gately, M.K., Schmitt, E. & Rude, E. (1995). Administration of IL-12 in combination with type II collagen induces severe arthritis in DBA/1 mice. *Proc. Natl. Acad. Sci., USA* 92: 4823–4827.

Glansbeek, H.L., van Beuningen, H.M., Vitters, E.L., Morris, E.A., van der Kraan, P.M. & van den Berg, W.B. (1997). Bone morphogenetic protein-2 stimulates articular cartilage proteoglycan synthesis in vivo but does counteract IL-1α effects on proteoglycan synthesis and content. *Arthritis Rheum.* 40: 1020–1028.

Guerne, P.A., Zuraw, B.L., Vaughan, J.H., Carson, D.A. & Lotz, M. (1989). Synovium as a source of interleukin 6 in vitro. Contribution to local and systemic manifestations of arthritis. *J. Clin. Invest.* 83: 585–592.

Guerne, P.A., Carson, D.A. & Lotz, M. (1990). IL-6 production by human articular chondrocytes. Modulation of its synthesis by cytokines, growth factors, and hormones in vitro. *J. Immunol.* 144: 499–505.

Henderson, B. & Pettipher, E.R. (1989). Arthritogenic actions of recombinant IL-1 and TNFα in the rabbit; evidence for synergistic interactions between cytokines in vivo. *Clin. Exp. Immunol.* 75: 306–310.

Hess, H., Gately, M.K., Rude, E., Schmitt, E., Szeliga, J. & German, T. (1996). High doses of IL-12 inhibit the development of joint disease in DBA/1 mice immunized with type II collagen in complete Freund's adjuvant. *Eur. J. Immunol.* 26: 177–191.

Houssiau, F.A. (1995). Cytokines in rheumatoid arthritis. *Clin. Immunol.* 14: 10–13.

Ishibashi, T., Kimura, H., Shikama, Y., Uchida, T., Kariyone, S., Hirano, T., Kishimoto, T., Takatsuki, F. & Akiyama, Y. (1989). Interleukin-6 is a potent thrombopoietic factor in vivo in mice. *Blood* 74: 1241–1244.

Ito, A., Itoh, Y., Sasaguri, Y., Morimatsu, M. & Mori, Y. (1992). Effects of interleukin-6 on the metabolism of connective tissue components in rheumatoid synovial fibroblasts. *Arthritis Rheum.* 35: 1197–1201.

Joosten, L.A.B., Helsen, M.M.A. & van den Berg, W.B. (1994). Accelerated onset of collagen-induced arthritis by remote inflammation. *Clin. Exp. Immunol.* 97: 204–211.

Joosten, L.A.B., Helsen, M.M.A., van de Loo, F.A.J. & van den Berg, W.B. (1996). Anticytokine treatment of established type II collagen-induced arthritis in DBA/1 mice: a comparative study using anti-TNFα, anti-IL-1α/β, and IL-1ra. *Arthritis Rheum.* 39: 797–809.

Joosten, L.A.B., Lubberts, E., Durez, P., Helsen, M.M.A., Jacobs, M.J.M., Goldman, M. & van den Berg, W.B. (1997a). Role of IL-4 and IL-10 in murine collagen-induced arthritis: protective effect of IL-4 and IL-10 treatment on cartilage destruction. *Arthritis Rheum.* 40: 249–260.

Joosten, L.A.B., Lubberts, E., Helsen, M.M.A. & van den Berg, W.B. (1997b). Dual role of IL-12 in early and late stages of murine collagen type II arthritis. *J. Immunol.* 159: 4094–4102.

Kasama, T., Strieter, R.M., Lukacs, N.W., Lincoln, P.M. & Burdick, M.D. (1995). IL-10 expression and chemokine regulation during the evolution of murine type II collagen-induced arthritis. *J. Clin. Invest.* 95: 2868–2876.

Katsikis, P., Chu, C.Q., Brennan, F.M., Maini, R.N. & Feldmann, M. (1994). Immunoregulatory role of IL-10 in RA. *J. Exp. Med.* 179: 1517–1527.

Keffer, J., Probert, L., Cazlaris, H., Georgopoulos, S., Kaslaris, E., Kioussis, D. & Kollias, G. (1991). Transgenic mice expressing human TNF: a predictive genetic model of arthritis. *EMBO J.* 10: 4025–4031.

Killar, L.M. & Dunn, C.J. (1989). IL-1 potentiates the development of collagen induced arthritis in mice. *Clin. Sci.* 76: 535–538.

Kishimoto, T., Akira, S. & Taga, T. (1992). Interleukin-6 and its receptor: a paradigm for cytokines. *Science* 258: 593–597.

Kotake, S., Sato, K., Kim, K.J., Takahashi, N., Udagawa, N., Nakamura, I., Yamaguchi, A., Kishimoto, T., Suda, T. & Kashiwazaki, S. (1996). Interleukin-6 and soluble interleukin-6 receptors in the synovial fluids from rheumatoid arthritis patients are responsible for osteoclast-like cell formation. *J. Bone Miner. Res.* 11: 88–95.

Ku, G., Faust, T., Lauffer, L.L., Livingston, D.J. & Harding, M.W. (1996). IL-1β converting enzyme inhibition blocks progression of type II collagen induced arthritis in mice. *Cytokine* 8: 377–386.

Lacraz, S., Isler, P., Vey, E., Welgus, H.G. & Dayer, J.M. (1994). Direct contact between T lymphocytes and monocytes is a major pathway for induction of metalloproteinase expression. *J. Biol. Chem.* 269: 22 027–22 033.

Lens, J.W., van den Berg, W.B., van de Putte, L.B.A. & Zwarts, W.A. (1986). Flare-up of antigen induced arthritis in mice after challenge with intravenous antigen: kinetic of antigen in the circulation and localization of antigen in the arthritic and noninflamed joint. *Arthritis Rheum.* 29: 665–674.

Lubberts, E., Joosten, L.A.B., Helsen, M.M.A. & van den Berg, W.B. (1998). More therapeutic benefit with IL-4/IL-10 combination therapy than with IL-10 treatment alone. *Cytokine*, 10: 361–369.

May, L.T., Neta, R., Moldawer, L.L., Kenney, J.S., Patel, K. & Sehgal, P.B. (1993). Antibodies chaperone circulating IL-6. Paradoxical effects of anti-IL-6 'neutralizing' antibodies in vivo. *J. Immunol.* 151: 3225–3236.

McInnes, I.B., Al-Mughales, J., Field, M., Leung, B.P., Huang, F.P., Dixon, R., Sturrock, R.D., Wilkinson, P.C. & Liew, F.Y. (1996). The role of IL-15 in T-cell migration and activation in rheumatoid arthritis. *Nature Med.* 2: 175–182.

McInnes, I.B., Leung, B.P., Sturrock, R.D., Field, M. & Liew, F.Y. (1997). IL-15 mediates T cell-dependent regulation of TNFα production in rheumatoid arthritis. *Nature Med* 3: 189–195.

Meyaard, L.E., Hovenkamp, S., Otto, A. & Miedema, F. (1996). IL-12 induced IL-10 production by human T cells as a negative feedback for IL-12 induced immune responses. *J. Immunol.* 156: 2776–2783.

Mori, L., Iselin, S., De Libero, G. & Lesslauer, W. (1996). Attenuation of collagen-induced arthritis in 55-kDa TNF receptor type 1 (TNFR1)-IgG$_1$-treated and TNFR1-deficient mice. *J. Immunol.* 157: 3178–3182.

Okamoto, H., Yamamura, M., Morita, Y., Harada, S., Makino, H. & Ota, Z. (1997). The synovial expression and serum levels of interleukin-6, interleukin-11, leukemia inhibitory factor, and oncostatin M in rheumatoid arthritis. *Arthritis Rheum.* 40: 1096–1105.

222　W. B. van den Berg and F. A. J. van de Loo

Paleolog, E.M., Hunt, M., Elliott, M.J., Feldmann, M., Maini, R.N. & Woody, J.N. (1996). Deactivation of vascular endothelium by monoclonal anti-TNFα antibody in rheumatoid arthritis. *Arthritis Rheum.* 39: 1082–1091.

Pasparakis, M., Alexopoulou, L., Episkopou, V. & Kollias, G. (1996). Immune and inflammatory responses in TNFα-deficient mice: a critical requirement for TNFα in the formation of primary B cell follicles, follicular dendritic cell networks and germinal centers, and in the maturation of the humoral immune response. *J. Exp. Med.* 184: 1397–1411.

Prieur, A.M., Roux-Lombard, P. & Dayer, J.M. (1996). Dynamics of fever and the cytokine network in systemic juvenile arthritis. *Rev. Rhum.* (English edn), 3: 163–170.

Probert, L., Plows, D., Kontogeorgos, G. & Kollias, G. (1995). The type I IL-1 receptor acts in series with TNFα to induce arthritis in TNFα transgenic mice. *Eur. J. Immunol.* 25: 1794–1797.

Romani, M., Sironi, M., Toniatti, C., Polentarutti, N., Fruscella, P., Ghezzi, P., Faggioni, R., Luini, W., van Hinsberg, V., Sozzani, S., Bussolino, F., Poli, V., Ciliberto, G. & Mantovani, A. (1997). Role of IL-6 and its soluble receptor in induction of chemokines and leukocyte recruitment. *Immunity* 6: 315–325.

Sugita, T., Furukawa, O., Ueno, M., Murakami, T., Takata, I. & Tosa, T. (1993). Enhanced expression of interleukin 6 in rat and murine arthritis models. *Int. J. Immunopharmac.* 15: 469–476.

Szeliga, J., Hess, H., Rude, E., Schmitt, E. & German, T. (1996). IL-12 promotes cellular but not humoral type II collagen specific Th1 type responses in C57B1/6 and B10.Q mice and fails to induce arthritis. *Int. Immunol.* 8: 1221–1227.

Tak, P.P., Smeets, T.J.M., Daha, M.R., Kluin, P.M., Meijers, K.A.E., Brand, R., Meinders, A.E. & Breedveld, F.C. (1997). Analysis of the synovial cell infiltrate in early rheumatoid synovial tissue in relation to local disease activity. *Arthritis Rheum.* 40: 217–225.

Tilg, H., Trehu, E., Atkins, M.B., Dinarello, C.A. & Mier, J.W. (1994). Interleukin-6 (IL-6) as an anti-inflammatory cytokine: induction of circulating IL-1 receptor antagonist and soluble tumor necrosis factor receptor p55. *Blood* 83: 113–118.

van Beuningen, H.M., van der Kraan, P.M., Arntz, O.J. & van den Berg, W.B. (1994a). In vivo protection against interleukin-1-induced articular cartilage damage by transforming growth factor-B1: age related differences. *Ann. Rheum. Dis.* 53: 593–600.

van Beuningen, H.M., van der Kraan, P.M., Arntz, O.J. & van den Berg, W.B. (1994b). Transforming growth factor-β1 stimulates articular chondrocyte proteoglycan synthesis and induces osteophyte formation in the murine knee joint. *Lab. Invest.* 71: 279–290.

van de Loo, A.A.J. & van den Berg, W.B. (1990). Effects of murine recombinant IL-1 on synovial joints in mice: measurement of patellar cartilage metabolism and joint inflammation. *Ann. Rheum. Dis.* 49: 238–245.

van de Loo, A.A.J., Arntz, O.J. & van den Berg, W.B. (1992a). Flare-up of experimental arthritis in mice with murine recombinant IL-1. *Clin. Exp. Immunol.* 87: 196–202.

van de Loo, F.A.J., Arntz, O.J., Otterness, I.G. & van den Berg, W.B. (1992b). Protection against cartilage proteoglycan synthesis inhibition by anti-interleukin 1 antibodies in experimental arthritis. *J. Rheumatol.* 19: 348–356.

van de Loo, A.A.J., Arntz, O.J., Bakker, A.C., van Lent, P.L.E.M., Jacobs, M.J.M. & van den Berg, W.B. (1995a). Role of interleukin-1 in antigen-induced exacerbations of murine arthritis. *Am. J. Pathol.* 146: 239–249.

van de Loo, A.A.J., Joosten, L.A.B., van Lent, P.L.E.M., Arntz, O.J. & van den Berg, W.B. (1995b). Role of interleukin-1, tumor necrosis factor α and interleukin-6 in cartilage proteoglycan metabolism and destruction. Effect of in situ cytokine blocking in murine antigen- and zymosan-induced arthritis. *Arthritis Rheum.* 38: 164–172.

van de Loo, F.A.J., Kuiper, S., van Enckevort, F.H.J., Arntz, O.J. & van den Berg, W.B. (1997). Interleukin-6 ameliorates cartilage destruction during experimental arthritis: a study in interleukin-6-deficient mice. *Am. J. Pathol.* 151: 177–191.

van den Berg, W.B. & van Lent, P.L.E.M. (1996). Role of macrophages in chronic arthritis. *Immunobiology* 195: 614–623.

van den Berg, W.B., Joosten, L.A.B., Helsen, M.M.A. & van de Loo, A.A.J. (1994). Amelioration of established murine collagen induced arthritis with anti-IL-1 treatment. *Clin. Exp. Immunol.* 95: 237–243.

van Leeuwen, M.A., Westra, J., Limburg, P.C., van Riel, P.L.C.M. & van Rijswijk, M.H. (1995). Clinical significance of interleukin-6 measurements in early rheumatoid arthritis: relation with laboratory and clinical variables and radiological progression in a three year prospective study. *Ann. Rheum. Dis.* 54: 674–677.

van Lent, P.L.E.M., van den Hoek, A.E.M., van den Bersselaar, L.A.M., van de Loo, F.A.J., Eykholt, H.E., Brouwer, W.F.M., van de Putte, L.B.A. & van den Berg, W.B. (1994). Early cartilage degradation in cationic immune complex arthritis in mice: relative role of interleukin 1, the polymorphonuclear cell (PMN) and PMN elastase. *J. Rheumatol.* 21: 321–329.

van Lent, P.L.E.M., Holthuysen, A.E.M., van den Bersselaar, L.A.M., van Rooijen, N., Joosten, L.A.B., van de Loo, F.A.J., van de Putte, L.B.A. & van den Berg, W.B. (1996). Phagocytic lining cells determine local expression of inflammation in type II collagen-induced arthritis. *Arthritis Rheum.* 39: 1545–1555.

Wagner, S., Fritz, P., Einsele, H., Sell, S. & Saal, J.G. (1997). Evaluation of synovial cytokine patterns in rheumatoid arthritis and osteoarthritis by quantitative reverse transcription polymerase chain reaction. *Rheumatol. Int.* 16: 191–196.

Walmsley, M., Katsikis, P.D., Abney, E., Parry, S., Williams, R.O., Maini, R.N. & Feldmann, M. (1996). IL-10 inhibition of the progression of established collagen induced arthritis. *Arthritis Rheum.* 39: 495–503.

Wendling, D., Racadot, E. & Wijdenes, J. (1993). Treatment of severe rheumatoid arthritis by anti-interleukin 6 monoclonal antibody. *J. Rheumatol.* 20: 259–262.

Williams, R.O., Feldmann, M. & Maini, R.N. (1992). Anti-TNF ameliorates joint disease in murine collagen induced arthritis. *Proc. Natl. Acad. Sci., USA* 89: 9784–9788.

Wood, N.C., Symons, J.A., Dickens, E. & Duff, G.W. (1992). In situ hybridization of IL-6 in rheumatoid arthritis. *Clin. Exp. Immunol.* 87: 183–189.

Wooley, P.H., Dutcher, J., Widmer, M.B. & Gillis, S. (1993). Influence of a recombinant human soluble TNF receptor Fc fusion protein on type II collagen induced arthritis in mice. *J. Immunol.* 151: 6602–6607.

11

T lymphocyte subsets in relation to autoimmune disease

F. RAMIREZ, B. SEDDON and D. MASON

Introduction

The immune system has evolved a wide variety of potent mechanisms for the elimination of pathogens. As these mechanisms are potentially damaging to the host, an essential feature of the adaptive immune response is that it should be able to distinguish self from non-self and respond, when appropriate, only to the latter. The failure of the immune system to make this distinction can result in autoreactive cells mounting immune responses against self tissues, causing life-threatening pathology. There are now an increasing number of diseases in which an autoimmune process has been implicated in the pathogenesis, including RA, insulin-dependent diabetes mellitus (IDDM), multiple sclerosis, thyrotoxicosis, systemic lupus erythematosus (SLE), autoimmune haemolytic anaemia and myasthenia gravis to name a few. In order to avoid the damaging reactions that can cause this type of disease, the immune system has evolved a number of strategies for preventing autoreactive cells from making responses against host tissues, thus maintaining a state of self-tolerance.

In broad terms, mechanisms of self-tolerance can be categorized into two different classes. In the first, tolerance is maintained by both intra- and extrathymic mechanisms. Autoreactive T cells that encounter self-antigen within the thymus are clonally deleted (Kappler, Roehm & Marrack, 1987) while autoreactive cells that escape this process are either rendered anergic (Mueller, Jenkins & Schwartz, 1989), a state thought to result from the non-immunogenic presentation of self-antigens, or simply fail to respond to self-antigens, a state known as clonal indifference (Ohashi et al., 1991). These mechanisms may be termed 'passive' since they rely upon the functional absence of autoreactive cells or the failure of the self-antigens to be presented in an immunogenic form. In recent years, it has become evident that these mechanisms are not sufficient to account for tolerance to all self-antigens. There is now compelling evidence for the existence of a

225

second class of mechanism for self-tolerance, in which autoimmunity is prevented by specific regulatory T cells. These mechanisms are termed 'active' since they rely upon the action of a regulatory population controlling autoreactive cells.

This chapter will discuss how T cell subsets have been implicated both in the cause and prevention of autoimmunity. T cell subsets will be defined by the pattern of cytokine secretion and their cell surface phenotype.

T_H1 and T_H2 subsets of peripheral T cells

Mouse CD4+ T cells

Although some CD4+ T cells can be cytotoxic, it seems that cells of this phenotype regulate the immune response predominantly through the production of cytokines. Long-term mouse CD4+ T cells clones can be divided on the basis of cytokine synthesis into two mutually exclusive subsets: T_H1 cells, secreting IFN-γ, IL-2 and TNF, and T_H2 cells, which secrete IL-4, IL-5, IL-6, IL-10 and IL-13 (Mosmann & Coffman, 1989). These cytokines activate different effector mechanisms on different target cells. For instance, IFN-γ is the major macrophage-activating factor and induces IgG2a antibody responses (Coffman *et al.*, 1988); IL-4 induces switching of B cells to IgE and IgG_1 production, and IL-5 is the principal eosinophil-differentiation factor. The activity of the cytokines produced make T_H1 cells primarily mediators of cell-mediated responses whereas T_H2 are preferentially mediators of humoral responses (Mosmann & Coffman, 1989). The existence of two different T helper populations that regulate independently cell-mediated and humoral immunities provides an explanation for the observed reciprocal regulation of these two responses *in vivo* (Parish, 1972).

The activation of murine T_H1 and T_H2 T cell subsets appears to be mutually antagonistic not only because the cytokines secreted by these subsets have distinct functional properties but also because they are often mutually inhibitory. For example, the synthesis and activation of IFN-γ is inhibited by the T_H2 cytokines IL-4 and IL-10 (Fiorentino, Bond & Mosmann, 1989; Powrie & Coffman, 1993). Conversely, IFN-γ inhibits both the action of IL-4 on IgE and IgG_1 synthesis and the proliferation of T_H2 cells (Fernandez-Botran *et al.*, 1988; Gajewski & Fitch, 1988).

Murine CD4 T cell clones have been isolated that do not fall into the T_H1/T_H2 classification but secrete both types of cytokine and are, therefore, described as T_H0 (Firestein *et al.*, 1989). The existence of these T_H0 clones suggests that CD4+ T cells pass through an intermediate stage of differentiation and these uncommitted cells can be induced to secrete either T_H1 or T_H2 cytokines on subsequent stimulations depending on the environment in which they were primarily activated. In strong immune responses characterized by repetitive stimulation, the T_H1 and T_H2 phenotypes may become dominant. Several factors have been shown to regulate the balance between T_H1 and T_H2 responses. The route of administration and physical state of the antigen (Asherson & Stone, 1965), dose of antigen (Hosken *et al.*, 1995), MHC (Murray *et al.*, 1989), antigen-presenting cell involved in the T cell activation (Chang *et al.*, 1990; Gajewski *et al.*, 1991; Stockinger *et al.*, 1996) and hormones present at the time of activation (Daynes & Araneo, 1989; Ramírez *et al.*, 1996) have all been shown to influence this balance in different experimental systems. However, the most important factors in determining the pattern of cytokines produced by T cells are the cytokines they themselves produce and those produced by the antigen-presenting cells. Early studies showed that IL-4 supports the development of T_H2 effector cells (Le-Gros *et al.*, 1990) whilst IFN-γ, IL-12 and TGFβ are strong inductors of T_H1 cell development (Swain, Weinberg & English, 1990; Hsieh *et al.*, 1993). It is widely accepted that macrophages and dendritic cells when activated by bacterial components produce IL-12, and this cytokine directs the development of T_H1 cells (Macatonia *et al.*, 1993). However, the *in vivo* source of IL-4 is a matter of controversy and several cell types have been proposed as candidates in different experimental systems: NK1.1+ CD4+ T cells (Yoshimoto & Paul, 1994), recent thymic emigrants (Bendelac & Schwartz, 1991), eosinophils/mast cells (Paul, Seder & Plaut, 1993; Sabin & Pearce, 1995) and CD4+ T cells (Launois *et al.*, 1997).

Human CD4+ T cells

Earlier studies analysing cytokine production by short-term human T cell clones failed to demonstrate segregation into T_H1 and T_H2 cells similar to that seen in murine T cell clones. The majority of these clones displayed a T_H0 phenotype (Maggi *et al.*, 1988). However, when CD4+ T cell clones were obtained from individuals with chronic inflammatory or allergic diseases and they were activated with the disease-inducing antigen, the division between T_H1 and T_H2 clones was observed. T cell clones from these patients probably represent T cells that have been repetitively stimulated *in vivo*, suggesting that the chronic antigen exposure leads to a more stable polarization than does short-term culture. A T_H2 pattern of cytokine production is observed in allergen-specific cells from atopic patients (Wierenga *et al.*, 1990). In contrast, T_H1 cytokines are synthesized by T cell clones specific for *Borrelia burdorgferi* antigens obtained from patients with Lyme arthritis and by *Mycobacterium leprae*-reactive T cell clones obtained from individuals with tuberculoid leprosy (Haanen *et al.*, 1991; Yssel *et al.*, 1991).

CD8+ T cells

Whereas CD8+ mouse T cells stimulated *in vitro* usually secrete a T_H1 pattern of cytokines (Fong & Mosmann, 1990), there is now increasing evidence that a T_H2-like pattern of cytokines is also inducible in these cells by IL-4 addition (Seder *et al.*, 1992). Recent studies have shown that alloantigen-activated mouse CD8+ T cells can be treated in a similar way to CD4+ T cells to generate T_H1 or T_H2 responses, the so-called T_C1 and T_C2 cells (Sad, Marcotte & Mosmann, 1995). Some human CD8+ T cell clones have been found to secrete a T_H0 pattern of cytokines (Paliard *et al.*, 1988).

T_H1 and T_H2 cells and autoimmune diseases

As discussed, T_H1 responses are characterized by the activation of the cellular component of the immune system and the synthesis of inflammatory cytokines. In contrast, some of the T_H2 cytokines display anti-inflammatory effects and inhibit the development of T_H1 responses, suggesting that T_H2 cells could be the physiological regulators of T_H1 cells. According to this hypothesis, the T_H1/T_H2 balance could be important in the induction and regulation of autoimmunity. T_H1 responses against self-antigens would provoke the autoimmune disease and T_H2 cells would have the potential to downregulate this autoimmune attack. This concept has been explored in several experimental autoimmune models, the best characterized being experimental allergic encephalomyelitis (EAE) and the spontaneous development of diabetes by the non-obese diabetic (NOD) mouse. It is also important to point out that some experimental autoimmune diseases are characterized by a dysregulated T_H2 response (Prigent *et al.*, 1995).

Experimental allergic encephalomyelitis

EAE is an experimental paralysing disease that is studied as a model for multiple sclerosis (Zamvil & Steinman, 1990). The disease is induced in the appropriate animal strains after immunization with CNS antigens emulsified in complete Freund's adjuvant (CFA). This procedure is termed 'active EAE' in contrast to the induction of 'passive EAE' by the injection into naive animals of CNS antigen-specific lymphocytes. Most rat and mouse strains are resistant to the induction of active EAE, but this disease can be induced in Lewis rats after immunization with myelin-basic protein (MBP) in CFA (Hughes & Stedronska, 1973) and in SJL/J mice after immunization with pertussis toxin (Levine & Sowinski, 1973).

Lewis rats are susceptible to the induction of many experimental autoimmune and inflammatory diseases such as EAE, mycoplasmosis (Davis *et al.*, 1982), experimental autoimmune myasthenia gravis (Biesecker & Koffler, 1988) and arthritis (Griffiths & DeWitt, 1984). The high susceptibility in Lewis rats has been related to the defective regulation of glucocorticoid hormone production. During immune or inflammatory responses, blood glucocorticoid concentration increases as a result of activation of the hypothalamic–pituitary–adrenal axis by inflammatory and immune mediators such as IL-1, IL-6 and TNF (Besedovsky *et al.*, 1986; Naitoh *et al.*, 1988; Warren *et al.*, 1988). The glucocorticoid hormones produced in this way have an inhibitory effect on the synthesis of these cytokines and, as a result, the amounts produced are regulated to avoid an excessive and dangerous immune and inflammatory response (Munck, Guyre & Holbrook, 1984). Lewis rats manifest a deficiency in this regulatory interaction between the immune and neuroendocrine systems (Sternberg *et al.*, 1989) and there is also evidence that patients with RA show a similar defective regulation of corticosteroid production (Chikanza *et al.*, 1992).

Similar to multiple sclerosis, certain forms of EAE in mice and rats are characterized by relapsing paralysis (Lublin *et al.*, 1981; Feurer, Prentice & Cammisuli, 1985), but EAE in Lewis rats is characterized by a single episode of paralysis followed by spontaneous recovery. The animals develop a transient paralysis caused by the action of CD4+ T lymphocytes that infiltrate the CNS (Sedgwick, Brostoff & Mason, 1987). Animals recover spontaneously and become refractory to attempts to induce further episodes of disease (MacPhee & Mason, 1990). Several mechanisms responsible for the spontaneous recovery from EAE and the maintenance of the refractory phase have been proposed, including different regulatory leukocyte populations and several cytokines and soluble factors (Lider *et al.*, 1988; Kennedy *et al.*, 1992; Santambrogio *et al.*, 1993). A role has been also suggested for neuroendocrine-mediated immunoregulation (Levine, Sowinski & Steinetz, 1980; MacPhee, Antoni & Mason, 1989). Blood corticosteroid concentration increases before the onset of paralysis, with its peak at the time of maximum clinical score. The animals start to recover from paralysis after the peak in serum corticosterone and when they recover fully the glucocorticoid levels fall to their normal values. The role of endogenously produced corticosterone was analysed by evaluating the effect of adrenalectomy in Lewis rats subjected to EAE. It was observed that adrenalectomized animals developed an unremitting and progressive paralysis with a fatal outcome. If these adrenalectomized rats were given corticosterone-replacement therapy at the onset of paralysis, they recovered within a few days and developed the refractory state like non-adrenalectomized animals (MacPhee *et al.*, 1989). These observations showed that endogenously produced corticosterone plays an essential role in the recovery of rats from EAE. The interpretation of these observations is that the spontaneous recovery occurs because corticosteroids acutely depress the auto-immune response through their immunosuppressive and anti-inflammatory effects. Once animals have recovered from EAE, adrenalectomy has no adverse effect and the refractory phase develops as it does in non-adrenalectomized controls. Evidently corticosteroids are not directly responsible for the maintenance of the refractory phase of the disease, but these observations do not exclude the possibility that the transiently elevated levels of glucocorticoid hormones during paralysis have long-term effects on the immune response to MBP.

The analysis of cytokines synthesized by animals with EAE during the different phases of the disease show a predominant production of Th1 cytokines previous to the onset of disease and predominance of IL-10 and TGF-β during and after the recovery from paralysis (Kennedy *et al.*, 1992; Issazadeh *et al.*, 1995). The studies performed employing MBP-specific lines has shown that EAE in Lewis rats is mediated by CD4$^+$ T cells that produce IL-2 and IFN-γ (Sedgwick, MacPhee & Puklavec, 1989) whilst IL-4-producing lines are not able to induce passive EAE (F. Ramírez, unpublished data). Similar findings have been described in the mouse EAE model: MBP-specific T_H1 clones can induce disease but T_H2 clones do not and, in some circumstances, can inhibit the development of EAE (Chen *et al.*, 1994; Kuchroo *et al.*, 1995). However, other authors have obtained encephalitogenic T_H1 lines that were not suppressed by T_H2 lines (Khoruts, Miller & Jenkins, 1995). Our experience with the Lewis rat model confirms this observation: rat T_H1 lines are encephalitogenic and T_H2 lines do not transfer disease; however, we do not observe any protective effect from the T_H2 lines when these are injected simultaneously with T_H1 lines (F. Ramírez, unpublished data).

From these observations it seems that EAE is provoked by a T_H1- or cell-mediated response but that after recovery the T_H1 reactivity may become dominated by T_H2 cytokines with the ability to downregulate cell-mediated responses. If glucocorticoids can tip the T_H1/T_H2 balance, favouring the latter, as suggested by the *in vitro* experiments (Daynes & Araneo, 1989; Ramírez *et al.*, 1996), then the refractory phase of EAE in Lewis rats can, in principle, be explained by endogenously produced glucocorticoids inducing a switch from a T_H1 to a T_H2 response to MBP (Mason, 1991). This hypothesis provides an explanation for the recovery and refractory periods, although a more detailed analysis is necessary to verify it.

NOD mice

NOD mice spontaneously develop insulitis that progresses into diabetes with a higher incidence amongst females. Studies have shown some evidence for a pathogenic role for T_H1 cells and a protective function for T_H2 cells in diabetes. The *in vivo* administration of antibodies against IFN-γ prevents the onset of diabetes in NOD mice (Debray-Sachs *et al.*, 1991) and systemic administration of IL-4 prevents the disease (Rapoport *et al.*, 1993). T cell clones with a T_H1 phenotype are able to accelerate the onset of disease and T_H2 T cell clones are innocuous but cannot prevent the damaging effects of the T_H1 clones (Katz, Benoist & Mathis, 1995). Recent data have indicated that the situation is very complex. For instance, IFN-γ knock-out NOD mice develop diabetes like normal NOD mice, indicating that this cytokine is not necessary for the induction of diabetes (Hultgren *et al.*, 1996). Another paradox is that IL-10 transgenes expressed in the pancreas of NOD mice rather that inhibiting actually promote the development of diabetes (Lee *et al.*, 1996). This result shows that in different *in vivo* systems, T_H2 cytokines can inhibit or promote the development of disease. It is apparent that a more detailed analysis is required to understand the aetiology of diabetes in NOD mice.

Subsets of peripheral CD4+ T cells identified by the expression of different CD45 isoforms

In the preceding discussion, subsets of T cells were characterized according to cytokine production following activation. An alternative approach is to examine the expression of cell-surface antigens by T lymphocytes. One marker that has proved useful in defining functionally distinct subsets of CD4+ T cells is the leukocyte common antigen (LCA or CD45). CD45 is expressed in a number of different isoforms, generated by the differential use of exons A, B and C at the amino terminus of the extracellular end of the molecule (Thomas, 1989). Any combination of these three exons may be used, resulting in theoretically eight different forms, including CD45 molecules lacking all three exons, denoted as CD45RO. The functional significance of the range of isoforms is unknown. However, the analysis of subsets of CD4+ peripheral T cells defined by the expression of different CD45 isoforms has provided clear evidence for functional specialization amongst these cells.

In the rat, a mouse mAb specific for the C exon of CD45 reveals two subsets of CD4+ T cells: one third CD45RC[low] and two thirds CD45RC[high]. Studies of these subsets reveal extensive functional differences. Responses to OVA-DNP made by nude rats reconstituted with different subsets of CD4+ T cells revealed that it was CD4+CD45RC[high] cells that provided helper activity for primary antibody responses (Powrie & Mason, 1989). In contrast CD4+CD45RC[low] cells were more potent at providing B cells with help for secondary antibody responses (Spickett *et al.*, 1983), suggesting that CD45RC[high] cells are the precursors of

CD45RC[low] memory cells. Further, CD45RC[high] cells were found to mediate lethal graft-versus-host (GVH) disease or local GVH responses in the popliteal lymph node assay (Spickett *et al.*, 1983).

In vitro experiments with these subsets both confirmed and extended the data from *in vivo* studies. CD45RC[low] but not CD45RC[high] cells were found to mediate secondary anti-hapten antibody responses when cultured with B cells. Activation of these subsets also revealed differences in the patterns of secreted cytokines: levels of IL-2 and IFN-γ were much higher in cultures of activated CD45RC[high] cells than in similar cultures of CD45RC[low] cells, but the latter expressed higher levels of IL-4 mRNA (Arthur & Mason, 1986; McKnight, Barclay & Mason, 1991). The repertoire of cytokines synthesized by these subsets *in vitro* is in broad agreement with their behaviour *in vivo*. However, while there are considerable functional differences between these subsets, neither is homogeneous and other markers subdivide them (Fowell & Mason, 1993). Further, there is evidence that the CD4+CD45RC[high] subset contains long-term memory cells (Bunce & Bell, 1997).

Subsets of mouse CD4+ lymphocytes based on the differential expression of the isoform CD45RB have been identified, and it is apparent that there are considerable similarities in the behaviour of these subsets with those of rat subsets defined by CD45RC expression (Bottomly *et al.*, 1989). In humans, there are two non-overlapping T cell subsets defined by the expression of the isoforms containing the CD45RA exon and an epitope characteristic of the CD45RO isoform, which are thought to correspond to the naive and memory T cell pool, respectively (Akbar *et al.*, 1988). However this conclusion has been reconsidered (Pilling *et al.*, 1996.)

Evidence for the presence of autoreactive cells in the T cell repertoire of normal rodents

There is now much evidence that overtly autoreactive cells are present in the normal repertoire of T cells and that they are prevented from mediating pathological responses to self-antigens through active regulation by other T cells. In particular, studies in which congenitally athymic (nude) rodents are reconstituted with congenic T cells or in which the T cell pool of normal rodents is perturbed by protocols rendering the host lymphopenic have provided convincing support.

Reconstitution of nude rodents with subsets of peripheral CD4+ lymphocytes

Previous studies have examined the behaviour of different T cell subsets following their adoptive transfer into nude rats. Nude rats receiving CD4+CD45RC^{low} cells isolated from congenic donors remained healthy and were more resistant to infection than unreconstituted rats. In contrast, rats injected with CD4+CD45RC^{high} cells from congenic donors developed a wasting disease with a fatal outcome. Examination of tissues from these rats revealed mononuclear cellular infiltrates in organs including liver, pancreas, stomach and thyroid. The development of the multiorgan pathology mediated by CD4+CD45RC^{high} cells could be completely prevented by the co-transfer of CD4+CD45RC^{low} cells from normal animals (Powrie & Mason, 1990).

Similar studies in the mouse have shown that reconstitution of C. B-17 *scid* mice with CD4+CD45RB^{high} lymphocytes from B*alb/c* mice caused the mice to develop a lethal wasting disease. Mice were found to be suffering from an inflammatory bowel disease (IBD) characterized by profound mononuclear infiltrates of the colon. Mice receiving injections of CD45RB^{low}, unfractionated CD4+ lymphocytes or co-transfer of CD4+CD45RB^{low} cells with CD4+CD45RB^{high} cells at a ratio of 1 : 2, respectively, remained healthy (Powrie *et al.*, 1993). Further studies of the mechanisms of pathology and disease control showed that *in vivo* blockade of IFN-γ by neutralising mAb and systemic administration of IL-10 but not IL-4 prevented colitis development in recipients of CD45RB^{high} cells (Powrie *et al.*, 1994) whilst anti-TGFβ blocking mAb prevented control of colitis in recipients receiving both CD45RB^{high} and CD45RB^{low} cells (Powrie *et al.*, 1996).

In both these sets of studies, a subset of T cells capable of causing lethal inflammatory responses was demonstrable amongst CD4+ lymphocytes of normal rodents and their pathological activity was controlled by a distinct subset of lymphocytes, providing clear evidence of regulatory interactions between these subsets.

Cyclophosphamide-induced lymphopenia in NOD mice

The effect of cyclophosphamide, a cytotoxic chemotherapeutic agent known to induce lymphopenia, on the development of diabetes in NOD mice has been the subject of several studies. NOD mice treated with cyclophosphamide developed diabetes at an accelerated rate and the drug also increased the incidence of disease amongst male mice (Yasunami & Bach, 1988). Adoptive transfer of mononuclear cells from non-diabetic NOD mice prevented the accelerated disease development. Cyclophosphamide was shown to be non-diabetogenic in other mouse strains and it was, therefore, concluded that it was not cytotoxic towards beta cells of the pancreas. The drug probably has an immunomodulatory action, allowing diabetogenic cells to act on beta cells (Charlton *et al.*, 1989). Studies of lymphocyte population dynamics of NOD mice treated with cyclophosphamide revealed an initial drop in cell numbers in all lymphoid organs followed by an excessive repopulation of the pancreatic lymph node coincident with development of insulitis (Zhang, Georgiou & Mandel, 1993). These data suggest that the immune response that results in the destruction of the beta cells of the pancreas may be initiated in the pancreatic lymph node, which may also be the site of regulation of diabetogenic T cells.

Autoimmune-like pathology in mice thymectomized neonatally

In particular mouse strains, thymectomy of 3-day-old mice results, several months later, in organ-specific cell-mediated immune responses. The organs affected depend on the mouse strain; BALB/c mice predominantly develop an auto-immune gastritis (AIG) while other strains have been shown to develop oophritis (Taguchi *et al.*, 1980), thyroiditis (Kojima *et al.*, 1976), orchitis (Taguchi & Nishizuka, 1981), prostatitis (Taguchi, Kojima & Nishizuka, 1985) and pancreatitis (Bonomo, Kehn & Shevach, 1995). Development of disease is highly dependent on thymectomy at 2–4 days, since mice thymectomized at birth or at 7 days are unaffected. The data suggest that the numbers of T lymphocytes exported in the first 3 days of life are not sufficient to allow regulatory cells to prevent autoimmune responses. An alternative explanation is that autoreactive cells that initially escape deletion in the neonatal thymus can be deleted when they recirculate to the thymus, a phenomenon described elsewhere (Surh, Sprent & Webb, 1993). However, this explanation is not compatible with studies on adult thymectomized rats (described below). Direct evidence that disease induced by neonatal thymectomy results from ineffective regulation comes from studies in which AIG transferred to nude recipients from neonatally thymectomized mice can be controlled by co-transfer of splenocytes from normal syngeneic euthymic donors (Nishio *et al.*, 1995). The protective population is contained in a subset of peripheral CD4+ T cells that express IL-2 receptor (Asano *et al.*, 1996). These CD4+IL-2R+ cells appear in the first days of life in normal animals but their number in the periphery decreases after thymectomy. Under normal circumstances, these cells express *in vivo* mRNAs for IL-4, IL-10 and TGFβ.

Autoimmunity in high-dose irradiated mice

Total lymphoid irradiation of mice causes various organ-specific autoimmune diseases, such as gastritis, thyroiditis and orchitis, depending on the irradiation regimen and the mouse strain. Radiation-induced tissue damage does not seem to be the cause of disease. Irradiated animals reconstituted with thymocytes, splenocytes or bone marrow cells from normal syngeneic animals do not develop the autoimmune syndrome. CD4+ T cells from irradiated animals induce autoimmunity in syngeneic nude mice and CD4+ T cells from normal animals prevent the development of autoimmunity (Sakaguchi, Miyai & Sakaguchi, 1994). These results suggest that irradiation perturbs the balance between an autoreactive T cell population and a regulatory one that normally prevents autoimmunity.

Autoimmunity in adult thymectomized irradiated rats

Autoimmunity can be induced in normal PVG rats by a protocol of thymectomy at a few weeks of age followed by four doses of γ-irradiation, rendering the rats lymphopenic. A significant proportion of rats treated in this way developed thyroiditis, with mononuclear infiltrates of the thyroid gland and high titres of antithyroglobulin antibody in their sera (Penhale *et al.*, 1973). Disease could be prevented by reconstituting treatment of the rats following their last irradiation with lymph node cells or splenocytes from congenic donors (Penhale *et al.*, 1976). A small proportion of the thyroiditis-prone rats also developed insulin-dependent diabetes (Penhale *et al.*, 1990).

Development of diabetes in thymectomized and irradiated rats

The same protocol of adult thymectomy and γ-irradiation induces a very high incidence of diabetes in PVG.RT1ᵘ rats. Three weeks after the final dose of irradiation, these animals start to develop the disease and by 12 weeks 70% of females and practically all male rats develop diabetes with selective destruction of the beta cells of the pancreas (Fowell & Mason, 1993). Disease development requires CD8+ cells, as is the case in the spontaneously diabetic NOD mouse (Bendelac *et al.*, 1987).

Reversal of the lymphopenia in prediabetic PVG.RT1ᵘ rats by their reconstitution with unfractionated lymphocytes prevented disease in approximately 50% of recipients, and this protective capacity was shown to result entirely from the CD4+ cells. Significantly development of disease could be prevented in all recipients by their reconstitution with CD4+CD45RClow cells (Fowell & Mason, 1993). The protective lymphocytes are a long-lived population of cells and not recent thymic emigrants, since prediabetic rats could also be protected by reconstitution with CD4+CD45RClow cells from long-term thymectomized congenic donors. Further studies of phenotype revealed that the protective population was amongst CD4+CD45RClow TCR αβ+RT6+ Thy-1- cells, which is also the phenotype of a memory cell. CD4+CD45RClow cells have been shown to be a potent source of IL-4 but not IFN-γ following activation and, therefore, resemble T$_H$2-like T cells (McKnight *et al.*, 1991). However, the importance of IL-4 in the protection of prediabetic rats from development of diabetes by CD4+CD45RClow lymphocytes has yet to be determined.

These studies in adult thymectomized irradiated rats demonstrate firstly that normal animals contain cells with the potential to cause autoimmunity and, secondly, that these cells are prevented from fulfilling their pathological potential by regulatory T cells. However, maintenance of self-tolerance by regulatory T cells can be compromised either genetically or by disruption of the peripheral T cell pool, resulting in development of autoimmunity.

CD4+CD8- thymocytes are a potent source of cells that prevent development of autoimmune diabetes in adult thymectomized irradiated rats

Since the phenotype of the regulatory population of peripheral T cells is also the phenotype of a long-lived memory cell, it was assumed that this regulatory population was generated from naive precursors following encounter with an unknown antigen in the periphery. It was, therefore, a surprise to find that low doses of CD4+CD8- thymocytes purified from normal donors, a naive population of cells, could also prevent development of diabetes, albeit in only a proportion of recipients. Comparisons of the potency of peripheral cells and thymocytes reveal that the latter population is far more potent at preventing diabetes. Furthermore, the potency of thymocytes upon adoptive transfer appears to be restricted to their ability to control autoimmune responses. When assayed for their ability to provide primed B cells with help for secondary antibody responses upon adoptive transfer, CD4+CD8- thymocytes are far less able to support such a humoral response than either antigen-primed or unprimed peripheral CD4+ cells (Saoudi *et al.*, 1996).

Significantly, even at the highest dose of CD4+CD8- thymocytes used, only a proportion of rats are protected from development of diabetes. This inability to protect all recipients resembles the protection observed in prediabetic rats reconstituted with unfractionated CD4+ peripheral cells. In this instance, the incomplete protection was attributed to an antagonism of the CD45RChigh cells upon the protective CD45RClow constituents of the inoculum. If this argument is applied to the protection by CD4+CD8- thymocytes, it implies that these cells, like peripheral CD4+ cells, are a functionally heterogeneous population containing both cells capable of promoting autoimmune responses and cells that regulate such responses. However, attempts to fractionate these cells into functionally distinct subsets phenotypically have so far been unsuccessful (Seddon *et al.*, 1996).

Conclusion

There is now strong support for the view that normal animals contain cells with the potential to cause autoimmunity and that these cells are under the control of regulatory T cells. The mechanism that underlies this phenomenon is mostly unknown and is the object of intense research. The T_H1/T_H2 paradigm does not satisfactorily account for the activity of regulatory cells since self-tolerance is associated with an absence of both cell-mediated (T_H1) and humoral (T_H2) autoreactive responses. It may be that the T cells that prevent autoimmunity in some of the systems described in this chapter produce a number of the cytokines characteristic of T_H2 cells, but if T_H2 cells are identified as those that promote humoral immune responses then regulatory T cells and T_H2 cells are not identical populations.

References

Akbar, A.N., Terry, L., Timms, A., Beverly, P.C.L. & Janossy, G. (1988). Loss of CD45R and gain of UCHL1 activity is a feature of primed T cells. *J. Immunol.* 140: 2171–2175.

Arthur, R.P. & Mason, D. (1986). T cells that help B cell responses to soluble antigen are distinguishable from those producing interleukin 2 on mitogenic or allogeneic stimulation. *J. Exp. Med.* 163: 774–786.

Asano, M., Toda, M., Sakaguchi, N. & Sakaguchi, S. (1996). Autoimmune disease as a consequence of developmental abnormality of a T cell subpopulation. *J. Exp. Med.* 184: 387–396.

Asherson, G.L. & Stone, S.H. (1965). Selective and specific inhibition of 24 hour skin reactions in the guinea pig. I Immune deviation: description of the phenomenon and the effect of splenecotomy. *Immunology* 9: 205–217.

Bendelac, A. & Schwartz, R.H. (1991). ThO cells in the thymus: the question of T-helper lineages. *Immunol. Rev.* 123: 169–188.

Bendelac, A., Carnaud, C., Boitard, C. & Bach, J.F. (1987). Syngeneic transfer of autoimmune diabetes from diabetic NOD mice to healthy neonates. Requirement for both L3T4+ and Lyt-2+ T cells. *J. Exp. Med.* 166: 823–832.

Besedovsky, H., del Rey, A., Sorkin, E. & Dinarello, C.A. (1986). Immunoregulatory feedback between interleukin-1 and glucocorticoid hormones. *Science* 233: 652–654.

Biesecker, G. & Koffler, D. (1988). Resistance to experimental autoimmune myasthenia gravis in genetically inbred rats. Association with decreased amounts of *in situ* acetylcholine receptor-antibody complexes. *J. Immunol.* 140: 3406–3410.

Bonomo, A., Kehn, P.J. & Shevach, E.M. (1995). Post-thymectomy autoimmunity: abnormal T-cell homeostasis. *Immunol. Today* 16: 61–67.

Bottomly, K., Luqman, M., Greenbaum, L., Carding, S., West, J., Pasqualini, T. & Murphy, D.B. (1989). A monoclonal antibody to murine CD45R distinguishes CD4 T cell populations that produce different cytokines. *Eur. J. Immunol.* 19: 617–623.

Bunce, C. & Bell, E.B. (1997). CD45RC isoforms define two types of CD4 memory T cells, one of which depends on persisting antigen. *J. Exp. Med.* 185: 767–776.

Chang, T.L., Shea, C.M., Urioste, S., Thompson, R.C., Boom, W.H. & Abbas, A.K. (1990). Heterogeneity of helper/inducer T lymphocytes. III. Responses of IL-2 and IL-4-producing (Th1 and Th2) clones to antigens presented by different accessory cells. *J. Immunol.* 145: 2803–2808.

Charlton, B., Bacelj, A., Slattery, R.M. & Mandel, T.E. (1989). Cyclophosphamide-induced diabetes in NOD/WEHI mice. Evidence for suppression in spontaneous autoimmune diabetes mellitus. *Diabetes* 38: 441–447.

Chen, Y., Kuchroo, V.K., Inobe, J., Hafler, D.A. & Weiner, H.L. (1994). Regulatory T cell clones induced by oral tolerance: suppression of autoimmune encephalomyelitis. *Science* 265: 1237–1240.

Chikanza, I.C., Petrou, P., Kingsley, G., Chrousos, G. & Panayi, G.S. (1992). Defective hypothalamic response to immune and inflammatory stimuli in patients with rheumatoid arthritis. *Arthritis Rheum.* 35: 1281–1288.

Coffman, R.L., Seymour, B.W.P., Lebman, D.A., Hiraki, D., Christiansen, J., Shrader, B., Cherwinski, H., Savelkoul, H., Finkelman, F., Bond, M. & Mosmann, T.R. (1988). The role of helper T cell products in mouse B cell differentiation and isotype regulation. *Immunol. Rev.* 102: 5–28.

Davis, J.K., Thorp, R.B., Maddox, P.A., Brown, M.B. & Cassell, G.H. (1982). Murine respiratory mycoplasmosis in F344 and LEW rats: evolution of lesions and lung lymphoid cell populations. *Infect. Immun.* 36: 720–729.

Daynes, R.A. & Araneo, B.A. (1989). Contrasting effects of glucocorticoids on the capacity of T cells to produce the growth factors interleukin 2 and interleukin 4. *Eur. J. Immunol.* 19: 2319–2325.

Debray-Sachs, M., Carnaud, C., Boitard, C., Cohen, H., Gresser, I., Bedossa, P. & Bach, J.F. (1991). Prevention of diabetes in NOD mice treated with antibody to murine IFN-gamma. *J. Autoimmun.* 4: 237–248.

Fernandez-Botran, R., Sanders, V.M., Mosmann, T.R. & Vitetta, E.S. (1988). Lymphokine-mediated regulation of the proliferative response of clones of T helper 1 and T helper 2 cells. *J. Exp. Med.* 168: 543–558.

Feurer, C., Prentice, D.E. & Cammisuli, S. (1985). Chronic relapsing experimental allergic encephalomyelitis in the Lewis rat. *J. Neuroimmunol.* 10: 159–166.

Fiorentino, D.F., Bond, M.W. & Mosmann, T.R. (1989). Two types of mouse T helper cell. IV. Th2 clones secrete a factor that inhibits cytokine production by TH1 clones. *J. Exp. Med.* 170: 2081–2095.

Firestein, G.S., Roeder, W.D., Laxer, J.A., Townsend, K.S., Weaver, C.T., Hom, J.T., Linton, J., Torbett, B.E. & Glasebrook, A.L. (1989). A new murine CD4+ T cell subset with an unrestricted cytokine profile. *J. Immunol.* 143: 518–525.

Fong, T.A. & Mosmann, T.R. (1990). Alloreactive murine CD8+ T cell clones secrete the Th1 pattern of cytokines. *J. Immunol.* 144: 1744–1752.

Fowell, D. & Mason, D. (1993). Evidence that the T cell repertoire of normal rats contains cells with the potential to cause diabetes. Characterization of the CD4+ T cell subset that inhibits this autoimmune potential. *J. Exp. Med.* 177: 627–636.

Gajewski, T.F. & Fitch, F. (1988). Anti-proliferative effect of IFN-γ in immune regulation. *J. Immunol.* 140: 4245–4252.

Gajewski, T.F., Pinnas, M., Wong, T. & Fitch, F.W. (1991). Murine Th1 and Th2 clones proliferate optimally in response to distinct antigen-presenting cell populations. *J. Immunol.* 146: 1750–1758.

Griffiths, M.M. & DeWitt, C.W. (1984). Genetic control of collagen-induced arthritis in rats: the immune response to type II collagen among susceptible and resistant strains and evidence for multiple gene control. *J. Immunol.* 132: 2830–2836.

Haanen, J.B., de-Waal-Malefijt, R., Kraakman, E.M., Ottenhoff, T.H., de-Vries, R.R. & Spits, H. (1991). Selection of a human T helper type 1-like T cell subset by *Mycobacteria. J. Exp. Med.* 174: 583–592.

Hosken, N.A., Shibuya, K., Heath, A.W., Murphy, K.M. & O'Garra, A. (1995). The effect of antigen dose on CD4+ T helper cell phenotype development in a T cell receptor-αβ-transgenic model. *J. Exp. Med.* 182: 1579–1584.

Hsieh, C.S., Macatonia, S.E., Tripp, C.S., Wolf, S.F., O'Garra, A. & Murphy, K.M. (1993). Development of TH1 CD4+ T cells through IL-12 produced by *Listeria*-induced macrophages. *Science* 260: 547–549.

Hughes, R.A.C. & Stedronska, J. (1973). The susceptibility of rat strains to experimental allergic encephalomyelitis. *Immunology* 24: 879–884.

Hultgren, B., Huang, X., Dybdal, N. & Stewart, T.A. (1996). Genetic absence of gamma-interferon delays but does not prevent diabetes in NOD mice. *Diabetes* 45: 812–817.

Issazadeh, S., Ljungdahl, A., Hojeberg, B., Mustafa, M. & Olsson, T. (1995). Cytokine production in the central nervous system of Lewis rats with experimental autoimmune encephalomyelitis: dynamics of mRNA expression for interleukin-10, interleukin-12, cytolysin, tumor necrosis factor alpha and tumor necrosis factor beta. *J. Neuroimmunol.* 61: 205–212.

Kappler, J.W., Roehm, N. & Marrack, P. (1987). T cell tolerance by clonal elimination in the thymus. *Cell* 49: 273–280.

Katz, J.D., Benoist, C. & Mathis, D. (1995). T helper cell subsets in insulin-dependent diabetes. *Science* 268: 1185–1188.

Kennedy, M.K., Torrance, D.S., Picha, K.S. & Mohler, K.M. (1992). Analysis of cytokine mRNA expression in the central nervous system of mice with experimental autoimmune encephalomyelitis reveals that IL-10 mRNA expression correlates with recovery. *J. Immunol.* 149: 2496–2505.

Khoruts, A., Miller, S.D. & Jenkins, M.K. (1995). Neuroantigen-specific Th2 cells are inefficient suppressors of experimental allergic encephalomyelitis induced by effector Th1 cells. *J. Immunol.* 155: 5011–5017.

Kojima, A., Tanaka-Kojima, Y., Sakakura, T. & Nishizuka, Y. (1976). Spontaneous development of autoimmune thyroiditis in neonatally thymectomized mice. *Lab. Invest.* 34: 550–557.

Kuchroo, V.K., Das, M.P., Brown, J.A., Ranger, A.M., Zamvil, S.S., Sobel, R.A., Weiner, H.L., Nabavi, N. & Glimcher, L.H. (1995). B7–1 and B7–2 costimulatory molecules activate differentially the Th1/Th2 developmental pathways: application to autoimmune disease therapy. *Cell* 80: 707–718.

Launois, P., Maillard, I., Pingel, S., Swihart, K.G., Xenarios, I., Acha-Orbea, H., Diggelmann, H., Locksley, R.M., MacDonald, H.R. & Louis, J.A. (1997). IL-4 rapidly produced by Vβ4 Vα8 CD4+ T cells instructs Th2 development and susceptibility to *Leishmania major* in BALB/c mice. *Immunity* 6: 541–549.

Lee, M., Mueller, R., Wickler, L.S., Peterson, L.B. & Sarvetnick, N. (1996). IL-10 is necessary and sufficient for autoimmune diabetes in conjunction with NOD MHC homozygosity. *J. Exp. Med.* 183: 2663–2668.

Le-Gros, G., Ben-Sasson, S.Z., Seder, R., Finkelman, F.D. & Paul, W.E. (1990). Generation of interleukin 4 (IL-4)-producing cells in vivo and in vitro: IL-2 and

IL-4 are required for in vitro generation of IL-4-producing cells. *J. Exp. Med.* 172: 921–929.

Levine, S. & Sowinski, R. (1973). Experimental allergic encephalomyelitis in inbred and outbred mice. *J. Immunol.* 110: 139–143.

Levine, S., Sowinski, R. & Steinetz, B. (1980). Effects of experimental allergic encephalomyelitis on thymus and adrenal: relation to remission and relapse. *Proc. Soc. Exp. Biol. Med.* 165: 218–224.

Lider, O., Reshef, T., Beraud, E., Ben-Nun, A. & Cohen, I.R. (1988). Anti-idiotypic network induced by T cell vaccination against experimental allergic encephalomyelitis. *Science* 239: 181–183.

Lublin, F.D., Maurer, P.H., Berry, R.G. & Tippett, D. (1981). Delayed, relapsing experimental allergic encephalomyelitis in mice. *J. Immunol.* 126: 819–822.

Macatonia, S.E., Hsieh, C.S., Murphy, K.M. & O'Garra, A. (1993). Dendritic cells and macrophages are required for Th1 development of CD4+ T cells from $\alpha\beta$ TCR transgenic mice: IL-12 substitution for macrophages to stimulate IFN-γ production is IFN-γ-dependent. *Int. Immunol.* 5: 1119–1128.

MacPhee, I.A.M. & Mason, D.W. (1990). Studies on the refractoriness to reinduction of experimental allergic encephalomyelitis in Lewis rats that have recovered from one episode of the disease. *J. Neuroimmunol.* 27: 9–19.

MacPhee, I.A.M., Antoni, F.A. & Mason, D.W. (1989). Spontaneous recovery of rats from experimental allergic encephalomyelitis is dependent on regulation of the immune system by endogenous adrenal corticosteroids. *J. Exp. Med.* 169: 431–445.

Maggi, E., Del Prete, G., Macchia, D., Parronchi, P., Tiri, A., Chretien, I., Ricci, M. & Romagnani, S. (1988). Profile of lymphokine activities and helper function for IgE in human T cell clones. *Eur. J. Immunol.* 18: 1045–1050.

Mason, D. (1991). Genetic variation in the stress response: susceptibility to experimental allergic encephalomyelitis and implications for human inflammatory disease. *Immunol. Today* 12: 57–60.

McKnight, A.J., Barclay, A.N. & Mason, D.W. (1991). Molecular cloning of rat interleukin 4 CDNA and analysis of the cytokine repertoire of subsets of CD4+ T cells. *Eur. J. Immunol.* 21: 1187–1194.

Mosmann, R.T. & Coffman, R.L. (1989). Th1 and Th2 cells: different patterns of lymphokine secretion lead to different functional properties. *Annu. Rev. Immunol.* 7: 145–173.

Mueller, D.L., Jenkins, M.K. & Schwartz, R.H. (1989). An accessory cell-derived costimulatory signal acts independently of protein kinase C activation to allow T cell proliferation and prevent the induction of unresponsiveness. *J. Immunol.* 142: 2617–2628.

Munck, A., Guyre, P. & Holbrook, N.J. (1984). Physiological functions of glucocorticoids in stress and their relation to pharmacological actions. *Endocr. Rev.* 5: 25–44.

Murray, J.S., Madri, J., Tite, J., Carding, S.R. & Bottomly, K. (1989). MHC control of CD4+ T cell subset activation. *J. Exp. Med.* 170: 2135–2140.

Naitoh, Y., Fukata, J., Tominaga, T., Nakai, Y., Tamai, S., Mori, K. & Imura, H. (1988). Interleukin-6 stimulates the secretion of adrenocorticotropic hormone in conscious, freely moving rats. *Biochem. Biophys. Res. Commun.* 155: 1459–1463.

Nishio, A., Katakai, T., Hosono, M., Inaba, M., Sakai, M., Okuma, M. & Kasakura, S. (1995). Breakdown of self-tolerance by intrathymic injection of a T-cell line inducing autoimmune gastritis in mice. *Immunology* 85: 270–275.

Ohashi, P.S., Oehen, S., Buerki, K., Pircher, H., Ohashi, C.T., Odermatt, B., Malissen, B., Zinkernagel, R.M. & Hengartner, H. (1991). Ablation of 'tolerance' and induction of diabetes by virus infection in viral antigen transgenic mice. *Cell* 65: 305–317.

Paliard, X., de-Waal-Malefijt, R., Yssel, H., Blanchard, D., Chretien, I., Abrams, J., de-Vries, J. & Spits, H. (1988). Simultaneous production of IL-2, IL-4, and IFN-gamma by activated human CD4+ and CD8+ T cell clones. *J. Immunol.* 141: 849–855.

Parish, C.R. (1972). The relationship between humoral and cell-mediated immunity. *Transplant. Rev.* 13: 35–66.

Paul, W.E., Seder, R.A. & Plaut, M. (1993). Lymphokine and cytokine production by FcεRI+ cells. *Adv. Immunol.* 53: 1–29.

Penhale, W.J., Farmer, A., McKenna, R.P. & Irvine, W.J. (1973). Spontaneous thyroiditis in thymectomized and irradiated Wistar rats. *Clin. Exp. Immunol.* 15: 225–236.

Penhale, W.J., Irvine, W.J., Inglis, J.R. & Farmer, A. (1976). Thyroiditis in T cell-depleted rats: suppression of the autoallergic response by reconstitution with normal lymphoid cells. *Clin. Exp. Immunol.* 25: 6–16.

Penhale, W.J., Stumbles, P.A., Huxtable, C.R., Sutherland, R.J. & Pethick, D.W. (1990). Induction of diabetes in PVG/c strain rats by manipulation of the immune system. *Autoimmunity* 7: 169–179.

Pilling, D., Akbar, A.N., Bacon, P.A. & Salmon, M. (1996). CD4+CD45RA+ T cells from adults respond to recall antigens after CD28 ligation. *Int. Immunol.* 8: 1737–1742.

Powrie, F. & Coffman, R. (1993). IL-4 and IL-10 inhibit DTH and IFN-γ production. *Eur. J. Immunol.* 23: 2223–2229.

Powrie, F. & Mason, D. (1989). The MRC OX-22−CD4+ T cells that help B cells in secondary immune responses derive from naive precursors with the MRC OX-22+CD4+ phenotype. *J. Exp. Med.* 169: 653–662.

Powrie, F. & Mason, D. (1990). OX-22highCD4+ T cells induce wasting disease with multiple organ pathology: prevention by the OX-22low subset. *J. Exp. Med.* 172: 1701–1708.

Powrie, F., Leach, M.W., Mauze, S., Caddle, L.B. & Coffman, R.L. (1993). Phenotypically distinct subsets of CD4+ T cells induce or protect from chronic intestinal inflammation in C. B-17 *scid* mice. *Int. Immunol.* 5: 1461–1471.

Powrie, F., Leach, M.W., Mauze, S., Menon, S., Caddle, L.B. & Coffman, R.L. (1994). Inhibition of Th1 responses prevents inflammatory bowel-disease in *scid* mice reconstituted with CD45RBhiCD4+ T cells. *Immunity* 1: 553–562.

Powrie, F., Carlino, J., Leach, M.W., Mauze, S. & Coffman, R.L. (1996). A critical role for transforming growth factor-β but not interleukin 4 in the suppression of T helper type 1-mediated colitis by CD45RBlow CD4+ T cells. *J. Exp. Med.* 183: 2669–2674.

Prigent, P., Saoudi, A., Pannetier, C., Graber, P., Bonnefoy, J.Y., Druet, P. & Hirsch, F. (1995). Mercuric chloride, a chemical responsible for T helper cell (Th)2-mediated autoimmunity in Brown Norway rats, directly triggers T cells to produce interleukin-4. *J. Clin. Invest.* 96: 1484–1389.

Ramírez, F., Fowell, D.J., Puklavec, M., Simmonds, S. & Mason, D. (1996). Glucocorticoids promote a Th2 cytokine response by CD4+ T cells in vitro. *J. Immunol.* 7: 2406–2412.

Rapoport, M.J., Jaramillo, A., Zipris, D., Lazarus, A.H., Serreze, D.V., Leiter, E.H., Cyopick, P., Danska, J.S. & Delovitch, T.L. (1993). Interleukin 4 reverses T cell proliferative unresponsiveness and prevents the onset of diabetes in nonobese diabetic mice. *J. Exp. Med.* 178: 87–99.

Sabin, E.A. & Pearce, E.J. (1995). Early IL-4 production by non-CD4+ T cells at the site of antigen deposition predicts the development of a T helper 2 response to *Schistosoma mansoni* eggs. *J. Immunol.* 155: 4844–4853.

Sad, S., Marcotte, R. & Mosmann, T.R. (1995). Cytokine-induced differentiation of precursor mouse CD8+ T cells into cytotoxic CD8+ T cells secreting Th1 or Th2 cytokines. *Immunity* 2: 271–279.

Sakaguchi, N., Miyai, K. & Sakaguchi, S. (1994). Ionizing radiation and autoimmunity. Induction of autoimmune disease in mice by high dose fractionated total lymphoid irradiation and its prevention by inoculating normal T cells. *J. Immunol.* 152: 2586–2595.

Santambrogio, L., Hochwald, G.M., Saxena, B., Leu, C.H., Martz, J.E., Carlino, J.A., Ruddle, N.H., Palladino, M.A., Gold, L.I. & Thorbecke, G.J. (1993). Studies on the mechanisms by which transforming growth factor-beta (TGF-beta) protects against allergic encephalomyelitis. Antagonism between TGF-beta and tumor necrosis factor. *J. Immunol.* 151: 1116–1127.

Saoudi, A., Seddon, B., Fowell, D. & Mason, D. (1996). The thymus contains a high frequency of cells that prevent autoimmune diabetes on transfer into pre-diabetic recipients. *J. Exp. Med.* 184: 2393–2398.

Seddon, B., Saoudi, A., Nicholson, M. & Mason, D. (1996). CD4+CD8− thymocytes that express L-selectin protect rats from diabetes upon adoptive transfer. *Eur. J. Immunol.* 26: 2702–2708.

Seder, R.A., Boulay, J.L., Finkelman, F., Barbier, S., Ben-Sasson, S.Z., Le-Gros, G. & Paul, W.E. (1992). CD8+ T cells can be primed in vitro to produce IL-4. *J. Immunol.* 148: 1652–1656.

Sedgwick, J., Brostoff, S. & Mason, D. (1987). Experimental allergic encephalomyelitis in the absence of a classical delayed-type hypersensitivity reaction. Severe paralytic disease correlates with the presence of interleukin 2 receptor-positive cells infiltrating the central nervous system. *J. Exp. Med.* 165: 1058–1075.

Sedgwick, J.D., MacPhee, I.A.M. & Puklavec, M. (1989). Isolation of encephalitogenic CD4+ T cell clones in the rat. Cloning methodology and interferon-γ secretion. *J. Immunol. Meth.* 121: 185–196.

Spickett, G.P., Brandon, M.R., Mason, D.W., Williams, A.F. & Woollett, G.R. (1983). MRC OX-22, a monoclonal antibody that labels a new subset of T lymphocytes and reacts with the high molecular weight form of the leukocyte-common antigen. *J. Exp. Med.* 158: 795–810.

Sternberg, E.M., Young III, W.S., Bernardini, R., Calogero, A.E., Chrousos, G.P., Gold, P.W. & Wilder, R.L. (1989). A central nervous system defect in biosynthesis of corticotropin-releasing hormone is associated with susceptibility to streptococcal cell wall-induced arthritis in Lewis rats. *Proc. Natl. Acad. Sci., USA* 86: 4771–4775.

Stockinger, B., Zal, T., Zal, A. & Gray, D. (1996). B cells solicit their own help from T cells. *J. Exp. Med.* 183: 891–899.

Surh, C.D., Sprent, J. & Webb, S.R. (1993). Exclusion of circulating T cells from the thymus does not apply in the neonatal period. *J. Exp. Med.* 177: 379–385.

Swain, S.L., Weinberg, A.D. & English, M. (1990). CD4+ T cell subsets. Lymphokine secretion of memory cells and of effector cells that develop from precursors in vitro. *J. Immunol.* 144: 1788–1799.

Taguchi, O. & Nishizuka, Y. (1981). Experimental autoimmune orchitis after neonatal thymectomy in the mouse. *Clin. Exp. Immunol.* 46: 425–434.

Taguchi, O., Nishizuka, Y., Sakakura, T. & Kojima, A. (1980). Autoimmune oophoritis in thymectomized mice: detection of circulating antibodies against oocytes. *Clin. Exp. Immunol.* 40: 540–553.

Taguchi, O., Kojima, A. & Nishizuka, Y. (1985). Experimental autoimmune prostatitis after neonatal thymectomy in the mouse. *Clin. Exp. Immunol.* 60: 123–129.

Thomas, M.L. (1989). The leukocyte common antigen family. *Annu. Rev. Immunol.* 7: 339–369.

Warren, R.S., Starness, H.F., Alcock, N., Calvano, S. & Brennam, M.F. (1988). Hormonal and metabolic response to recombinant human tumor necrosis factor in rat: in vivo and in vitro. *Am. J. Physiol.* 255: E206–E212.

Wierenga, E.A., Snoek, M., de-Groot, C., Chretien, I., Bos, J.D., Jansen, H.M. & Kapsenberg, M.L. (1990). Evidence for compartmentalization of functional subsets of CD4+ T lymphocytes in atopic patients. *J. Immunol.* 144: 4651–4656.

Yasunami, R. & Bach, J.F. (1988). Anti-suppressor effect of cyclophosphamide on the development of spontaneous diabetes in NOD mice. *Eur. J. Immunol.* 18: 481–484.

Yoshimoto, T. & Paul, W.E. (1994). CD4[pos] NK1.1[pos] T cells promptly produce interleukin 4 in response to in vivo challenge with anti-CD3. *J. Exp. Med.* 179: 1285–1295.

Yssel, H., Shanafelt, M.C., Soderberg, C., Schneider, P.V., Anzola, J. & Peltz, G. (1991). *Borrelia burgdorferi* activates a T helper type 1-like T cell subset in Lyme arthritis. *J. Exp. Med.* 174: 593–601.

Zamvil, S.S. & Steinman, L. (1990). The T lymphocyte in experimental allergic encephalomyelitis. *Annu. Rev. Immunol.* 8: 579–621.

Zhang, Z.L., Georgiou, H.M. & Mandel, T.E. (1993). The effect of cyclophosphamide treatment on lymphocyte subsets in the nonobese diabetic mouse: a comparison of various lymphoid organs. *Autoimmunity* 15: 1–10.

12

Complement receptors

J. M. AHEARN and A. M. ROSENGARD

Complement receptor type 1

The primary function of complement receptor (CR) type 1 (CR1, CD35) is phagocytosis and clearance of immune complexes, which is mediated by its capacity to bind complement ligands C3b, iC3b, C4b and C1q and its capacity to inactivate the C3 and C5 convertases of the alternative and classical complement pathways through decay-accelerating and cofactor functions (Fearon, 1979; Iidia & Nussenzweig, 1981; Medof *et al.*, 1982; Klickstein *et al.*, 1997). CR1 is expressed primarily by haematopoietic cells, including erythrocytes, mononuclear phagocytes, eosinophils, B lymphocytes and T lymphocytes. It is also present on glomerular podocytes and follicular dendritic cells (Fearon, 1980; Wilson, Tedder & Fearon, 1983; Gelfand, Frank & Green, 1975; Kazatchkine *et al.*, 1982; Reynes *et al.*, 1985).

Structurally, CR1 is a type I transmembrane glycoprotein (Fig. 12.1). Four CR1 allotypes have been identified (Dykman *et al.*, 1983a,b; 1985; Wong, Wilson & Fearon, 1983; Dykman, Hatch & Atkinson, 1984), with M_r under reducing/non-reducing conditions of ~250 000/190 000 (A, F), 290 000/220 000 (B, S), 210 000/160 000 (C, F') and >290 000/250 000 (D) (Wong & Fearon, 1987). All CR1 allotypes share the same transmembrane domain of 25 amino acid residues and a 43 residue cytoplasmic tail. All allotypes have extracytoplasmic domains composed entirely of structural motifs, referred to as short consensus repeats (SCR), or complement control protein (CCP) modules, arranged in tandem. The A(F) allotype comprises 2039 residues, including a 41 residue signal peptide and a 1930 residue extracellular domain composed entirely of 30 SCRs (Klickstein *et al.*, 1988; Hourcade *et al.*, 1988). The amino terminal 28 SCRs are arranged in four long homologous repeats (LHRs) (A–D) of seven SCRs each; two additional SCRs link LHR-D with a 25 residue transmembrane region and a 43 residue cytoplasmic domain (Klickstein *et al.*, 1988).

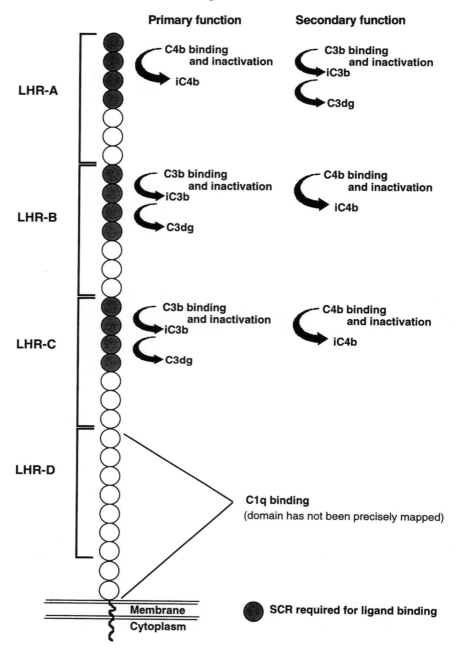

Fig. 12.1. Structure and function of complement receptor type 1 (CR1, CD35).

The other CR1 allotypes differ from one another structurally by an integral number of LHRs (Klickstein *et al.*, 1987). Allotypes A(F), B(S), and C(F') have extracytoplasmic domains that consist of four, five and three LHRs, respectively, as well as two additional SCRs that separate the last LHR from the transmembrane domain in each allotype. The D allotype has not yet been cloned and characterized, but it presumably consists of six LHRs. The frequencies of the A(F), B(S), C(F') and D allotypes are 0.82, 0.18, <0.01 and <0.01, respectively (Dykman *et al.*, 1984).

A single copy gene encoding CR1 maps to band q32 of chromosome 1, within the 750 kb regulators of complement activation (RCA) gene cluster, which also includes genes encoding CR type 2 (CR2, CD21), decay accelerating factor (DAF, CD55), membrane cofactor protein (MCP, CD46), factor H and C4-binding protein (Weis *et al.*, 1987; Rodriguez *et al.*, 1985; Lublin *et al.*, 1988; Bora *et al.*, 1989; Carroll *et al.*, 1988; Rey-Campos, Rubinstein & Rodriguez de Cordoba, 1988). The S allele of CR1 spans 158 kb and contains 47 exons (Vik & Wong, 1993; Wong *et al.*, 1989). The F allele, which does not contain the genomic region of the S allele that encodes LHR-B/A, spans 133 kb and is composed of 39 exons (Vik & Wong, 1993). The F' allele differs from the F allele in that it lacks LHR-B (Wong & Farrell, 1991).

The tandem alignment of 30 SCRs in the F allotype of CR1 creates a flexible, filamentous structure 80–90 nm in length, as determined by electron microscopic analysis (Weisman *et al.*, 1990).

Amino acid sequence homologies between SCRs that occupy the same relative positions in two different LHRs range from 56 to 100% identity (Klickstein *et al.*, 1987; 1988). The sequence of SCR-3 through SCR-7 of LHR-A differs from the sequence of SCR-10 through SCR-14 of LHR-B by only 1 of 327 residues. SCR-8 through SCR-11 of LHR-B and SCR-15 through SCR 18 of LHR-C differ at 3 of 253 positions.

There are 25 potential N-linked glycosylation sites in the F allotype (Klickstein *et al.*, 1988), of which six to eight appear to be modified by tri- and tetra-antennary complex-type oligosaccharides (Sim, 1985; Lublin, Griffith & Atkinson, 1986). Variable glycosylation is responsible for differences in CR1 size observed between erythrocytes and polymorphonuclear leukocytes in the same individual (Sim, 1985). A naturally occurring soluble form of CR1 has been demonstrated in serum and plasma of normal individuals (17.8–55.7 μg/l) (Yoon & Fearon, 1985; Pascual *et al.*, 1993), and serum levels have been demonstrated to fluctuate widely in a variety of pathological states (Pascual *et al.*, 1993); however, it has not been determined whether levels correlate with *in vivo* complement activation. It has also not been determined whether this soluble form of the receptor is secreted or shed from plasma membranes. The ligand-binding domains of

CR1 have been mapped through deletion mutagenesis (Klickstein *et al.*, 1988), substitution mutagenesis (Krych, Hourcade & Atkinson, 1991; Krych *et al.*, 1994) and creation and characterization of chimaeric receptors (Kalli *et al.*, 1991b). Together, these studies have identified three distinct and independent ligand-binding domains within the F allotype of CR1, each of which is capable of binding both C3 and C4 fragments (Klickstein *et al.*, 1988). SCR-1 and SCR-2 of LHR-A form a primary C4-binding site and a secondary C3-binding site, and the amino terminal pair of SCRs within both LHR-B and LHR-C are primary C3-binding sites and secondary C4-binding sites. One report was unable to detect binding of C3b dimers to receptors containing SCR1–4 of LHR-A, suggesting that this secondary affinity may be considerably lower than that of the primary recognition sites (Makrides *et al.*, 1992). The nine SCRs common to all CR1 allotypes lack an intact C3/C4-binding domain.

Although the amino terminal pair of SCRs within LHR-A-C were initially shown to determine ligand specificity, it was subsequently recognized that the first four SCRs of an LHR are required to bind C3b with an affinity indistinguishable from that of the wild-type receptor (Kalli *et al.*, 1991b). The dissociation constants for polymeric C3b of wild-type CR1 and recombinant chimaeric receptors bearing LHR-BD and LRH-CD were 1.0–2.7 nM, and chimaeric receptors that contained SCRs 1–4, 1–3 or 2–4 of LHR-B or LHR-C had K_d of 1.8–2.4, 6–9 and 22–36 nM, respectively (Kalli *et al.*, 1991b; Seya, Holers & Atkinson, 1985).

The entire C4b ligand-binding domain of CR1 also consists of four SCRs. SCRs 1–4 of LHR-A bind C4b dimers with an affinity (K_d ~4×10^{-7} M) similar to wild-type receptor, whereas SCRs 1–2 alone bind C4b dimers with lower affinity (K_d 1.4×10^{-6} M) (Reilly *et al.*, 1994). The first four SCRs of LHR-C (SCRs 15–18) are less effective in binding C4b dimers (K_d 1.2×10^{-6} M) compared with the first four SCRs of LHR-A (SCRs 1–4).

Potential functional differences among the CR1 allotypes have been investigated through studies of soluble, recombinant forms of the F, S and F' allotypes (Wong & Farrell, 1991). All three soluble forms of the receptor were shown to be equally capable of binding monomeric C3b and serving as cofactors for factor-I-mediated conversion of C3b to iC3b and C3dg (Wong & Farrell, 1991). In contrast to these observations using monomeric C3b, the three variant forms of CR1 (which contain zero, one, and two LHR-B domains, respectively) differed considerably in their capacities to bind dimeric C3b (Wong & Farrell, 1991) and in their capacities to inhibit the alternative pathway C3 and C5 convertases, with the ABBCD and the ABCD forms being 30-fold more effective than the ACD form of soluble CR1 (Wong & Farrell, 1991). Together, these investigations have led to a model in which tandem ligand-binding domains contained within adjacent LHRs of a single CR1 molecule promote multivalent receptor–ligand inter-actions (Wong *et al.*, 1985).

Current efforts are focused upon identification of amino acids within these four SCR domains that determine ligand specificity. One strategy has involved sub-stitution of residues from C3-binding sites for those in analogous positions of C4-binding sites and vice versa (Krych *et al.*, 1991). The most interesting and informative results of these studies to date involved characterization of a mutant in which five amino acid residues at the carboxyl terminus of SCR-2 (DNET-PICD) were replaced by the five corresponding residues of SCR-9 (STKP-PICQ). These substitutions resulted in the acquisition of iC3 binding without alteration of C4b binding. This is one of only two model systems in which the sequences of individual SCRs have been manipulated to result in a gain of func-tion, and the results suggest that these residues are critical in determining the C3-binding specificity of LHR-B and LHR-C. These amino acid positions in general may be critical in ligand discrimination. Similar studies have demonstrated the potential to enhance the ligand-binding capacity of CR1 beyond that of the endogenous receptor (Subramanian *et al.*, 1996). In these investigations, transfer of four amino acids – glycine from SCR-1 and arginine, asparagine and tyrosine from SCR-2 – to corresponding locations in SCR-8 and SCR-9 created a ligand-binding domain with greater iC3- and C4b-binding activity than any wild-type site and enhanced cofactor activity for both ligands. Furthermore, replacement of serine-37 of SCR-1 with tyrosine from the homologous position of SCR-9 and replacement of glycine-79 of SCR-2 with aspartate from the corresponding posi-tion of SCR-16 resulted in acquisition of C3b binding by the C4b-binding site of CR1, whereas neither substitution alone had this effect.

Most recently, it has been reported that CR1 binds specifically to complement component C1q (Klickstein *et al.*, 1997). This interaction involves the collagen-like tail domain of C1q and LHR-D of CR1. Therefore, CR1 is capable of specifically binding to all opsonic ligands of the complement system, namely C3-derived ligands, C4-derived ligands and C1q. The functional consequences of C1q binding to CR1 remain to be determined.

Complement receptor type 2

The type 2 receptor (CR2, CD21) is expressed on B lymphocytes and cell lines (Ross *et al.*, 1973; Eden, Miller & Nussenzweig, 1973; Bhan *et al.*, 1981; Nadler *et al.*, 1981; Iida, Nadler & Nussenzweig, 1983; Tedder, Clement & Cooper, 1984; Weis, Tedder & Fearon, 1984), some T cell lines (Fingeroth, Clabby & Strominger, 1988; Tsoukas & Lambris, 1993; Sinha *et al.*, 1993), thymocytes (Tsoukas & Lambris, 1988), peripheral blood T cells (Fischer, Delibrias &

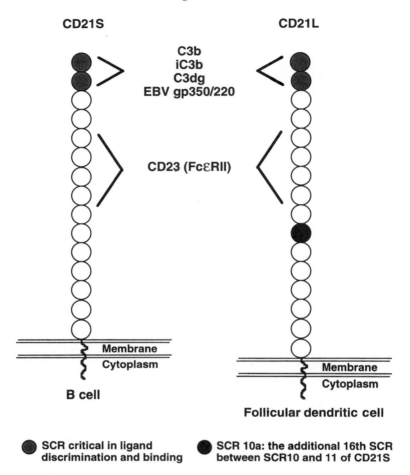

Fig. 12.2. Structure and function of complement receptor type 2 (CR2, CD21).

Kazatchkine, 1991), and follicular dendritic cells (Reynes *et al.*, 1985; Liu *et al.*, 1997). Structurally, CR2 is a 140 kDa type I transmembrane glycoprotein (Fig. 12.2). Short (CD21$_S$) and long (CD21$_L$) forms of CR2 share the same 24 residue transmembrane region and 34 residue cytoplasmic tail; they differ only in their extracellular domains (Liu *et al.*, 1997; Weis *et al.*, 1986; 1988; Moore *et al.*, 1987). The extracellular domains are composed entirely of either 15 (CD21S) or 16 (CD21L) SCR tandem repeats of approximately 60 amino acid residues. Functionally, CR2 is a receptor for the C3b, iC3b and C3dg cleavage fragments of C3 (Ross *et al.*, 1973; Eden *et al.*, 1973; Ross & Polley, 1975; Lambris, Dobson & Ross, 1975; Weis *et al.*, 1984; Frade *et al.*, 1985b; Mold, Cooper & Nemerow, 1986), the B lymphocyte receptor for Epstein–Barr virus (EBV) (Jondal & Klein, 1973; Fingeroth *et al.*, 1984; Frade *et al.*, 1985a; Mold *et al.*, 1986) and a receptor for CD23 (Aubry *et al.*, 1992; 1994; Bonnefoy *et al.*, 1993). Interferon α (Delcayre *et al.*, 1991) has also been reported to be a ligand for CR2.

A single copy gene encoding CR2 spans 35 kb (Yang, Behrens & Weis, 1991) within the 750 kb RCA gene cluster (see above). Restriction fragment length polymorphisms (RFLPs) of the gene have been identified for *Taq*I and *Hae*III (Fujisaku *et al.*, 1989). Two *Taq*I allelic fragments have frequencies of 0.7 and 0.3 in normal Caucasians (Fujisaku *et al.*, 1989), and three *Hae*III allelic fragments have frequencies of 0.93, 0.05, and 0.02 in normal Caucasians (Rey-Campos *et al.*, 1988).

Structurally, the short form of CR2 consists of a 20 amino acid residue signal peptide, a 954 residue extracellular domain organized into 15 SCRs of 57 to 74 residues each, a 24 residue transmembrane region and a 34 residue cytoplasmic tail (Weis *et al.*, 1988). The long form of CR2 also contains a 16th SCR referred to as 10a because of its location between SCR-10 and SCR-11 of the 15 SCR form of CR2 (Weis *et al.*, 1988). The 15 SCR (CD21$_s$) and 16 SCR (CD21$_l$) forms of CR2 are products of alternative splicing (Toothaker, Henjes & Weis, 1989). Functionally, the 16th SCR (10a) does not participate in binding ligands iC3b or gp350/220 (Kalli, Ahearn & Fearon, 1991a). However, it has recently been demonstrated that follicular dendritic cells selectively express the 16 SCR form while B cells selectively express the 15 SCR form of CR2 (Liu *et al.*, 1997), making CR2 the first human molecule specific to follicular dendritic cells to be characterized. The functional significance of this interesting and unexpected observation has not been determined. Hydrodynamic and electron microscopic studies of CR2 have demonstrated that the receptor is a highly extended, highly flexible molecule (Moore *et al.*, 1989).

The cytoplasmic domain of CR2 contains four tyrosine, four serine and two threonine residues (Moore *et al.*, 1987; Weis *et al.*, 1988). CR2 is phosphorylated in tonsillar B cells and in Raji cells following exposure to PMA (Changelian & Fearon, 1986). Glycosylation is required for CR2 stability but not for the receptor to bind C3–Sepharose (Weis & Fearon, 1985). There are 11 potential N-linked glycosylation sites in the 15 SCR form of CR2 and two additional sites in SCR 10a (Weis *et al.*, 1988; Moore *et al.*, 1987). Of these sites, 8–11 bear oligosaccharides on mature CR2 polypeptides in B lymphoblastoid cells (Weis & Fearon, 1985).

Soluble forms of CR2 have been identified in culture supernatants of Raji B lymphoblastoid cells, HPB-ALL acute leukemia T cells, and in normal human serum (Myones & Pross, 1987; Fremeaux-Bacchi *et al.*, 1996).

Four specific functions have been mapped to different structural domains of CR2. First, SCR-1 and SCR-2 are both necessary (Lowell *et al.*, 1989) and together sufficient (Lowell *et al.*, 1989; Carel *et al.*, 1990) for binding ligands

C3b, iC3b and C3dg. Second, SCR-1 and SCR-2 are both necessary (Lowell *et al.*, 1989) and together sufficient (Lowell *et al.*, 1989; Carel *et al.*, 1990) for binding and EBV ligand gp350/220. Soluble recombinant full-length CR2 (Nemerow *et al.*, 1990), as well as soluble, recombinant forms of the ligand-binding domain of CD21 (Hebell, Ahearn & Fearon, 1991; Moore *et al.*, 1991) block binding of gp350/220 to the receptor and the infection of B cells by EBV. Consistent with these observations, it has been determined that SCR-1 and SCR-2 are both necessary (Lowell *et al.*, 1989) and together sufficient (Lowell *et al.*, 1989; Carel *et al.*, 1990) for binding mAb OKB7 (Rao *et al.*, 1985), which blocks binding of CR2 to C3d and to EBV (Nemerow *et al.*, 1985). Anti-CR2 mAb HB-5, which does not block binding of either ligand to the receptor, binds to an epitope within SCR-3 and SCR-4. Third, CD23 (FcεR2), a low-affinity receptor for IgE, binds to CD21 (Aubry *et al.*, 1992); SCRs 5–8 of CR2 may be involved in this interaction, and N-linked oligosaccharides within this domain may participate (Aubry *et al.*, 1994). This interaction between CR2 and CD23 may influence the survival of B cells in germinal centres. Fourth, CD21 and CD19 participate in a multimolecular B cell membrane complex (Matsumoto *et al.*, 1991) in which CD21 interacts with CD19 on the B cell membrane via its transmembrane and extracellular domains (Matsumoto *et al.*, 1993). CR2 also forms a bimolecular complex with CD35 on B lymphocytes (Tuveson *et al.*, 1991) via the extracellular domains of the two receptors (Matsumoto *et al.*, 1993).

Although SCR-1 and SCR-2 of CR2 contain the binding sites for natural ligands derived from C3, the viral ligand gp350 and the mAb OKB7, the requirements for binding C3dg versus gp350 versus OKB7 are actually distinct. Studies that led to this conclusion took advantage of the differential capacities of murine CD21 and human CD21 to bind EBV. Murine CR2 and human CR2 are both composed of 15 SCRs, and the ligand-binding domains of the two receptors (SCR-1 and SCR-2) share 61% amino acid identity (Molina *et al.*, 1990); both receptors bind human C3dg (Molina *et al.*, 1991). However, murine CD21 and human CD21 are functionally distinct in that only the human receptor is capable of binding EBV. Characterization of the ligand-binding capacities of a panel of 24 human–murine CD21 chimaeric receptors demonstrated that preferential binding of EBV to human CR2 occurs because of the distinct conformation of the human receptor, which can be achieved in murine CR2 with single amino acid substitutions in two discontinuous regions of the primary structure: replacement of proline at position 15 with the corresponding serine from human CR2, and elimination of a potential N-linked glycosylation site between SCR-1 and SCR-2 (Martin *et al.*, 1991).

Finally, the role of CR2 in determining tropism of EBV for B lymphoblastoid cells appears to be limited to capture of virions at the cell surface, after which cofactors not associated with CR2-mediated postbinding events (Martin, Marlowe & Ahearn, 1994). This conclusion is based upon studies in which the ligand-binding domain of the rhinovirus receptor, ICAM-1 (CD54), was replaced with SCR-1 and SCR-2, the EBV gp350/220-binding domain of CR2. This CR2–ICAM-1 chimaeric receptor mediated EBV infection of three B lymphoblastoid cell lines, demonstrating that the extracytoplasmic, transmembrane and cytoplasmic non-ligand-binding domains of CR2 are not required for EBV infection of these B lymphoblastoid cells. This conclusion has not yet been extended to include primary B lymphocytes.

Complement receptor type 3

Complement receptor type 3 (CR3, CD11b/CD18, Mac-1, Mo1, OKM-1 α_m/β_2), an α/β heterodimeric adhesion molecule, is a member of the leukocyte-restricted integrin family (Springer *et al.*, 1979). CR3 shares a common 95 kDa β subunit with CD11a/CD18 (LFA-1, α_l/β_2) and CD11c/CD18 (CR4, p150, 95, α_x/β_2). It is the α subunits that distinguish the three heterodimers from one another. CR3 is expressed primarily by mononuclear phagocytes and natural killer (NK) cells, and expression of CR3 on activated granulocytes is considerably higher than on either of the other two leukocyte-restricted heterodimers. Expression of CR3 is greater than expression of CR4 in resting monocytes, whereas in tissue macrophages the opposite is true (Miller, Schwarting & Springer, 1986; Freyer *et al.*, 1988).

Functionally, CR3 is the most versatile complement receptor. Although iC3b is the only complement ligand for CR3 (Beller, Springer & Schreiber, 1982; Arnaout, Todd & Dana *et al.*, 1983; Micklem & Sim, 1985), CR3 is also a receptor for coagulation factor X (Altieri & Edgington, 1988a), fibrinogen (Wright *et al.*, 1988; Altieri *et al.*, 1988; Trezzini *et al.*, 1988), lipopolysaccharide (Wright & Jong, 1986), zymosan (Ross, Cain & Lachmann, 1985), soluble Fcγ receptor type III (FcγRIII, CD16) (Galon *et al.*, 1996), the counter-receptor ICAM-1 (CD54) (Smith *et al.*, 1989; Diamond *et al.*, 1990), filamentous haemagglutinin of *Bordetella pertussis* (Relman *et al.*, 1990), *Leishmania* promastigote surface glycoprotein gp63 (Russell & Wright, 1988) and for the acute phase protein haptoglobin (El Ghmati *et al.*, 1996). CR3 participates in a variety of cellular functions including adhesion of mononuclear phagocytes to endothelial cells (Anderson *et al.*, 1986; Arnaout, Lanier & Faller, 1988b; Lo *et al.*, 1989; Smith *et al.*, 1989), cellular extravasation and chemotaxis to sites of inflammation (Smith *et al.*, 1989), phagocytosis of CR3-ligand opsonized particles (Ezekowitz *et al.*, 1983) and enhancement of NK cell activity for C3-coated targets (Ramos *et al.*, 1988).

The single copy CD11b gene spans 55 kb on chromosome 16, band p11–p11.2 (Corbi *et al.*, 1988b; Arnaout *et al.*, 1988c), clustered with the other CD11 α subunits. Structurally, CR3 is a type I transmembrane glycoprotein with a 1 : 1 stoichiometry of α (CD11b) (165 000 M_r) and β (CD18) (95 000 M_r) subunits that associate non-covalently. Structurally, CD11b consists of a 16 residue signal peptide, a 1092 (or 1091) residue extracellular domain, a 26 residue transmembrane region and a 19 residue cytoplasmic tail (Arnaout *et al.*, 1988a; Corbi *et al.*, 1988a; Hickstein *et al.*, 1989). The one residue difference in the extracellular domain is a glutamine, located between two conserved cysteines at 478 and 489, which is of unknown functional significance. The single serine residue present in the cytoplasmic domain is constitutively phosphorylated in resting human leukocytes (Chatila, Geha & Arnaout, 1989; Buyon *et al.*, 1990).

The extracellular domain of CD11b contains seven homologous tandem repeats of ~60 residues. Repeats V through VII contain the consensus sequence DXDXDGXXDXXE, characteristic of EF-loop metal-binding proteins. Repeats I–IV lack this consensus sequence but contain the sequences YFGAS/AL and LVTVGAP, which are conserved in other integrins (Corbi *et al.*, 1988a). An I domain, consisting of 187 residues (150–338), inserted between repeats II and III, is homologous to the A domains of von Willebrand factor, factor B and C2.

There are 19 potential N-linked glycosylation sites in the CD11b sequence. The mature α_M subunit of ~167 000 is partially sensitive to Endo H (M_r ~153 000) and completely susceptible to N-glycanase (M_r ~137 000) (Miller & Springer, 1987).

CD11b shares approximately 25% amino acid identity (Corbi *et al.*, 1988a) with the α subunits of platelet glycoprotein IIb/IIIa (Poncz *et al.*, 1987), vitronectin receptor (Suzuki *et al.*, 1987) and fibronectin receptor (Argraves *et al.*, 1987). CD11b is specifically distinguished structurally from the last three receptors by the absence of a cleavage site that is involved in proteolytic processing of the α subunits into light chains, which are membrane anchored, and heavy chains, which are entirely extracellular and linked by disulphide bond to the α chains. The amino acid sequences of the transmembrane domains of CD11b and CD11c are 88% identical (Corbi *et al.*, 1987; 1988a). This observation suggests that these hydrophobic sequences may serve an important functional role in addition to simply providing a membrane anchor for the proteins.

CD18 is a type I transmembrane protein consisting of a 22 residue signal peptide, an extracellular domain of 678 residues, a 23 residue transmembrane domain and a 46 residue cytoplasmic tail (Kishimoto *et al.*, 1987; Law *et al.*, 1987). The cytoplasmic domain contains one tyrosine, three threonine and four serine residues. Induction with either PMA or FMLP generates primarily phosphoserine, with small amounts of phosphothreonine and phosphotyrosine (Chatila *et al.*,

1989; Buyon *et al.*, 1990). The extracellular domain of CD18 contains six potential N-linked glycosylation sites and 56 cysteine residues. One cysteine-rich (20%) region, extending from residues 445 to 631, contains four tandem repeats of an eight cysteine residue motif that is thought to be involved in extensive intrachain disulphide bond formation (Kishimoto *et al.*, 1987).

Binding sites for the numerous CR3 ligands have been partially characterized as follows. ICAM-1 (CD54), a counter-receptor for both LFA-1 (CD11a/CD18) (Marlin & Springer, 1987) and CR3 (CD11b/CD18) (Diamond *et al.*, 1990), has an extracellular region that consists of five tandem immunoglobulin-like domains (Simmons, Makgoba & Seed, 1988; Staunton *et al.*, 1988), and CR3 binds to the third immunoglobulin-like domain (Diamond *et al.*, 1991). Competitive inhibition studies have suggested that the binding sites for fibrinogen, iC3b, factor X and gp63 on CR3 are overlapping, if not identical (Altieri & Edgington, 1988a,b; Wright *et al.*, 1988).

Homologous sequences in human C3 (LEICTRYRGD) (1386–1395), fibrinogen (LGGAKQAGD) (402–410), leishmania gp63 (367–376) and filamentous haemagglutinin of *Bordetella pertussis* (TVGRGDPHQ) (1094–1102) were initially thought to mediate these CR3 – ligand interactions, based upon the capacity of peptides containing these sequences to inhibit binding of the respective ligands to CR3 (Wright *et al.*, 1987; 1988; Russell & Wright, 1988; Relman *et al.*, 1990). However, subsequent studies suggested that these RGD peptides indirectly affect CR3 function by binding to leukocyte response integrin (LRI), a β_3 integrin that is known to enhance the phagocytic capacity of polymorphonuclear cells (Brown & Goodwin, 1988; Gresham *et al.*, 1989; Altieri *et al.*, 1990; Taniguchi-Sidle & Isenman, 1992; van Strijp *et al.*, 1993). CR3 appears to be expressed in an inactive state on resting leukocytes, and high-avidity ligand binding by CR3 occurs only following stimulation of cells via heterologous receptors such as LRI (Altieri & Edgington, 1988b; Buyon *et al.*, 1988; Diamond & Springer, 1993; Stockl *et al.*, 1995). Additional structure–function studies based upon CR3/CR4 chimaeric receptors have demonstrated that the I domain is a major recognition site for iC3b, ICAM-1 and fibrinogen (Diamond *et al.*, 1993). In contrast, sCD16 is thought to bind outside the I domain, near the lectin-like region of CR3 (Galon *et al.*, 1996). The binding site for lipopolysaccharide (Wright & Jong, 1986) is also distinct from the iC3b/fibrinogen/gp63-binding domain (Wright *et al.*, 1989).

The capacity of CR3 to bind β glucan is controversial (van Strijp *et al.*, 1993); however, one study has suggested that CR3 is probably the only leukocyte β glucan receptor. CR3 has only one type of lectin site; this ligand-binding domain has broad sugar specificity, is cation independent and one or two such sites are located at the carboxy terminal area to the I domain (Thornton *et al.*, 1996). CR3 requires calcium or magnesium for ligand binding. A novel divalent cation-binding site has been identified in the A (I) domain of CR3, suggesting that the capacity of CD11b to bind iC3b, and perhaps other ligands, is dependent upon divalent cation binding to the A domain (Michishita, Videm & Arnaout, 1993). Determination of the secondary structure and the crystal structure of the A domain has confirmed and extended these observations (Perkins *et al.*, 1994; Lee *et al.*, 1995). Crystallographic studies have demonstrated that the A domain consists of one antiparallel and five parallel β strands that form a central sheet, surrounded by seven α helices, a classic 'Rossmann' fold (Lee *et al.*, 1995). A single metal-binding site, termed the metal ion-dependent adhesion site (MIDAS) motif (Lee *et al.*, 1995) sits at the top of the β sheet, on the surface of the A domain. The MIDAS consensus sequence is DXSXS (residues 140–144 in CD11b), and T^{209} and D^{242} from discontinuous regions of the polypeptide.

Recent data suggest that CR3 may form a membrane complex with glyco-phosphatidylinositol (GPI)-anchored FcγRIIIB (CD16) on human granulocytes (Stockl *et al.*, 1995). The carboxy terminal domain (which contains 15 of the 19 potential N-linked glycosylation sites in CD11b) has been implicated in this inter-action, and a lectin-like interaction between these two molecules has been pro-posed (Zhou *et al.*, 1993).

Complement receptor type 4

Complement receptor type 4 (CR4; CD11c/CD18; p150,95; α_x/β_2) α/β hetero-dimeric adhesion molecule is a member of the leukocyte-restricted integrin family (Sanchez-Madrid *et al.*, 1983; Lanier *et al.*, 1985; Springer, Miller & Anderson, 1986). CR4 shares a common 95 kDa β subunit with CD11a/CD18 (LFA α_L/β_2) and CD11b/CD18 (Mac-1, α_M/β_2), whereas the α subunit distinguishes the three heterodimers from one another. CR4 expression is restricted to leukocytes, including myeloid cells (Miller *et al.*, 1986), dendritic cells (Freudenthal & Steinman, 1990), NK cells (Werfel, Witter & Gotze, 1991), activated B lympho-cytes (Postigo *et al.*, 1991), some cytotoxic T cells (Miller *et al.*, 1986; Keizer *et al.*, 1987) and platelets (Vik & Fearon, 1987). Functionally, iC3b is the pri-mary complement ligand for CR4. Although it is not reported to be as versatile as CR3, CR4 also serves as a receptor for fibrinogen (Loike *et al.*, 1991), lipopolysaccharide (Wright & Jong, 1986), soluble FcγRIII (Galon *et al.*, 1996) and CD23 (Lecoanet-Henchoz *et al.*, 1995).

The single copy gene encoding CD11c is located on the short arm of chro-mosome 16, between 16p11 and 16p13.1, together with the genes encoding CD11a and CD11b (Corbi *et al.*, 1988b; Marlin *et al.*, 1986). The CD18 gene is located on chromosome 21, band q22.3 (Corbi *et al.*, 1988b; Marlin *et al.*, 1986).

Structurally, CD11c is a type I transmembrane glycoprotein, consisting of a 1081 residue extracellular domain, a 26 residue transmembrane region and a 30 residue cytoplasmic tail (Corbi *et al.*, 1987). The extracellular domain contains three tandem repeated sequences of 58, 70 and 68 residues, respectively. Centred in each of the repeats is a putative divalent cation-binding motif that has been determined to form a helix-loop-helix conformation, referred to as an 'EF hand' (Kretsinger & Nockolds, 1973). In this configuration, the calcium-binding domain resembles a right hand with the thumb (helix f) and the forefinger (helix E) extended, and fingers three through five clenched. The middle finger represents the calcium-binding loop.

Residues 125 to 318 of CD11c form an I domain, as described above for CR3, and there are 10 N-X-S/T sites (Corbi *et al.*, 1987), of which five or six appear to be glycosylated (Miller & Springer, 1987).

CD11c shares 35 and 67% amino acid identity with CD11a and CD11b, respectively (Corbi *et al.*, 1987), and approximately 25% amino acid identity with the α subunits of platelet glycoprotein IIb/IIIa (Poncz *et al.*, 1987), vitronectin receptor (Suzuki *et al.*, 1987) and fibronectin receptor (Argraves *et al.*, 1987). As described above for CD11b, the structure of CD11c is distinguished from the structures of these three RGD receptors by the absence of the cleavage sites that are involved in the proteolytic processing of each of the other three integrin α subunits (into a light chain that is membrane anchored and a heavy chain that is entirely extracellular, linked by disulphide bond to the α chain).

The structure of CD18 has been described above for CR3. There is no homology between CD11c and CD18.

Functionally, CR4 shares with CD11a/CD18 and CD11b/CD18 the capacity to mediate adhesion of leukocytes to endothelium (Anderson *et al.*, 1986; Stacker & Springer, 1991). CR4 has a counter-receptor on human umbilical vein endothelial cells, and the capacity of mAbs that recognize different regions of CR4 to inhibit the interaction between leukocytes and endothelial cells suggests that more than one ligand mediates the interaction (Stacker & Springer, 1991).

The role of CR4 as a complement receptor has been somewhat controversial. Early studies suggested that CR4 had the capacity to bind iC3b (Micklem & Sim, 1985; Anderson *et al.*, 1986; Malhotra, Hogg & Sim, 1986; Myones *et al.*, 1988). CD11c/CD18 was actually identified via iC3b–Sepharose chromatography (Micklem & Sim, 1985). However, cells expressing recombinant CD11c/CD18 failed to bind iC3b (van Strijp *et al.*, 1993). Subsequent studies suggested that the I domain of the α subunit, CD11c, must adopt a particular conformation to acquire the capacity to bind iC3b (Bilsland, Diamond & Springer, 1994).

Soluble FcγRIII, a putative ligand for CR4, appears to bind outside of the I domain (Galon *et al.*, 1996). CR4 is also reported to serve as a monocyte receptor for CD23 (Lecoanet-Henchoz *et al.*, 1995), and ligation of CR4 activates neutrophil spreading and neutrophil respiratory burst (Berton *et al.*, 1989).

Complement receptor C1qR

Activation of the classical pathway of complement begins with C1, which is a multimolecular complex in which one C1q subunit is complexed with two C1r and two C1s molecules ($C1qC1r_2C1s_2$). The single C1q subunit, comprising 18 polypeptides, has been described structurally as a bouquet of six 'tulips' in which each of the six stalks comprises three distinct polypeptide chains that are arranged in a collagen-like triple helix and in which each 'flower' is formed when the carboxyl terminal portions of these three associated strands expand into globular domains. The first stage of the classical pathway begins when the globular domain of C1q becomes bound to the Fc portion of an antibody that has attached to antigen. These antigen–antibody complexes that activate the classical pathway via C1q may be soluble, bound to the surface of cells or trapped in interstitial spaces. This activation process is tightly regulated to ensure that it is set into motion only under certain appropriate conditions. Once C1q has attached to an immune complex via its globular (head) domains, the collagen-like (tail) domains of C1q stimulate a variety of cellular responses through interaction with numerous cell types including mononuclear phagocytes, lymphocytes, fibroblasts and endothelial cells.

The first phagocytic cell surface protein conclusively shown to modulate C1q-triggered responses was C1qRp (Nepomuceno *et al.*, 1997). The mature receptor consists of a 559 residue extracellular domain, a 25 residue transmembrane region and a 47 residue cytoplasmic tail that contains the sequence RAMENQY (638–644), which represents a tyrosine kinase recognition motif. The amino terminus of the extracellular region contains a 156 residue sequence that resembles a calcium-dependent carbohydrate recognition domain (CRD) (Nepomuceno *et al.*, 1997; Drickamer, 1987; 1988). This domain contains the sequence FWIGLQREK, which is similar to sequences present in membrane receptors believed to modulate endocytosis, including the human mannose macrophage receptor (Nepomuceno *et al.*, 1997; Ezekowitz *et al.*, 1990). Carboxyl terminal of the CRD are five epidermal growth factor (EGF)-like domains (Cooke *et al.*, 1987). Within each of the third, fourth and fifth EGF-like domains is an asparagine hydroxylation motif: $D/N-X-D/N-Q/E-C-X_{4-7}-C-X_3-C-X-D*/N*-X_4-Y/F$, in which the asterisks represent hydroxylated residues. Similar EGF-like domains are present in a variety of extracellular proteins, such as the vitamin K-dependent plasma proteins factors IX and X, protein C and protein S, the connective tissue component fibrillin-1, and the complement proteins C1r and C1s

(Rees *et al.*, 1988). X-ray crystallographic studies of a calcium-binding EGF-like domain from factor IX have suggested that calcium bound to EGF-like domains functions both to stabilize the structure of the domain and to mediate protein–protein interactions directly. These interactions can be between EGF-like domains or between EGF domains and other domain types, which many be diverse among this structurally related but functionally diverse group of proteins (Rao *et al.*, 1995). Based upon these data, the multiple tandem EGF-like domains of C1qRp are unlikely to function independently of one another (Rao *et al.*, 1995).

Modification of the single potential N-linked glycosylation site at position 325 as well as extensive O-linked glycosylation appear to be responsible for the discrepancy between the predicted molecular mass (66 495 Da) of C1qR$_p$ and the apparent molecular mass of the receptor as determined by SDS–PAGE (126 000 Da) (Nepomuceno *et al.*, 1997). C1qR$_p$ is a recently characterized membrane receptor with an extracellular domain characterized by a calcium-dependent carbohydrate recognition domain, five EGF domains, of which three are likely to bind calcium, and a cytoplasmic domain that contains a tyrosine phosphorylation motif. Demonstration of the capacity of C1qR$_p$ to enhance phagocytosis following cellular capture of C1q-containing complexes, in addition to the recent demonstration of the capacity of CR1 to bind C1q (Klickstein *et al.*, 1997), will undoubtedly generate additional important and unanticipated insights into multiple inflammatory processes.

Participation of the complement system in rheumatic diseases

The complement system plays a fundamental role during inflammatory and innate immune responses. As such, complement ligands and complement receptors are likely to participate in the pathogenesis of most, if not all, rheumatic diseases. For example, complement activation has been demonstrated in arthritides, immune complex vasculitides, glomerulonephritides, demyelinating disorders, coagulopathies, immune thrombocytopenias and cutaneous inflammation manifested by a variety of rashes. The role of complement in the pathogenesis of specific rheumatic disease has been preliminarily investigated in disorders such as RA, dermatomyositis, systemic lupus erythematosus (SLE), Henoch–Schonlein purpura, Goodpasture's syndrome, idiopathic thrombocytopenic purpura, autoimmune cutaneous diseases such as pemphigus and bullous pemphigoid, and multiple sclerosis. For most of these conditions, studies have focused on determining whether the complement system is activated during the disease process and which complement ligands are deposited in affected tissues. In general, these studies have indicated that the fundamental molecular mechanisms responsible for initiating rheumatic diseases do not involve the complement system. Rather, complement activation appears to participate downstream of causative molecular events. Therefore, the complement system serves to amplify inflammation, coagulation and immune responses in these diseases, and thereby contribute to disease pathogenesis. A detailed review of these studies is beyond the scope of this chapter, and recent excellent reviews of this subject are available (e.g. Holers, 1996).

Although complement activation appears to play a secondary role in the pathogenesis of most rheumatic diseases, there is one exception. The complement system serves a critical role in maintaining immune tolerance and protecting against the development of SLE. Specifically, complement ligands generated by the classical pathway of complement, and CR1 (CD35), appear to protect against the development of SLE. This observation is the most intriguing relationship between complement receptors and rheumatic diseases described to date. Clues to the molecular mechanism(s) by which the complement system protects against the development of SLE will be the focus of the remainder of this chapter.

The clinical phenotype of SLE is generally considered to represent several diseases that result from multiple genetic factors interacting with one or more environmental agents. Some of the genetic risk factors that have been defined influence the disease phenotype rather than actually cause the disease. For example, class II alleles of the MHC have been shown to be closely associated with production of specific autoantibodies by patients with SLE, but these loci do not appear to actually increase the risk of developing lupus itself (Arnett, 1994). In contrast, studies of monozygotic twins, in which the concordance rate for SLE ranges between 24% and 69%, suggest that there are hereditary factors that are actually causative (Arnett & Reveille, 1992). The strongest genetic risk factor for the development of human SLE is complete deficiency of one of the components of the classical pathway of complement (C1q, C1r, C1s, C4 and C2) (Nishino *et al.*, 1981; Meyer *et al.*, 1985; Agnello, 1986; Arnett & Moulds, 1991; Colten & Rosen, 1992; Suzuki *et al.*, 1992; Bowness *et al.*, 1994; Morgan & Walport, 1994). In fact, an individual with complete deficiency of one of these proteins is nearly guaranteed to develop SLE. For example, of 32 patients with homozygous genetic deficiency of C1q reported in the literature, 30 have developed SLE, and one has developed discoid lupus (Shibuya & Nishida *et al.*, 1981; Suxuki *et al.*, 1992; Bowness *et al.*, 1994; Nishino *et al.*, 1981; Slingsby *et al.*, 1996). An individual with C1q deficiency has a greater risk of developing lupus than an individual who has a monozygotic twin affected by the disease. This suggests that in those patients with complement-deficient lupus, no other genetic factor is involved. This is supported by the nearly complete penetrance of the defective gene together with the observation that such individuals have been reported throughout the world from different ethnic and genetic backgrounds. There is no reason to suspect other shared genetic defects among this group of patients. Therefore, although the aetiology and immunopathogenesis of SLE in general is most likely multifactorial, lupus that results from complement deficiency is most likely a single disease. It either results from the single genetic defect alone or a combination with one or more relatively ubiquitous environment agents such as ultraviolet light or a common virus. The classical pathway of complement plays a fundamental role during immune complex solubilization and clearance, primarily via CR1. Therefore, it has been generally presumed that complete deficiency of one of the classical pathway components causes lupus because of an impaired capacity to clear aggregates of antibody and antigen. However, this hypothesis has not been proved and there are surprisingly few data to support it. Alternatively, there are several reasons for suspecting that complement deficiency causes lupus through a molecular mechanism other than failure to clear antigen–antibody complexes.

First, patients who develop SLE as a result of complement deficiency have a relatively homogeneous, characteristic and specific syndrome. The nearly invariant feature of the disease is a severe photosensitive skin rash, which is frequently accompanied by high titres of anti-Ro(SSA) antibody (Meyer *et al.*, 1985). Patients tend to develop the disease at a younger age than other forms of lupus, and there is no female predominance, again supporting the idea that no other genetic factors are involved. There is no reason to believe that a general failure to clear immune complexes should lead to development of a consistent and specific disease phenotype compared with any other autoimmune disease. Why do patients with complement deficiency usually develop lupus with cutaneous photosensitivity and anti-Ro antibody instead of RA, Sjögren's syndrome, etc.?

Second, patients who develop SLE as a result of complement deficiency do not have greater difficulties with immune complex deposition in tissues as compared with SLE patients in general. If anything, this is less a feature of their clinical syndrome. The 'lupus band test', which many consider to represent immune complex deposition in the skin, is often negative in these patients.

Third, most antigen–antibody complexes can be activated and cleared by the alternative pathway, which is intact in all of these patients.

Fourth, patients with complete deficiency of C2 develop lupus even though they are capable of activating the classical pathway and coating circulating antigen–antibody complexes with C4b, a ligand that is readily recognized and cleared by CR1-bearing erythrocytes.

Fifth, numerous non-immunoglobulin activators of C1q *in vitro* have been described, including cardiolipin, DNA, RNA, cytoskeletal intermediate filaments, decorin, phosphatidylglycerol and C-reactive protein (Cooper, 1985; Krumdieck *et al.*, 1992). Most of these have a relatively high density of negative charges carried by phosphate or sulphate groups, and there are some suggestions that an appropriate mix of anions and cations will activate C1q. Although the *in vivo* relevance of these interactions has not been elucidated, these observations suggest that the role of C1q *in vivo* may not be limited to interaction with the Fc domain of specific immunoglobulin isotypes. Primarily for these reasons, alternative explanations for the molecular immunopathogenesis of complement-deficient lupus are being explored. One alternative hypothesis with supporting evidence will be presented here.

As discussed above, a common feature of SLE in patients with normal complement levels, but particularly in those with complement deficiency, is cutaneous photosensitivity. Recent observations suggest that the skin may not only be a primary immune target in SLE but it may also be the site at which tolerance is initially broken. Keratinocytes exposed to ultraviolet light undergo apoptosis, a programmed form of cell death in which cytoplasmic and nuclear condensation and blebbing are prominent features. Cytoplasmic and nuclear blebs that form on the surfaces of apoptotic cells have recently been shown to contain several autoantigens that are common targets of autoantibodies in lupus, including DNA, Ro, La and snRNP (Casciola-Rosen, Anhalt & Rosen, 1994). These packages not only contain higher concentrations of autoantigens that might be encountered elsewhere *in vivo*, but there is also evidence that the self-antigens within the blebs may be cleaved by intracellular proteases specific to the apoptotic process, thereby revealing cryptic epitopes (Casciola-Rosen, Anhalt & Rosen, 1995; Casiano *et al.*, 1996). In addition, it has been demonstrated that when apoptosis of human keratinocytes is induced by virus infection, viral antigens and autoantigens co-cluster in specific subsets within surface blebs and may present a novel challenge to self-tolerance if not cleared and processed properly (Rosen, Casciola-Rosen & Ahearn, 1995). It has also been demonstrated that C1q, the first component of the classical complement pathway, specifically and directly binds to blebs generated from human keratinocytes (Korb & Ahearn, 1997). This capacity to bind C1q appears to occur in focal patches on the plasma membrane early during the course of apoptosis, and it does not appear to involve nuclear constituents. Later during the course of apoptosis, these membrane patches surround packages of cytoplasm, and eventually these blebs are released. *In vivo*, these blebs are likely to consist of high concentrations of self-antigen that may be packaged with viral antigen or may bear cryptic epitopes generated by novel apoptotic proteases. C1q and the classical pathway may be required for proper clearance of these blebs from the skin to maintain immune tolerance (Fig. 12.3). A complete deficiency of C1q may lead to immunization with autoantigens of cutaneous origin. This scenario may also explain the observation that individuals with lower levels of CR1 expression are at greater risk for developing SLE. As described earlier in

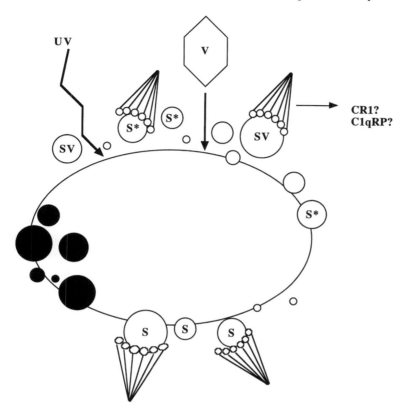

Fig. 12.3. Opsonization of apoptotic blebs by complement ligands. Shown is a cell undergoing apoptosis as a result of exposure to ultraviolet light (UV) or virus (V). Apoptosis leads to generation of nuclear (solid circles) and cytoplasmic (clear circles) blebs. One subset of blebs contains self-antigen (S). One subset of blebs contains self-antigen that has been modified to reveal immunocryptic epitopes, as might occur from proteolysis (S*). One subset of blebs contains self in a novel context, as might occur following viral infection and co-clustering of self-antigen and viral antigen (SV). Direct binding of C1q to the bleb surfaces may be the initial event in a molecular pathway by which the classical pathway of complement and receptors such as CR1 or C1qR$_p$ maintain immune tolerance.

this chapter, CR1 has traditionally been recognized as a primary receptor for C3- and C4-derived ligands. The recent demonstration that CR1 also serves as a receptor for C1q suggests that CR1 can bind all opsonic ligands generated by the classical pathway of complement (Klickstein *et al.*, 1997). It remains to be determined if CR1 may participate in the clearance of apoptotic blebs derived from keratinocytes or other tissue sources.

Other complement receptors, such as CR2, CR3, CR4, and C1qR must also be considered as potential participants in a molecular mechanism responsible for clearance of apoptotic blebs containing autoimmunogens. Recent observations that complement ligands and receptors can influence cytokine production and T_H1–T_H2 polarization (Karp, Wysocka & Wahl, 1996) have provided further incentive to revisit the relationship between the complement-deficient state and the development of SLE.

In summary, studies of the participation of the complement system in rheumatic diseases have primarily focused on secondary events that lead to deposition of complement ligands in affected tissues and organs. The one exception to this pattern has involved investigation of the role of complement deficiency in the aetiology and pathogenesis of SLE. Although it has been presumed that this is associated with an impaired capacity to clear immune complexes, evidence in support of this hypothesis has not accumulated and clues to alternative explanations have mounted. The complexity of the complement system suggests that many of its functions remain to be discovered. In parallel, the role of complement receptors in the aetiology and pathogenesis of rheumatic diseases is just beginning to surface.

References

Agnello, V. (1986). Lupus diseases associated with hereditary and acquired deficiencies of complement. *Springer Semin. Immunopathol.* 9: 161–178.

Altieri, D.C. & Edgington, T.S. (1988a). The saturable high affinity association of factor X to ADP-stimulated monocytes defines a novel function of the Mac-1 receptor. *J. Biol. Chem.* 263: 7007–7015.

Altieri, D.C. & Edgington, T.S. (1988b). A monoclonal antibody reacting with distinct adhesion molecules defines a transition in the functional state of the receptor CD11b/CD18 (Mac-1). *J. Immunol.* 141: 2656–2660.

Altieri, D.C., Bader, R., Mannucci, P.M. & Edgington, T.S. (1988). Oligospecificity of the cellular adhesion receptor MAC-1 encompasses an inducible recognition specificity for fibrinogen. *J. Cell. Biol.* 107: 1893–1900.

Altieri, D.C., Agbanyo, F.R., Plescia, J., Ginsberg, M.H., Edgington, T.S. & Plow, E.F. (1990). A unique recognition site mediates the interaction of fibrinogen with the leukocyte integrin Mac-1 (CD11b/CD18). *J. Biol. Chem.* 265: 12119–12122.

Anderson, D.C., Miller, L.J., Schmalstieg, F.C., Rothlein, R. & Springer, T.A. (1986). Contributions of the Mac-1 glycoprotein family to adherence-dependent granulocyte functions: structure function assessments employing subunit-specific monoclonal antibodies. *J. Immunol.* 137: 15–27.

Argraves, W.S., Suzuki, S., Arai, H., Thompson, K., Pierschbacher, M.D. & Ruoslahti, E. (1987). Amino acid sequence of the human fibronectin receptor. *J. Cell. Biol.* 105: 1183–1190.

Arnaout, M.A., Todd, R.F., Dana, N., Melamed, J., Schlossman, S.F. & Colten, H.R. (1983). Inhibition of phagocytosis of complement C3- or immunoglobulin G-coated particles and of C3bi binding by monoclonal antibodies to a monocyte-granulocyte membrane glycoprotein (Mo1). *J. Clin. Invest.* 72: 171–179.

Arnaout, M.A., Gupta, S.K., Pierce, M.W. & Tenen, D.G. (1988a). Amino acid sequence of the alpha subunit of human leukocyte adhesion receptor Mo1 (complement receptor type 3). *J. Cell. Biol.* 106: 2153–2158.

Arnaout, M.A., Lanier, L.L. & Faller, D.V. (1988b). Relative contribution of the leukocyte molecules Mo1, LFA-1, and p150,95 (LeuM5) in adhesion of granulocytes and monocytes to vascular endothelium is tissue- and stimulus-specific. *J. Cell. Physiol.* 137: 305–309.

Arnaout, M.A., Remold-Donnell, E., Pierce, M.W., Harris, P. & Tenen, D.G. (1988c). Molecular cloning of the α subunit of human and guinea pig leukocyte adhesion glycoprotein Mo1: chromosomal localization and homology to the α subunits of integrins. *Proc. Natl. Acad. Sci., USA* 85: 2776–2780.

Arnett, F.C. (1994). Histocompatibility typing in the rheumatic diseases. *Rheum. Dis. Clin. N. Am.* 20: 371–390.

Arnett, F.C. & Moulds, J.M. (1991). HLA class III molecules and autoimmune rheumatic diseases. *Clin. Exp. Rheum.* 9: 289–296.

Arnett, F.C. & Reveille, J.D. (1992). Genetics of systemic lupus erythematosus. *Rheum. Dis. Clin. N. Am.* 4: 865–891.

Aubry, J.P., Pochon, S., Graber, P., Jansen, K.U. & Bonnefoy, J.Y. (1992). CD21 is a ligand for CD23 and regulates IgE production. *Nature* 358: 505–507.

Aubry, J.P., Pochon, S., Gauchat, J.F., Nueda-Marin, A., Holers, V.M., Graber, P., Siegfried, C. & Bonnefoy, J.Y. (1994). CD23 interacts with a new functional extracytoplasmic domain involving N-linked oligosaccharides on CD21. *J. Immunol.* 152: 5806–5813.

Beller, D.I., Springer, T.A. & Schreiber, R.D. (1982). Anti-Mac-1 selectively inhibits the mouse and human type three complement receptor. *J. Exp. Med.* 156: 1000–1009.

Berton, G., Laudanna, C., Sorio, C. & Rossi, F. (1989). Generation of signals activating neutrophil functions by leukocyte integrins: LFA-land gp150/95, but not CR3, are able to stimulate the respiratory burst of human neutrophils. *J. Cell. Biol.* 109: 1341–1349.

Bhan, A.K., Nadler, L.M., Stashenko, P., McCluskey, R.T. & Schlossman, S.F. (1981). Stages of B cell differentiation in human lymphoid tissue. *J. Exp. Med.* 154: 737–749.

Bilsland, C.A.G., Diamond, M.S. & Springer, T.A. (1994). The leukocyte integrin p150,95 (CD11c/CD18) as a receptor for iC3b. Activation by a heterologous β subunit and localization of a ligand recognition site to the I domain. *J. Immunol.* 152: 4582–4589.

Bonnefoy, J.Y., Henchoz, S., Hardie, D., Holder, M.J. & Gordon, J. (1993). A subset of anti-CD21 antibodies promote the rescue of germinal center B cells from apoptosis. *Eur. J. Immunol.* 23: 969.

Bora, N.S., Lublin, D.M., Kumar, B.V., Hockett, R.D., Holers, V.M. & Atkinson, J.P. (1989). Structural gene for human membrane cofactor protein (MCP) of complement maps to within 100 kb of the 3' end of the C3b/C4b receptor gene. *J. Exp. Med.* 169: 597–602.

Bowness, P., Davies, K.A., Norsworthy, P.J., Athanassiou, P., Taylor Wiedeman, J., Borysiewicz, L.K., Meyer, P.A.R. & Walport, M.J. (1994). Hereditary C1q deficiency and systemic lupus erythematosus. *Q. J. Med.* 87: 455–464.

Brown, E.J. & Goodwin, J.L. (1988). Fibronectin receptors of phagocytes. Characterization of the Arg–Gly–Asp binding proteins of human monocytes and polymorphonuclear leukocytes. *J. Exp. Med.* 167: 777–793.

Buyon, J.P., Abramson, S.B., Philips, M.R., Slade, S.G., Ross, G.D., Weissman, G. & Winchester, R.J. (1988). Dissociation between increased surface expression of Gp165/95 and homotypic neutrophil aggregation. *J. Immunol.* 140: 3156–3160.

Buyon, J.P., Slade, S.G., Reibman, J., Abramson, S.B., Philips, M.R., Weissmann, G. & Winchester, R. (1990). Constitutive and induced phosphorylation of the α- and β-chains of the CD11/CD18 leukocyte integrin family. Relationship to adhesion-dependent functions. *J. Immunol.* 144: 191–197.

Carel, J.C., Myones, B.L., Frazier, B. & Holers, V.M. (1990). Structural requirements for C3dg/Epstein–Barr virus receptor (CR2/CD21) ligand binding, internalization, and viral infection. *J. Biol. Chem.* 265: 12 293–12 299.

Carroll, M.C., Alicot, E.M., Katzman, P.J., Klickstein, L.B., Smith, J.A. & Fearon, D.T. (1988). Organization of the genes encoding complement receptors type 1 and 2, decay-accelerating factor, and C4-binding protein in the RCA locus on human chromosome 1. *J. Exp. Med.* 167: 1271–1280.

Casciola-Rosen, L.A., Anhalt, G.J., & Rosen, A. (1994). Autoantigens targeted in systemic lupus erythematosus are clustered in two populations of surface structures on apoptotic keratinocytes. *J. Exp. Med.* 179: 1317–1330.

Casciola-Rosen, L.A., Anhalt, G.J. & Rosen, A. (1995). DNA dependent protein kinase is one of a subset of autoantigens specifically cleaved early during apoptosis. *J. Exp. Med.* 182: 1625.

Casiano, C.A., Martin, S.J., Green, D.R. & Tan, E.M. (1996). Selective cleavage of nuclear autoantigens during CD95 (Fas/APO 1)-mediated T cell apoptosis. *J. Exp. Med.* 184: 765–770.

Changelian, P.S. & Fearon, D.T. (1986). Tissue-specific phosphorylation of complement receptors CR1 and CR2. *J. Exp. Med.* 163: 101–115.

Chatila, T.A., Geha, R.S. & Arnaout, M.A. (1989). Constitutive and stimulus-induced phosphorylation of CD11/CD18 leukocyte adhesion molecules. *J. Cell. Biol.* 109: 3435–3444.

Colten, H.R. & Rosen, F.S. (1992). Complement deficiencies. *Annu. Rev. Immunol.* 10: 809–834.

Cooke, R.M., Wilkinson, A.J., Baron, M., Pastore, A., Tappin, M.J., Campbell, I.D., Gregory, H. & Sheard, B. (1987). The solution structure of human epidermal growth factor. *Nature* 327: 339–341.

Cooper, N.R. (1985). The classical complement pathway: activation and regulation of the first complement component. *Adv. Immunol.* 37: 151–216.

Corbi, A.L., Miller, L.J., Connor, K., Larson, R.S. & Springer, T.A. (1987). cDNA cloning and complete primary structure of the α subunit of a leukocyte adhesion glycoprotein, p150,95. *EMBO J.* 6: 4023–4028.

Corbi, A.L., Kishimoto, T.K., Miller, L.J. & Springer, T.A. (1988a). The human leukocyte adhesion glycoprotein Mac-1 (complement receptor type 3, CD11b) α subunit. Cloning, primary structure, and relation to the integrins, von Willebrand factor and factor B. *J. Biol. Chem.* 263: 12403–12411.

Corbi, A.L., Larson, R.S., Kishimoto, T.K., Springer, T.A. & Morton, C.C. (1988b). Chromosomal location of the genes encoding the leukocyte adhesion receptors LFA-1, Mac-1, and p150,95. Identification of a gene cluster involved in cell adhesion. *Exp. Med.* 167: 1597–1607.

Delcayre, A.X., Salas, F., Mathur, S., Kovats, K., Lotz, M. & Lernhardt, W.W. (1991). Epstein Barr virus/complement C3d receptor is an interferon α receptor. *EMBO. J.* 10: 919–926.

Diamond, M.S. & Springer, T.A. (1993). A subpopulation of Mac-1 (CD11b/CD18) molecules mediates neutrophil adhesion to ICAM-1 and fibrinogen. *J. Cell. Biol.* 120: 545–556.

Diamond, M.S., Staunton, D.E., de Fougerolles, A.R., Stacker, S.A., Garcia-Aguilar, J., Hibbs, M.L. & Springer, T.A. (1990). ICAM-1 (CD54): a counter-receptor for

Mac-1 (CD11b/CD18). *J. Cell. Biol.* 111: 3129–3139.

Diamond, M.S., Staunton, D.E., Marlin, S.D. & Springer, T.A. (1991). Binding of the integrin Mac-1 (CD11b/CD18) to the third immunoglobulin-like domain of ICAM-1 (CD54) and its regulation by glycosylation. *Cell* 65: 961–971.

Diamond, M.A., Garcia-Aguilar, J., Bickford, J.K., Corbi, A.L. & Springer, T.A. (1993). The I domain is a major recognition site on the leukocyte integrin Mac-1 (CD11b/CD18) for four distinct adhesion ligands. *J. Cell. Biol.* 120: 1031–1043.

Drickamer, K. (1987). Membrane receptors that mediate glycoprotein endocytosis: structure and biosynthesis. *Kidney Int.* 32: S167.

Drickamer, K. (1988). Two distinct classes of carbohydrate recognition domains in animal lectins. *J. Biol. Chem.* 263: 9557.

Dykman, T.R., Cole, J.L., Iida, K. & Atkinson, J.P. (1983a). Polymorphism of human erythrocyte C3b/C4b receptor. *Proc. Natl. Acad. Sci., USA* 80: 1698–1702.

Dykman, T.R., Cole, J.L., Iida, K. & Atkinson, J.P. (1983b). Structural heterogeneity of the C3b/C4b receptor (CR1) on human peripheral blood cells. *J. Exp. Med.* 157: 2160–2165.

Dykman, T.R., Hatch, J.A. & Atkinson, J.P. (1984). Polymorphism of the human C3b/C4d receptor. Identification of a third allele and analysis of receptor phenotypes in families and patients with systemic lupus erythematosus. *J. Exp. Med.* 159: 691–703.

Dykman, T.R., Hatch, J.A., Aqua, M.S. & Atkinson, J.P. (1985). Polymorphism of the C3b/C4b receptor (CR1): characterization of a fourth allele. *J. Immunol.* 134: 1787–1789.

Eden, A., Miller, G.W. & Nussenzweig, V. (1973). Human lymphocytes bear membrane receptors for C3b and C3d. *J. Clin. Invest.* 52: 3239.

El Ghmati, S.M., van Hoeyveld, E.M., van Strijp, J.A.G., Ceuppens, J.L. & Stevens, E.A.M. (1996). Identification of haptoglobin as an alternative ligand for CD11b/CD18. *J. Immunol.* 156: 2542–2552.

Ezekowitz, R.A.B., Sim, R.B., Hill, M. & Gordon, S. (1983). Local opsonization by secreted macrophage complement components. *J. Exp. Med.* 159: 244–260.

Ezekowitz, R.A.B., Sastry, K., Bailly, P. & Warner, A. (1990). Molecular characterization of the human macrophage mannose receptor: Demonstration of multiple carbohydrate recognition-like domains and phagocytosis of yeasts in cos-1 cells. *J. Exp. Med.* 172: 1785–1794.

Fearon, D.T. (1979). Regulation of the amplification C3 convertase of human complement by an inhibitory protein isolated from the human erythrocyte membrane. *Proc. Natl. Acad. Sci., USA* 76: 5867.

Fearon, D.T. (1980). Identification of the membrane glycoprotein that is the C3b receptor of human erythrocyte, polymorphonuclear leukocyte, B lymphocyte, and monocyte. *J. Exp. Med.* 152: 20–30.

Fingeroth, J.D., Weis, J.J., Tedder, T.F., Strominger, J.L., Biro, P.A. & Fearon, D.T. (1984). Epstein-Barr virus receptor of human B lymphocytes is the C3d receptor CR2. *Proc. Natl. Acad. Sci., USA* 81: 4510–4514.

Fingeroth, J.D., Clabby, M.L. & Strominger, J.D. (1988). Characterization of a T-lymphocyte Epstein–Barr virus/C3d receptor (CD21). *J. Virol.* 62: 1442–1447.

Fischer, E., Delibrias, C. & Kazatchkine, M.D. (1991). Expression of CR2 (the C3dg/EBV receptor, CD21) on normal human peripheral blood T lymphocytes. *J. Immunol.* 146: 865–869.

Frade, R., Barel, M., Ehlin-Henriksson, B. & Klein. (1985a). gp140: the C3d receptor of human B lymphocytes, is also the Epstein–Barr virus receptor. *Proc. Natl. Acad. Sci., USA* 82: 1490–1493.

Frade, R., Myones, B.L., Barel, M., Krikorian, L., Charriaut, C. & Ross, G.D. (1985b). Gp140, a C3b-binding membrane component of lymphocytes, is the B cell C3dg/C3d receptor (CR2) and is distinct from the neutrophil C3dg receptor (CR4). *Eur. J. Immunol.* 15: 1192.

Fremeaux-Bacchi, V., Bernard, I., Maillet, F., Mani, J.C., Fontaine, M., Bonnefoy, J.Y., Kazatchkine, M.D. & Fisher, E. (1996). Human lymphocytes shed a soluble form of CD21 (the C3dg/Epstein–Barr virus receptor, CR2) that binds iC3b and CD23. *Eur. J. Immunol.* 26: 1497–1503.

Freudenthal, P.S. & Steinman, R.M. (1990). The distinct surface of human blood dendritic cells, as observed after an improved isolation method. *Proc. Natl. Acad. Sci., USA* 87: 7698–7702.

Freyer, D.R., Morganroth, M.L., Rogers, C.E., Arnaout, M.A. & Todd, R.F. III (1988). Regulation of surface glycoproteins CD11/CD18 (Mo1, LFA-1, p150,95) by human mononuclear phagocytes. *Clin. Immunol. Immunopathol.* 46: 272–283.

Fujisaku, A., Harley, J.B., Frank, M.B., Gruner, B.A., Frazier, B. & Holers, V.M. (1989). Genomic organization and polymorphisms of the human C3d/Epstein–Barr virus receptors. *J. Biol. Chem.* 264: 2118.

Galon, J., Gauchat, J.F., Mazieres, N., Spagnoli, R., Storkus, W., Lotze, M., Bonnefoy, J.Y., Fridman, W.H. & Sautes, C. (1996). Soluble Fcγ receptor type III (FcγRIII,CD16) triggers cell activation through interaction with complement receptors. *J. Immunol.* 157: 1184.

Gelfquand, M.D., Frank, M.M. & Green, I. (1975). A receptor for the third component of complement in the human renal glomerulus. *J. Exp. Med.* 142: 1029–1034.

Gresham, H.D., Goodwin, J.L., Allen, P.M., Anderson, D.C. & Brown, E.J. (1989). A novel member of the integrin receptor family mediates Arg–Gly–Asp-stimulated neutrophil phagocytosis. *J. Cell. Biol.* 108: 1935–1943.

Hebell, T., Ahearn, J.M. & Fearon, D.T. (1991). Suppression of the immune response by a soluble complement receptor of B lymphocytes. *Science* 254: 102–105.

Hickstein, D.D., Hickey, M.J., Ozols, J., Baker, D.M., Back, A.L. & Roth, G.J. (1989). cDNA sequence for the α M subunit of the human neutrophil adherence receptor indicates homology to integrin α subunits. *Proc. Natl. Acad. Sci., USA* 86: 257–261.

Holers, V.M. (1996). Complement. In *Clinical Immunology: Principles and Practice.* ed. Rich, R.R., pp. 363–391. Mosby, St Louis.

Hourcade, D., Miesner, D.R., Atkinson, J.P. & Holers, V.M. (1988). Identification of an alternative polyadenylation site in the human C3b/C4b receptor (complement receptor type 1) transcriptional unit and prediction of a secreted form of complement receptor type 1. *J. Exp. Med.* 168: 1255–1270.

Iida, K. & Nussenzweig, V. (1981). Complement receptor is an inhibitor of the complement cascade. *J. Exp. Med.* 153: 1138–1150.

Iida, K., Nadler, L. & Nussenzweig, V. (1983). Identification of the membrane receptor for the complement fragment C3d by means of a monoclonal antibody. *J. Exp. Med.* 158: 1021–1033.

Jondal, M. & Klein, G. (1973). Surface markers on human B and T lymphocytes. II. Presence of Epstein–Barr virus receptors on B lymphocytes. *J. Exp. Med.* 138: 1365–1378.

Kalli, K.R., Ahearn, J.M. & Fearon, D.T. (1991a). Interaction of iC3b with recombinant isotypic and chimeric forms of CR2. *J. Immunol.* 147: 590–594.

Kalli, K.R., Hsu, P., Bartow, D.J., Ahearn, J.M., Matsumoto, A.K., Klickstein, L.B. & Fearon, D.T. (1991b). Mapping of the C3b-binding site of CR1 and construction of a (CR1)2-F(ab)2 chimeric complement inhibitor. *J. Exp. Med.* 174: 1451–1460.

Karp, C.L., Wysocka, M., Wahl, L.M., Ahearn, J.M., Cuomo, P.J., Sherry, B., Trinchieri, G. & Griffin, D.E. (1996). Inhibition of interleukin 12 production by viral and complement ligands for CD46. *Science* 273: 228–231.

Kazatchkine, M.D., Fearon, D.T., Appay, M.D., Mandet, C. & Bariety, J. (1982). Immunohistochemical study of the human glomerular C3b receptor in normal kidney and in seventy-five cases of renal diseases. *J. Clin. Invest.* 69: 900–912.

Keizer, G.D., Borst, J., Visser, W., Schwarting, R., de Vries, J.E. & Figdor, C.G. (1987). Membrane glycoprotein p150,95 of human cytotoxic T cell clones is involved in conjugate formation with target cells. *J. Immunol.* 138: 3130–3136.

Kishimoto, T.K., Connor, K., Lee, A., Roberts, T.M. & Springer, T.A. (1987). Cloning of the α subunit of the leukocyte adhesion proteins: homology to an extracellular matrix receptor defines a novel supergene family. *Cell* 48: 681–690.

Klickstein, L.B., Wong, W.W., Smith, J.A., Weis, J.H., Wilson, J.G. & Fearon, D.T. (1987). Demonstration of long homologous repeating domains that are composed of short consensus repeats characteristic of C3/C4 binding proteins. *J. Exp. Med.* 165: 1095.

Klickstein, L.B., Bartow, T.J., Miletic, V., Rabson, L.D., Smith, J.A. & Fearon, D.T. (1988). Identification of distinct C3b and C4b recognition sites in the human C3b/C4b receptor (CR1; CD35) by deletion mutagenesis. *J. Exp. Med.* 168: 1699–1717.

Klickstein, L.B., Barbashov, S.F., Liu, T., Jack, R.M. & Nicholson Weller, A. (1997). Complement receptor type 1 (CR1, CD35) is a receptor for C1q. *Immunity* 7: 345–355.

Korb, L.C. & Ahearn, J.M. (1997). C1q binds directly and specifically to surface blebs of apoptotic human keratinocytes. *J. Immunol.* 158: 4525–4528.

Kretsinger, R.H. & Nockolds, C.E. (1973). Carp muscle calcium binding protein. II. Structure determination and general description. *J. Biol. Chem.* 248: 3313–3326.

Krumdieck, R., Hook, M., Rosenberg, L.C. & Volanakis. (1992). The proteoglycan decorin binds C1q and inhibits the activity of the C1 complex. *J. Immunol.* 148: 3695–3701.

Krych, M., Hourcade, D. & Atkinson, J.P. (1991). Sites within the complement C3b/C4b receptor important for the specificity of ligand binding. *Proc. Natl. Acad. Sci., USA* 88: 4353–4357.

Krych, M., Clemenza, L., Howdeshell, D., Hauhart, R., Hourcade, D. & Atkinson, J.P. (1994). Analysis of the functional domains of complement receptor type 1 (C3b/C4b receptor; CD35) by substitution mutagenesis. *J. Biol. Chem.* 269: 13273–13278.

Lambris, J.D., Dobson, N.J. & Ross, G.D. (1975). Isolation of lymphocyte membrane complement receptor type two (the C3d receptor) and preparation of receptor-specific antibody. *Proc. Natl. Acad. Sci., USA* 78: 1828–1832.

Lanier, L.L., Arnaout, M.A., Schwarting, R., Warner, N.L. & Ross, G.D. (1985). P150/95: third member of the LFA-1/CR3 polypeptide family identified by anti-Leu M5 monoclonal antibody. *Eur. J. Immunol.* 15: 713–718.

Law, S.K.A., Gagnon, J., Hildreth, J.E.K., Wells, C.E., Willis, A.C. & Wong, A.J. (1987). The primary structure of the β-subunit of the cell surface adhesion glycoproteins LFA-1, CR3 and p150,95 and its relationship to the fibronectin receptor. *EMBO J.* 6: 915–919.

Lecoanet-Henchoz, S., Gauchat, J.F., Aubry, J.P. *et al.* (1995). CD23 regulates monocyte activation through a novel interaction with the adhesion molecules CD11b-CD18 and CD11c-CD18. *Immunity* 3: 119–125.

Lee, J.O., Rieu, P., Arnaout, M.A. & Liddington, R. (1995). Crystal structure of the A domain from the α subunit of integrin CR3 (CD11b/CD18). *Cell* 80: 631–638.

Liu, Y.J., Xu, J., de Bouteiller, O., Parham, C.L., Grouard, G., Djossou, O., de Saint-Vis, B., Lebecque, S., Banchereau, J. & Moore, K.W. (1997). Follicular dendritic cells specifically express the long CR2/CD21 isoform. *J. Exp. Med.* 185: 165–170.

Lo, S.K., van Seventer, G.A., Levin, S.M. & Wright, S.D. (1989). Two leukocyte receptors (CD11a/CD18 and CD11b/CD18) mediate transient adhesion to endothelium by binding to different ligands. *J. Immunol.* 143: 3325–3329.

Loike, J.D., Sodeik, B., Cao, L., Leucona, S., Weitz, J.I., Detmers, P.A., Wright, S.D. & Silverstein, S.C. (1991). CD11c/CD18 on neutrophils recognizes a domain at the N terminus of the Aa chain of fibrinogen. *Proc. Natl. Acad. Sci., USA* 88: 1044–1048.

Lowell, C.A., Klickstein, L.B., Carter, R.H., Mitchell, J.A., Fearon, D.T. & Ahearn, J.M. (1989). Mapping of the Epstein–Barr virus and C3dg binding sites to a common domain on complement receptor type 2. *J. Exp. Med.* 170: 1931–1946.

Lublin, D.M., Griffith, R.C. & Atkinson, J.P. (1986). Influence of glycosylation on allelic and cell-specific M_r variation, receptor processing and ligand binding of the human complement C3b/C4b receptor. *J. Biol. Chem.* 261: 5736–5744.

Lublin, D.M., Liszewski, M.K., Post, T.W., Acre, M.A., LeBeau, M.M., Rebentisch, M.B., Lemons, R.S., Seya, T. & Atkinson, J.P. (1988). Molecular cloning and chromosomal localization of human membrane cofactor protein (MCP). *J. Exp. Med.* 168: 181–194.

Makrides, S.C., Scesney, S.M., Ford, P.J., Evans, K.S., Carson, G.R. & Marsh, H.C. (1992). Cell surface expression of the C3b/C4b receptor (CR1) protects Chinese hamster ovary cells from lysis by human complement. *J. Biol. Chem.* 267: 24 754–24 761.

Malhotra, V., Hogg, N. & Sim, R.B. (1986). Ligand binding by the p150,95 antigen of U937 cells: properties in common with complement receptor type 3 (CR3). *Eur. J. Immunol.* 16: 1117–1123.

Marlin, S.D. & Springer, T.A. (1987). Purified intercellular adhesion molecule-1 (ICAM-1) is a ligand for lymphocyte function associated antigen 1 (LFA-1). *Cell* 51: 813–819.

Marlin, S.D., Morton, C.C., Anderson, D.C. & Springer, T.A. (1986). LFA-1 immunodeficiency disease: definition of the genetic defect and chromosomal mapping of alpha and beta subunits of the lymphocyte function-associated antigen 1 (LFA-1) by complementation in hybrid cells. *J. Exp. Med.* 164: 855–867.

Martin, D.R., Yuryev, A., Kalli, K.R., Fearon, D.T. & Ahearn, J.M. (1991). Determination of the structural basis for selective binding of Epstein–Barr virus to human complement receptor type 2. *J. Exp. Med.* 174: 1299–1311.

Martin, D.R., Marlowe, R.L. & Ahearn, J.M. (1994). Determination of the role for CD21 during Epstein–Barr virus infection of B lymphoblastoid cells. *J. Virol.* 68: 4716–4726.

Matsumoto, A.K., Kopicky-Burd, J., Carter, R.H., Tuveson, D.A., Tedder, T.F. & Fearon, D.T. (1991). Intersection of the complement and immune systems: a signal transduction complex of the B lymphocyte-containing complement receptor type 2 and CD19. *J. Exp. Med.* 173: 55–64.

Matsumoto, A.K., Martin, D.R., Carter, R.H., Klickstein, L.B., Ahearn, J.M. & Fearon, D.T. (1993). Functional dissection of the CD21/CD19/TAPA-1/Leu-13 complex of B lymphocytes. *J. Exp. Med.* 178: 1407–1417.

Medof, M.E., Iida, K., Mold, C. & Nussenzweig, V. (1982). Unique role of the complement receptor CR1 in the degradation of C3b associated with immune complexes. *J. Exp. Med.* 156: 1739–1754.

Meyer, O., Hauptmann, G., Tappenier, G., Ochs, H.D. & Mascart Lemone, F. (1985). Genetic deficiency of C4, C2, or C1q and lupus syndromes. Association with anti-Ro (SS-A) antibodies. *Clin. Exp. Immunol.* 62: 678–684.

Michishita, M., Videm, V. & Arnaout, M.A. (1993). A novel divalent cation binding site in the A domain of the β_2 integrin CR3 (CD11b/CD18) is essential for ligand binding. *Cell* 72: 857–867.

Micklem, K.J. & Sim, R.B. (1985). Isolation of complement fragment-iC3b-binding proteins by affinity chromatography. *Biochem. J.* 231: 233–236.

Miller, L.J. & Springer, T.A. (1987). Biosynthesis and glycosylation of p150,95 and related leukocyte adhesion proteins. *J. Immunol.* 139: 842–847.

Miller, L.J., Schwarting, R. & Springer, T.A. (1986). Regulated expression of the Mac-1, LFA-1, p150,95 glycoprotein family during leukocyte differentiation. *J. Immunol.* 137: 2891–2900.

Mold, C., Cooper, N.R. & Nemerow, G.R. (1986). Incorporation of the purified Epstein Barr virus/C3d receptor (CR2) into liposomes and demonstration of its dual ligand binding functions. *J. Immunol.* 136: 4140–4145.

Molina, H., Kinoshita, T., Inoue, K., Carel, J.C. & Holers, V.M. (1990). A molecular and immunochemical characterization of mouse CR2. *J. Immunol.* 145: 2974–2983.

Molina, H., Brenner, C., Jacobi, S., Gorka, J., Carel, J.C., Kinoshita, T. & Holers, V.M. (1991). Analysis of Epstein–Barr virus-binding sites on complement receptor 2 (CR2/CD21) using human-mouse chimeras and peptides. *J. Biol. Chem.* 266: 12 173–12 179.

Moore, M.D., Cooper, N.R., Tack, B.F. & Nemerow, G.R. (1987). Molecular cloning of the cDNA encoding the Epstein–Barr virus/C3d receptor (complement receptor type 2) of human B lymphocytes. *Proc. Natl. Acad. Sci., USA* 84: 9194–9198.

Moore, M.D., DiScipio, R.G., Cooper, N.R. & Nemerow, G.R. (1989). Hydrodynamic, electron microscopic, and ligand-binding analysis of the Epstein–Barr virus/C3dg receptor (CR2). *J. Biol. Chem.* 264: 20 576–20 582.

Moore, M.D., Cannon, M.J., Sewall, A., Finlayson, M., Okimoto, M. & Nemerow, G.R. (1991). Inhibition of Epstein–Barr virus infection in vitro and in vivo by soluble CR2 (CD21) containing two short consensus repeats. *J. Virol.* 65: 3559–3565.

Morgan, B.P. & Walport, M.J. (1994). Complement deficiency and disease. *Immunol. Today* 12: 301–306.

Myones, B.L. & Pross, G.D. (1987). Identification of a spontaneously shed fragment of B cell complement receptor type two (CR2) containing the C3d-binding site. *Complement* 4: 87–98.

Myones, B.L., Dalzell, J.G., Hogg, N. & Ross, G.D. (1988). Neutrophil and monocyte cell surface p150,95 has iC3b-receptor (CR4) activity resembling CR3. *J. Clin. Invest.* 82: 640–651.

Nadler, L.M., Stashenko, P., Hardy, R., van Agthoven, A., Terhorst, C. & Schlossman, S.F. (1981). Characterization of a human B cell specific antigen (B2) distinct from B1. *J. Immunol.* 126: 1941–1947.

Nemerow, G.R., Wolfert, R., McNaughton, M.E. & Cooper, N.R. (1985). Identification and characterization of the EBV receptor on human B lymphocytes and its relationship to the C3d receptor (CR2). *J. Virol.* 55: 347–351.

Nemerow, G.R., Mullen, J.J., Dickson, P.W. & Cooper, N.R. (1990). Soluble recombinant CR2 (CD21) inhibits Epstein–Barr virus infection. *J. Virol.* 64: 1348–1352.

Nepomuceno, R.R., Henschen-Edman, A.H., Burgess, W.N.H. & Tenner, A.J. (1997).

cDNA cloning and primary structure analysis of C1qRP, the human C1q/MBL/SPA receptor that mediates enhanced phagocytosis in vitro. *Immunity* 6: 119–129.

Nishino, H., Shibuya, K., Nishida, Y. & Mushimoto, M. (1981). Lupus erythematosus-like syndrome with selective complete deficiency of C1q. *Ann. Int. Med.* 95: 322–324.

Pascual, M., Duchosal, M.A., Steiger, G., Giostra, E., Pechere, A., Paccaud, J.P., Danielsson, C. & Schifferli, J.A. (1993). Circulating soluble CR1 (CD35): serum levels in diseases and evidence for its release by human leukocytes. *J. Immunol.* 151: 1702–1711.

Perkins, S.J., Smith, K.F., Williams, S.C., Harris, P.I., Chapman, D. & Sim, R.B. (1994). The secondary structure of the von Willebrand factor type A domain in factor B of human complement by Fourier transform infrared spectroscopy. Its occurrence in collagen types VI, VII, XII, and XIV, the integrins and other proteins by averaged structure predictions. *J. Mol. Biol.* 238: 104–119.

Poncz, M., Eisman, R., Heidenreich, R., Silver, S.M., Vilaire, G., Surrey, S., Schwartz, E. & Bennett. (1987). Structure of the platelet membrane glycoprotein IIb. *J. Biol. Chem.* 262: 8476–8482.

Postigo, A.A., Corbi, A.L., Sanchez-Madrid, F. & de Landazuri, M.O. (1991). Regulated expression and function of CD11c/CD18 integrin on human B lymphocytes. Relation between attachment to fibrinogen and triggering of proliferation through CD11c/CD18. *J. Exp. Med.* 174: 1313–1322.

Ramos, O.F., Kai, C., Yefenof, E. & Klein, E. (1988). The elevated natural killer sensitivity of targets carrying surface-attached C3 fragments require the availability of the iC3b receptor (CR3) on the effectors. *J. Immunol.* 140: 1239–1243.

Rao, P.E., Wright, S.D., Westberg, E.F. & Goldstein, G. (1985). OKB7, a monoclonal antibody that reacts at or near the C3d binding site of human CR2. *Cell Immunol.* 93: 549–555.

Rao, Z., Handford, P., Mayhew, M., Knott, V., Brownlee, G.G. & Stuart, D. (1995). The structure of a Ca²⁺-binding epidermal growth factor like domain: its role in protein-protein interactions. *Cell* 82: 131–141.

Rees, D.J.G., Jones, I.M., Handford, P.A., Walter, S.J., Esnouf, M.P., Smith, K.J. & Brownlee, G.G. (1988). The role of β-hydroxyaspartate and adjacent carboxylate residues in the first EGF domain of human factor IX. *EMBO J.* 7: 2053–2061.

Reilly, B.D., Makrides, S.C., Ford, P.J., Marsh, H.C. & Mold, C. (1994). Quantitative analysis of C4b dimer binding to distinct sites on the C3b/C4b receptor (CR1). *J. Biol Chem.* 269: 7696–7701.

Relman, D., Tuomanen, E., Falkow, S., Golenbock, D.T., Saukkonen, K. & Wright, S.D. (1990). Recognition of a bacterial adhesin by an integrin: macrophage CR3 (aMb2, CD11b/CD18) binds filamentous hemagglutinin of *Bordetella pertussis*. *Cell* 61: 1375–1382.

Rey-Campos, J., Rubinstein, P. & Rodriquez de Cordoba. (1988). A physical map of the human regulator of complement activation gene cluster linking the complement genes CR1, CR2, DAF, and C4BP. *J. Exp. Med.* 167: 664–669.

Reynes, M., Aubert, J.P., Cohen, J.H.M., Audoin, J., Tricottet, V., Diebold, J. & Kazatchkine, M.D. (1985). Human follicular dendritic cells express CR1, CR2, and CR3 complement receptor antigens. *J. Immunol.* 135: 2687–2694.

Rodriquez de Cordoba, S., Lublin, D.M., Rubinstein, P. & Atkinson, J.P. (1985). Human genes for the three complement components that regulate the activation of C3 are tightly linked. *J. Exp. Med.* 161: 1189–1195.

Rosen, A, Casciola-Rosen, L., & Ahearn, J.M. (1995). Novel packages of viral and self antigens are generated during apoptosis. *J. Exp. Med.* 181: 1557–1561.

Ross, G.D. & Polley, M.J. (1975). Specificity of human lymphocyte complement receptors. *J. Exp. Med.* 141: 1163–1180.

Ross, G.D., Polley, M.J., Rabellino, E.M. & Grey, H.M. (1973). Two different complement receptors on human lymphocytes: one specific for C3b and one specific for C3b inactivator-cleaved C3b. *J. Exp. Med.* 138: 798–811.

Ross, G.D., Cain, J.A. & Lachmann, P.J. (1985). Membrane complement receptor type three (CR3) has lectin-like properties analogous to bovine conglutinin and functions as a receptor for zymosan and rabbit erythrocytes as well as a receptor for iC3b. *J. Immunol.* 134: 3307–3315.

Russell, D.G. & Wright, S.D. (1988). Complement receptor type 3 (CR3) binds to an Arg-Gly-Asp-containing region of the major surface glycoprotein, gp63, of *Leishmania* promastigotes. *J. Exp. Med.* 168: 279–292.

Sanchez-Madrid, F., Nagy, J.A., Robbins, E., Simon, P. & Springer, T.A. (1983). A human leukocyte differentiation antigen family with distinct α-subunits and a common β-subunit: the lymphocyte function associated antigen (LFA-1), the C3bi complement receptor (OKM1/Mac-1), and the p150,95 molecule. *J. Exp. Med.* 158: 1785.

Seya, T., Holers, V.M. & Atkinson, J.P. (1985). Purification and functional analysis of the polymorphic variants of the C3b/C4b receptor (CR1) and comparison with H, C4-binding protein (C4bp), and decay accelerating factor (DAF). *J. Immunol.* 135: 2661–2667.

Sim, R.B. (1985). Large scale isolation of complement receptor type 1 (CR1) from human erythrocytes. Proteolytic fragmentation studies. *Biochem. J.* 232: 883–889.

Simmons, D., Makgoba, M.W. & Seed, B. (1988). ICAM1, an adhesion ligand of LFA-1, is homologous to the neural cell adhesion molecule NCAM. *Nature* 331: 624–627.

Sinha, S.K., Todd, S.C., Hedrick, J.A., Speiser, C.L., Lambris, J.D. & Tsoukas, C.O. (1993). Characterization of the EBV/C3d receptor on the human Jurkat T cell line: evidence for a novel transcript. *J. Immunol.* 150: 5311–5320.

Slingsby, J.H., Norsworthy, P., Pearce, G., Vaishnaw, A.K., Issler, H., Morley, B.J. & Walport, M.J. (1996). Homozygous hereditary C1q deficiency and systemic lupus erythematosus. A new family and the molecular basis of Clq deficiency in three families. *Arthritis Rheum.* 39: 663–670.

Smith, C.W., Marlin, S.D., Rothlein, R., Toman, C. & Anderson, D.C. (1989). Cooperative interactions of LFA-1 and Mac-1 with intercellular adhesion molecule-1 in facilitating adherence and transendothelial migration of human neutrophils in vitro. *J. Clin. Invest.* 83: 2008–2017.

Springer, T., Galfre, G., Secher, D.S. & Milstein, C. (1979). Mac-1: a macrophage differentiation antigen identified by monoclonal antibody. *Eur. J. Immunol.* 9: 301–306.

Springer, T.A., Miller, L.J. & Anderson, D.C. (1986). P150,95: the third member of the MAC-1, LFA-1 human leukocyte adhesion glycoprotein family. *J. Immunol.* 136: 240–245.

Stacker, A.S.A. & Springer, T.A. (1991). Leukocyte integrin p150,95 (CD11c/CD18) functions as an adhesion molecule binding to a counter-receptor on stimulated endothelium. *J. Immunol.* 146: 648–655.

Staunton, D.E., Marlin, S.D., Stratowa, C., Dustin, M.L. & Springer, T.A. (1988). Primary structure of intercellular adhesion molecule 1 (ICAM1) demonstrates interaction between members of the immunoglobulin and integrin supergene families. *Cell* 52: 925.

Stockl, J., Majdic, O., Pickl, W.F., Rosenkranz, A, Prager, E., Schwantler, E. & Knapp, W. (1995). Granulocyte activation via a binding site near the C-terminal region of complement receptor type α-chain (CD11b) potentially involved in intramembrane complex formation with glycosylphosphatidylinositol-anchored FcαRIIIB (CD16) molecules. *J. Immunol.* 154: 5452–5463.

Subramanian, V.B., Clemenza, L., Krych, M. & Atkinson, J.P. (1996). Substitution of two amino acids confers C3b binding to the C4b binding site of CR1 (CD35): analysis based on ligand binding by chimpanzee erythrocyte complement receptor. *J. Immunol.* 157: 1242–1247.

Suzuki, S., Argraves, W.S., Arai, H., Languino, L.R., Pierschbacher, M.D. & Ruoslahti, E. (1987). Amino acid sequence of the vitronectin receptor a subunit and comparative expression of adhesion receptor mRNAs. *J. Biol. Chem.* 262: 14080–14085.

Suzuki, Y., Ogura, Y., Otsubo, O., Akagi, K., & Fujita, T. (1992). Selective deficiency of C1s associated with a systemic lupus erythematosus-like syndrome. *Arthritis Rheum.* 35: 576–578.

Taniguchi-Sidle, A. & Isenman, D.E. (1992). Mutagenesis of the Arg–Gly–Asp triplet in human complement component C3 does not abolish binding of iC3b to the leukocyte integrin complement receptor type III (CR3, CD11b/CD18). *J. Biol. Chem.* 267: 635–643.

Tedder, T.F., Clement, L.T. & Cooper, M.D. (1984). Expression of C3d receptors during human B cell differentiation: immunofluorescence analysis with the HB-5 monoclonal antibody. *J. Immunol.* 133: 678–683.

Thornton, B.P., Vetvicka, V., Pitman, M., Goldman, R.C. & Ross, G.D. (1996). Analysis of the sugar specificity and molecular location of the α-glucan-binding lectin site of complement receptor type 3 (CD11b/CD18). *J. Immunol.* 156: 1235–1246.

Toothaker, L.E., Henjes, A.J. & Weis, J.J. (1989). Variability of CR2 gene products is due to alternative exon usage and different CR2 alleles. *J. Immunol.* 142: 3668–3675.

Trezzini, C., Jungi, T.W., Kuhnert, P. & Peterhans, E. (1988). Fibrinogen association with human monocytes: evidence for constitutive expression of fibrinogen receptors and for involvement of Mac-1 (CD18, CR3) in the binding. *Biochem. Biophys. Res. Commun.* 156: 477–484.

Tsoukas, C.D. & Lambris, J.D. (1988). Expression of CR2/EBV receptors on human thymocytes detected by monoclonal antibodies. *Eur. J. Immunol.* 18: 1299–1302.

Tsoukas, C.D. & Lambris, J.D. (1993). Expression of EBV/C3d receptors on T cells: biological significance. *Immunol. Today* 14: 56.

Tuveson, D.A., Ahearn, J.M., Matsumoto, A.K. & Fearon, D.T. (1991). Molecular interactions of complement receptors on B lymphocytes: a CR1/CR2 complex distinct from the CR2/CD19 complex. *J. Exp. Med.* 173: 1083–1089.

van Strijp, J.A.G., Russell, D.G., Tuomanen, E., Brown, E.J. & Wright, S.D. (1993). Ligand specificity of purified complement receptor type three (CD11b/CD18, aMb2,Mac-1). Indirect effects of an ARG-GLY-ASP (RGD) sequence. *J. Immunol.* 151: 3324–3336.

Vik, D.P. & Fearon, D.T. (1987). Cellular distribution of complement receptor type 4 (CR4): expression on human platelets. *J. Immunol.* 138: 254–258.

Vik, D.P. & Wong, W.W. (1993). Structure of the gene for the F allele of complement receptor type 1 and sequence of the coding region unique to the S allele. *J. Immunol.* 151: 6214–6224.

Weis, J.H., Morton, C.C., Bruns, G.A.P., Weis, J.J., Klickstein, L.B., Wong, W.W. & Fearon, D.T. (1987). A complement receptor locus: genes encoding C3b/C4b receptor and C3d/Epstein-Barr virus receptor maps to 1q32. *J. Immunol.* 138: 312–315.

Weis, J.J. & Fearon, D.T. (1985). The identification of N-linked oligosaccharides on the human CR2/Epstein–Barr virus receptor and their function in receptor metabolism, plasma membrane expression, and ligand binding. *J. Biol. Chem.* 260: 13 824–13 830.

Weis, J.J., Tedder, T.F. & Fearon, D.T. (1984). Identification of a 145,000 M_r membrane protein as the C3d receptor (CR2) of human B lymphocytes. *Proc. Natl. Acad. Sci., USA* 81: 881–885.

Weis, J.J., Fearon, D.T., Klickstein, L.D., Wong, W.W., Richards, S.A., de Bruyn Kops, A., Smith, J.A. & Weis, J.H. (1986). Identification of a partial cDNA clone for the C3d/Epstein–Barr virus receptor of human B lymphocytes: homology with the receptor for fragments C3b and C4b of the third and fourth components of complement. *Proc. Natl. Acad. Sci., USA* 83: 5639–5643.

Weis, J.J., Toothaker, L.E., Smith, J.A., Weis, J.H. & Fearon, D.T. (1988). Structure of the human B lymphocyte receptor for C3d and the Epstein–Barr virus and relatedness to other members of the family of C3/C4 binding proteins. *J. Exp. Med.* 167: 1047–1066.

Weisman, H.F., Bartow, T., Leppo, M.K., Marsh, H.C., Carson, G.R., Concino, M.F., Boyle, M.P., Roux, K.H., Weisfeldt, M.L. & Fearon, D.T. (1990). Soluble human complement receptor type 1: an in vivo inhibitor of complement suppressing post-ischemic myocardial inflammation and necrosis. *Science* 249: 146–151.

Werfel, T., Witter, W. & Gotze, O. (1991). CD11b and CD11c antigens are rapidly increased on human natural killer cells upon activation. *J. Immunol.* 147: 2423–2427.

Wilson, J.G., Tedder, T.F. & Fearon, D.T. (1983). Characterization of human T lymphocytes that express the C3b receptor. *J. Immunol.* 131: 684–689.

Wong, W.W. & Farrell, S.A. (1991). Proposed structure of the F allotype of human CR1. Loss of a C3b binding site may be associated with altered function. *J. Immunol.* 146: 656–662.

Wong, W.W. & Fearon, D.T. (1987). Human receptor for C3b/C4b: complement receptor type I. *Meth. Enzymol.* 150: 579–585.

Wong, W.W., Wilson, J.G. & Fearon, D.T. (1983). Genetic regulation of a structural polymorphism of human C3b receptor. *J. Clin. Invest.* 72: 685–693.

Wong, W.W., Klickstein, L.B., Smith, J.A., Weis, J.H. & Fearon, D.T. (1985). Identification of a partial cDNA clone for the human receptor for complement fragment C3b/C4b. *Proc. Natl. Acad. Sci., USA* 82: 7711–7715.

Wong, W.W., Cahill, J.M., Rosen, M.D., Kennedy, C.A., Bonaccio, E.T., Morris, M.J., Wilson, J.G., Klickstein, L.B. & Fearon, D.T. (1989). Structure of the human CR1 gene. Molecular basis of the structural and quantitative polymorphisms and identification of a new CR1-like allele. *J. Exp. Med.* 169: 847–863.

Wright, S.D. & Jong, M.T.C. (1986). Adhesion-promoting receptors on human macrophages recognize *Escherichia coli* by binding to lipopolysaccharide. *J. Exp. Med.* 164: 1876–1888.

Wright, S.D., Reddy, P.A., Jong, M.T.C. & Erickson, B.W. (1987). C3bi receptor (complement receptor type 3) recognizes a region of complement protein C3 containing the sequence Arg-Gly-Asp. *Proc. Natl. Acad. Sci., USA* 84: 1965–1968.

Wright, S.D., Weitz, J.I., Huang, A.J., Levin, S.M., Silverstein, S.C. & Loike, J.D. (1988). Complement receptor type three (CD11b/CD18) of human polymor-phonuclear leukocytes recognizes fibrinogen. *Proc. Natl. Acad. Sci., USA* 85: 7734–7738.

Wright, S.D., Levin, S.M., Jong, M.T.C., Chad, Z. & Kabbash, L.G. (1989). CR3 (CD11b/CD18) expresses one binding site for Arg–Gly–Asp-containing peptides and a second site for bacterial lipopolysaccharide. *J. Exp. Med.* 169: 175–183.

Yang, L., Behrens, M. & Weis, J.J. (1991). Identification of 5 regions affecting the expression of the human CR2 gene. *J. Immunol.* 147: 2404–2410.

Yoon, S.H. & Fearon, D.T. (1985). Characterization of a soluble form of the C3b/C4b receptor (CR1) in human plasma. *J. Immunol.* 134: 3332–3338.

Zhou, M.J., Todd, R.F., van de Winkel, J.G.J. & Petty, H.R. (1993). Cocapping of the leukoadhesion molecules complement receptor type 3 and lymphocyte function-associated antigen-1 with Fcγ receptor III on human neutrophils. Possible role of lectin-like interactions. *J. Immunol.* 150: 3030–3041.

Index

Note: page numbers in *italics* refer to figures and tables